POLLY'S BIRTH BOOK

Obstetrics for the Home

POLLY'S BIRTH BOOK

Obstetrics for the Home

by

Polly Block

Polly's Birth Book: Obstetrics for the Home

Copyright © 1984 by Mattie Eula Webb Block

ALL RIGHTS RESERVED.

No part of this book may be photocopied or reproduced in any form whatsoever without prior written permission of the author or publisher, except in the case of brief passages embodied in critical reviews and articles where the ISBN, author and publisher are mentioned.

Any and all herbal recipes are under copyright and may be produced only "exactly" as recipes are given in book, in the form given in the book. For *personal use only* and never to be sold for profit without prior written permission from the author, publisher and/or owner of *Polly's Birth Book*.

Published by:
HEARTHSPUN PUBLISHERS
775 North 300 East
Pleasant Grove, UT 84062

Join, Like, and Follow us:
Facebook: Pollys Birth Book
Twitter: Jeanette@pollysbirthbook
LinkedIn: Jeanette Lasson
and on the web: pollysbirthbook.com

First Printing; 1984
Second Printing; 1996
Third - Seventh Printing to-date in 2020

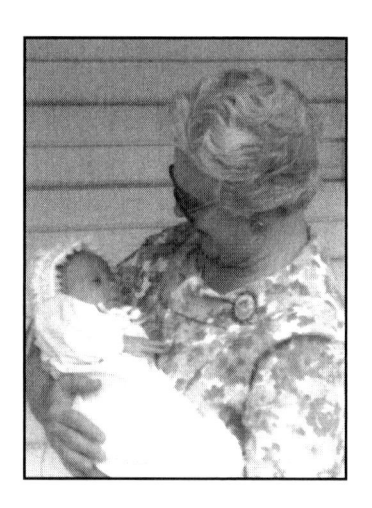

Other books by Polly Block:
  A Coal of Fire from the Hearth
  A Superior Alternative: Childbirth at Home
  Aaron, You're Awesome
  Nurturing the Spirit Vol. 1
   • *The Crossing*
   • *Beneath a Prairie Bush*
  Tell Me
  The Song of A Volunteer
  O Jerusalem, Jerusalem

  Nurturing the Spirit Vol. 2
   • *She Carried Me All the Way*
   • *The Fastest Buggy Horse in Alpine*

Cover Design and Production: SunrisePublishing@gmail.com
ISBN: 1-57636-019-9
Library of Congress Catalog Card Number: 96-68998

DEDICATION

To all who hold in reverence the gift of life.

*** * * ***

To my beautiful, gifted firstborn, Vivian, who after five losses filled my empty arms. To my talented and loving son, Bruce, who believes in me. To our special bonuses who stay close to us: lovely Jeanette and handsome Aaron. They were sent to be a comfort and a joy to us in our old age! And to my sweetheart husband, Andy, who gives me so much in life.

ACKNOWLEDGMENTS

My deepest gratitude goes to those who have sacrificed, been inconvenienced, and labored with love and patience for a few centuries to help bring this volume to you! These special people include my dear husband, Andy, my son, Aaron, the whole Mortenson family, and my devoted editor, Kathryn Burton. As editor and designer, Kathryn worked on the unfamiliar material of a difficult subject and developed a clean, readable format.

Special thanks also go to Darlene and Byron Okada for their word processing expertise and skillful preparation of the manuscript. The serenity of their "Taj Mahal" became a haven to me in times of discouragement. It was so because of their sweet spirits.

Jeanne Johnson and many, many others are also remembered with a grateful heart for the encouragement and support given in this undertaking.

TABLE OF CONTENTS

Illustrations by the Author xvii-xviii
Preface xix
"Birth" xx
"The Midwife" xxi

UNIT I ATTITUDES AND PERSPECTIVES

1. **Introduction** 3
   A Word to Midwives 8
   Women and Midwifery 11
   How to Choose a Midwife 13
   Selected References 14
2. **Legislation Regarding Midwifery** 17
3. **Abortion** 25
4. **Better Sit Down for This One** 30
   Misunderstanding the Marriage Act 30
   Marriage Counseling 33
   A Word to Husbands 34
   Intercourse During Pregnancy 37
   Family Planning and Birth Control 38
   The Eternal Perspective 42
5. **Medication and the Midwife** 45
   Drug Use in Pregnancy and Childbirth 45
   Inducing Labor 51
   Natural Management of Pregnancy 54

UNIT II PRENATAL

6. **Obstetrical Anatomy** 59
   The Birth Canal 59
     The Pelvis 59
     The Vagina 62
     The Perineum 62

viii POLLY'S BIRTH BOOK

  The Vulva 64
  The Bladder 64
  The Uterus 65
  The Conceptus 68
   The Placenta 70
   The Amniotic Sac and Fluid 71
   The Umbilical Cord 72
   Development of the Embryo 73
7. Determining Home Birth Feasibility 76
  Ascertaining Pregnancy 76
  Determining a Due Date 81
  Initial Screening 82
   Prenatal Questionnaire 83
   Commentary on Prenatal Questionnaire 87
   Pelvic and Vaginal Assessment 102
8. Prenatal Tests and Visits 108
  Nature of Prenatal Care 108
  Prenatal Tests 109
   Laboratory Tests 109
   Ultrasound 110
   Amniocentesis 114
  Prenatal Visits 116
   Blood Pressure 118
   Urinalysis 120
   Weight 122
   Fundal Height 123
   Fetal Heart Rate 123
   Vaginal Exams 125
  Diagnosis of Multiple Pregnancy 125
  Diagnosis of Death in Utero 126
  Diagnosis of Pre-eclampsia (Toxemia) 127
9. The Good Program 133
  Nutrition 133
   Vegetarianism 137
   Diet 138
   Seasons Point the Way 143
   Avoid Harmful Substances 144
   Water 148
  Herbs and Supplements 149
   Preventive Supplementation 151

Hormone Helpers 153
Polly-Jean Five-Week Antenatal Formula 155
Exercise 158
  Walking 160
  Pelvic Floor Exercise 161
  Abdominal Breathing Exercise 161
  Stomach and Back Exercises 162
  Pelvic Rocks 163
  Sitting and Squatting 163
The Sitz Bath 165

10. Changes During Pregnancy 168
Physical Changes 168
  Breast Changes 168
  Stretch Marks 168
  Weight Gain 169
Physical Complaints 170
  Drowsiness 170
  Nausea 171
  Constipation 171
  Diarrhea 172
  Frequent Urination 172
  Fainting 173
  Back Ache 174
  Leg Cramps 174
  Heartburn 175
  Excessive Hunger 175
  Anemia, Other Deficiencies 175
  Hemorrhoids, Other Varicosities 178
  Vaginal Discharge 182
  Yeast Infection 182
Psyche 183

11. Disorders in Pregnancy 185
Danger Signals 185
Vaginal Bleeding, Abdominal Pain 186
  Abruptio Placenta 186
  Placenta Previa 187
  Ectopic Pregnancy 189
  Unexplained Spontaneous Abortion 191
  Threatened Spontaneous Abortion 192

Conditions Mistaken for Threatened
     Miscarriage   194
Edema   195
Severe, Continuous Headache   195
Visual Disturbances   196
Persistent Vomiting   196
Premature Membrane Rupture   199
Chills and Fever   200
12. Conditions Affecting Pregnancy   204
Rh Factor and Hemolytic Disease   204
Diabetes Mellitus   208
Rubella   212
Venereal Disease   212
13. Birthing Supplies   214
Portable Maternity Kit for the Car   214
Home Birth Supplies   216
The Midwife's Kit   221
14. Antenatal Preparation for Birth   228
Preparing for Controlled Crowning   228
Determining Fetal Position   229
Determining Engagement   233
Understanding the Process of Labor   236
Mechanism of Labor: Vertex Presentations   238

UNIT III   PARTURITION

15. First Stage of Labor: Begins with the Onset of Labor and Ends with Full Dilation   251
When to Call the Midwife   251
The Midwife Arrives   255
  Keeping a Labor Log   256
  Timing Contractions   257
  Noting Vital Signs   257
  Position and Engagement   258
  Dilation and Effacement   258
  Enemas and "Prepping"   261
  Setting the (First) Stage   262
Aids for the Laboring Mother   264
  Femoral Pressure Points   265
  Sacral Pressure Points   266

Back Adjustments 268
Cervical Rimming 271
Hydrotherapy 272
Foot Therapy: The Uterine Reflex 273
Lobelia Tincture 278
Resting Between Contractions 278
Coaching: The Relax-Rhythm Method 280
Progression of Labor 283
Uterine Inertia 284
Obstructed Labor 288

16. Second Stage of Labor: Begins with Full Dilation of the Cervix and Ends with the Birth of the Baby 293
Early Second Stage 293
Therapies for Birth Canal Expansion 294
Pelvic (-0- Station) Expansion 295
Cervical and Perineal Expansion 297
Anticipating, Preventing, and Correcting Problems 297
Anterior Lip 298
Narrow Build 299
Meconium Staining 300
Eclampsia 301
Excessive Bleeding 305
Transverse Head Arrest 307
Shoulder Arrest 309
Cord Stress 310
Cord Knots 314
Prolapsed Cord 314
Delivery Positions for the Mother 321
Late Second Stage 324
Pushing 324
Coaching 325
Rupturing the Amniotic Sac 327
About Tearing 329
Episiotomies 330
Controlled Crowning and Delivery 332

17. Third Stage of Labor: Begins with the Birth of the Baby and Ends with Delivery of the Placenta 341

xii   POLLY'S BIRTH BOOK

    Early Third Stage   341
       Suctioning the Baby   341
       Apgar Evaluation   342
       Establishing Respiration   342
       Cutting the Umbilical Cord   349
       Bonding   355
    Delivering the Placenta   355
    Possible Third Stage Complications   360
       Retained Placenta   360
       Uterine Retraction Ring   363
       Adhered Placenta   367
    Hemorrhage   367
       Avoiding Hemorrhage: Points to
          Memorize   369
       Kinds and Causes of Bleeding   370
       Summary: Kinds and Causes of Bleeding   373
       Controlling Postpartum Hemorrhage: Points
          to Memorize   375
       Transporting   381
       Treatment Following Postpartum
          Hemorrhage   381
    Evaluating the Placenta and Membrane   382
18. Fourth Stage of Parturition   388
    Keeping the Fundus Hard   388
    Lacerations   389
    Suturing   390
       Suturing Materials   391
       Suturing Techniques   392
       Wound Healing   396
       Pericare   397
       Removing Stitches   398
    Care of the Mother   399
    Care of the Baby   400
       Weighing and Measuring the Baby   400
       Examining and Dressing the Baby   401
       Newborn Evaluation   408
19. Postpartum   412
    Postpartum Instructions   412
    Lochia   414
    Afterpains   415

Breast-Feeding 417
   Milk Loss 419
   Excess Milk 420
   Let-Down Reflex 421
   Mastitis 421
   Sore Nipples 422
   Illness 422
   Weaning 423
Suggestions for the Newborn's Care and
     Comfort 423
   Circumcision 423
   Care of the Umbilical Stump 424
   Jaundice 425
   Crying 426
   Colic 427
   Solid Foods 428
   Constipation 428
   Diarrhea 429
   Unusual Baby Odors 429
   Umbilical Hernia 430
   Yeast Infection (Thrush) 430
Healing and Security Benefits of Bonding 431
Postnatal Exercises 433
Feeling Beautiful Because You Are 435

UNIT IV   SPECIAL SITUATIONS

20. Higher Risk Deliveries 439
Using Landmarks 439
Breech Births 440
   Breech Version (Turning the Fetus) 444
   Some Important Points 445
   Delivery Management of Breech Births 449
Multiple Births 456
   Some Important Points 456
   Delivery Management of Multiple
      Births 458
   Triplets (Or More!) 460
Uncommon Presentations 461
   Arm and Shoulder Presentations 461

Face Presentations   463
21. **Malformations, Injuries, and Abnormalities** 467
    Birth Defects   467
        Cleft Palate and Cleft Lip   468
        Retardation   469
        Spinal Defects   469
    Birth Injuries   470
        Swelling   470
        Laceration of the Liver   471
        Erb's Paralysis (Erb's Palsy)   472
    Uterine Abnormalities   474
        Anteflected Uterus   474
        Prolapsed Uterus   476
        Inverted Uterus   479
    "Hyaline Membrane Disease" (Respiratory
        Distress Syndrome)   481
22. **Cesarean Sections**   484

APPENDICES

A. **Aseptic Technique**   491
B. **Vital Signs**   496
    Respiration   496
    Vascular and Circulatory Systems   497
        Heart and Pulse Rates   497
        Blood Pressure   499
    Temperature   500
    Shock: Symptoms and Treatment   501
C. **Sample Recipes for the Good Program**   504
    Transition Diet   504
    Breakfasts Will Never Be the Same Again!   505
        Petra's Auflauf   505
        Whole Grain Cereals   505
        Grapenut Crunch   506
        Apple Topping   506
        Pancake Toppings   506
        Maple Syrup   507
    Fruits are Fun!   507
        Extravaganza   507
        Pineapple Gondola   507

Watermelon Basket 508
Fruit Malts 509
Main Dishes 510
  Lentil Loaf 510
  Cooking With Soybeans 510
  Baked Soybeans 511
  Tomato Cups 512
  Green Pepper Cups (Raw) 512
  Green Pepper Cups (Cooked) 512
  Vegetable Plate Pinwheel 513
  Summer Fair Salad 514
  Ruby Delight Salad 514
  Tossed Salad Supreme 514
Dressings 515
  Basic Recipe for Soy Mayonnaise 515
  Golden Harvest Salad Dressing 515
  Thousand Island Dressing 515
  Mustard Variation 516
  Avocado Dip 516
  Oil and Vinegar Dressing 516
Treats 516
  Carob Nut Log 516
  Carob Bread Pudding 517
  Candy Bars 517
  Trail Mix 518
  Shortcake 518
Green Drinks 518
  Basic Green Drink 518
  Jeanne's Blend Green Drink 518
Canning Recipes 520
  Freezer Jams and Jellies 520
  Iris's Home Canning Method 521

D. Herbal Preparations 522
Herbs for Female Problems 522
  Female Corrective Formula 522
  To Rebuild an Unhealthy Vaginal Floor 523
  For Varicosities of the Vulva 524
Herbs for Illness, Infection 524
  Herbal Composition Powder 524
  Black Walnut Tincture 525

Garlic Powder Douche   525
Garlic and Cayenne Enema   525
LB Formula   526
For Bladder and Kidney Ailments,
    Toxemia   526
For Mastitis   527
Herbs for Hydrotherapy   527
Herbs for Childbirth   528
    For with the Five-Week Antenatal
        Formula   528
    For Use with Pressure Points   529
    Antispasmodics   529
Herbs for the Newborn   531
    Mucus-Cutting Formula, Stools   531
    Mucus-Cutting Formula, Nose and
        Throat   531
    For Hematomas   531
    For Feeding Problems   532
    Sore Baby Bottoms   532

Index   533

ILLUSTRATIONS
By the Author

1. Female Pelvis, Front View 60
2. Inlet and Outlet of the Bony Birth Canal 61
3. Pelvic Cavity Divisions 63
4. Female Reproductive Organs, Side View 63
5. The Vulva 65
6. The Uterus 67
7. Cervical Os, Bottom View 68
8. The Conceptus 69
9. Internal Anatomy of a Pregnant Uterus 69
10. The Umbilical Cord (Funis) 73
11. Internal Ballottement 77
12. External Pelvimetry 103
13. First Vaginal Exam 103
14. Internal Pelvimetry 105
15. Fundal Height Measurement 124
16. Breakfast Plate Volume 139
17. Dinner Plate Volume 139
18. Prenatal Exercises 159
19. Pelvic Rock 164
20. The Sitz Bath 166
21. The Birthing Bed 217
22. Instruments from the Midwife's Kit 224
23. The Fetal Head, Side and Top Views 230
24. Occipital Positions 233
25. Mechanism of Labor: LOA Position 240-41
26. Directional Force of Contractions 242
27. Stations of Progress in the Birth Canal 243
28. Anterior Rotation: ROP Position 245
29. The Curve of Carus 246
30. The Mucous Plug 252
31. Forewaters Assist Dilation 252
32. Effacement of the Cervix 259
33. Measuring Dilation of the Cervix 259
34. The Drive Angle in Labor 263
35. Femoral Pressure Points 265

36. Sacral Pressure Points   267
37. Upper Back Adjustment   269
38. Foot Therapy   275
39. Inferior Symphysis Pubis Touch   295
40. Inferior Sacral Pressure Points   296
41. Knee-Chest Position   316
42. Catheter for Reinserting Prolapsed Cord   318
43. Transporting Support for Prolapsed Cord   320
44. Squat Position in Parturition   322
45. Left Lateral Position in Parturtion   323
46. Controlled Crowning: Preventing Premature Extension   336
47. Controlled Crowning: Anal Push Technique   336
48. Controlled Crowning: Perineal Press Technique   337
49. Apgar Scoring System   343
50. Establishing Respiration: Thorax Rub   344
51. Establishing Respiration: Byrd's Method   348
52. Fetal Circulation   353
53. Cutting the Umbilical Cord   354
54. Fundal Mobility   356
55. Placental Abnormality   359
56. Retained Placenta   360
57. Uterine Retraction Ring   364
58. Uterine Activity in Parturition   365
59. Examining the Afterbirth   383
60. "Shiny" Schultze Placental Separation   385
61. "Dirty" Duncan Placental Separation   385
62. Suturing Techniques   395
63. Swaddling   403
64. Care of the Newborn's Scalp   405
65. Hip Dislocation   410
66. Uterine Reflex Points (Neuro-Vascular Dynamics)   417
67. Postnatal Exercises   434
68. Breech Presentations   441
69. Management of Breech Birth   452
70. Face Presentation   464
71. Erb's Paralysis and Treatment   473

PREFACE

By the time the material for most publications has been assembled and organized, some of the information has become obsolete. Other ways will have been found to manage some phase of the work so carefully written about. Birth, nevertheless, is a natural course in life, and ways to manage or assist in its happening will continue to vary as long as people and birth exist. Outcomes, no doubt, will vary also with and without the application of assistance. I can take no responsibility for the outcomes developed through the options or choices of others, in myriad circumstances, or the application of various principles found herein.

Some of the materials from my six-day seminars have also been circulated in various forms. I do not assume responsibility for possible deviations or misdirections disseminated in those materials.

It is hoped, instead, that students of obstetrics will remember one piece of advice from an ancient physician: "Above all else, do no harm."

BIRTH

Quieted hearts!
Quickened ears!
Deliberately stilled, in tune.
Heaven's signs tapped on doors,
It's now, it will be soon!

Angels summoned angels,
Through windows now obscure,
To coach, support and mingle
Round parents by the score.

Movement upon movement,
Wait! Don't breathe in yet!
'Tis but another moment,
Child, this you'll ne'er forget.

Now earthlings hover o'er thee,
Charmed by your presence there,
Waiting for the message
You must have brought to share.

Time hastens for your learning,
Experiences or replays
Of which a former training
Prepared you for your stay.

Child, teach them,
Some will listen.
You too must bear remembering
I want you back someday.

    --Polly Block

THE MIDWIFE

Who am I to have taken part
    In such wonderful earthbound schemes,
To have found a place, a welcoming place
    To serve little kings and queens?

One thing is very certain,
    Each tiny one always knew
'Twas my heart, not my hands that swaddled,
    And cuddled and communed anew.

              --Polly Block

UNIT I
Attitudes & Perspectives

CHAPTER 1

INTRODUCTION

A **midwife** is anyone, male or female, who assists in the delivery of a newborn. Midwifery calls for knowledge and skills that encourage and protect life. The ability to instill confidence in the mother regarding her labor is the epitome of the midwife's tasks and pleasure. Healthy attitudes toward childbirth itself, toward the family, other midwives, and back-up personnel are vital to a midwife's success. A midwife must be teachable and willing to teach correct principles. The primary duty of a midwife is to assist in childbirth with competence, reverence, and sensitivity, ever mindful of the Giver of Life, His power and direction.

I have written this book because I want people who have chosen home birth to know what they are undertaking. I am concerned about the untrained couple who have safely had one baby at home without competent help and decide that, because everything went well the first time, they will attempt it alone again. I am concerned about the couple who plan a home birth entirely for economic reasons. I am concerned about the woman who hemorrhages during a home birth and must be transported to a hospital, where she is forced to wait for treatment because of paperwork, or is treated badly because she has not chosen a method of childbirth preferred by established medicine. I am concerned about the woman who chooses home birth and expects all to go well, but does not prepare her body through good nutrition and exercise, or neglects regular prenatal checkups!

More and more couples are choosing home birth in spite of attempts to persuade them that it is not safe. Home birth CAN be safe, and parents who want to give birth at home are entitled to competent, experienced help, both during pregnancy and during delivery. In order for there to be competent help available, birth attendants must have somewhere to go for reliable information, outside the sources and philosophies from which they are turning. I would rather teach them than criticize, suppress, or otherwise hinder their fine intentions. I would rather befriend and help midwives and parents to understand home birth than force them underground, making it less likely that they will be able to manage the event safely. There must be a starting place, a beginning, and so I offer this volume.

If you are excited about home birth, you are not alone. The number of parents who want to have a birth THEIR way--without intervention, without unnecessary medication, WITH herbal therapy, without being told what is best for them--is growing constantly.

Whether you are an expectant parent wanting to know more about birth, a person interested in becoming a midwife, or just someone interested in the miracle of life, this book has been written to give you more than the basics. It is not, however, a replacement for practical experience. Many of the skills I talk about are learned only through careful observation and on-the-job instruction over a period of time. No one should feel she can read this book and safely go out and deliver her first baby alone.

For those who are serious about learning the skills of midwifery, this book is a companion to experiential learning. These skills are especially valuable in an emergency situation, perhaps when a physical disaster has crippled hospitals and communication and you are the only person available to help. This book takes you through a birth, from the first signs of pregnancy through prenatal care, delivery, and postpartum care, in chronological order; possible complications in each phase are explained.

A word here about complications and problems: they don't always arise. Yet, in any birth situation some decisions may have to be made that have life-or-death consequences. Those who attempt home birth should have training, experience, and another quality, which I call "faith." It would be difficult to preside in situations where decisions may occasionally result in death or impaired quality of life, unless you were convinced of a divine power or plan governing the processes of life and birth. I have provided instructions for handling most situations, but a willingness to seek and be aware of higher guidance is also paramount.

Parents who are planning a home birth should be advised that their conscious choice of this alternative carries with it a great responsibility. Home births are for low risk pregnancies; a mother who has not been properly screened or who has not properly taken care of herself during her entire pregnancy has no right to endanger the life of her child or her own life by choosing home birth. If the birth is not planned for home, but happens to occur at home because of uncontrollable circumstances, you can be sure the Lord will be with you. But if you deliberately set out to give birth at home and you have not seen to it that you are properly screened or you have not conscientiously followed a careful nutritional and exercise regimen, then if something goes wrong at the birth--well, as an old saying goes, I don't know how many times the Lord will pull your chestnuts out of the fire.

This is NOT to say that home birth is not safe, given the proper circumstances. For reasons outlined extensively in **A Superior Alternative: Childbirth at Home,** I believe home birth is safer than hospital birth for low risk mothers. But you are only low risk if you take the responsibility for home birth seriously and see to it that you are fully prepared. This includes full preparation in the area of faith as well. Whether you are a parent or a midwife in a home birth situation, I hope you will feel totally and honestly convinced that your Heavenly Father is with you, guiding and approving your decisions every step of the way. If you can say you feel this conviction, then no so-called authority has any right to berate, harass, or intimidate you for going through with your home birth, WHATEVER the outcome.

With that caveat, read my book and consider it a launching pad from which to continue to learn about birth. You will find here guidance in natural methods and birthing techniques, including ways to prepare for childbirth, to alleviate pain and curb bleeding (without side effects), and ways to promote safety. As a rule, nurses, Emergency Medical Technicians, and other paramedical personnel will have had much less instruction about

Introduction 7

childbirth, unless they have also had midwifery training.

As you read and continue to learn and experience, take advantage of open-minded experts such as your back-up doctors. Learn from them and make use of their skills. Adapt their procedures to what you find works so that your own expertise in natural methods will grow. You will find that they will also have much to learn from you, if you strive to be competent and aware of ways to improve your skills.

Work with those in the medical profession in a spirit of cooperation. Befriend them and be grateful that their alternatives exist in addition to yours. Their emergency equipment and medical interventions are blessings when they are necessary, just as your natural remedies are blessings to those who do not need drastic interference.

Work hard and be well-read, so that you understand thoroughly the biological norms and can recognize which variants are within manageable limits and which are complications. There is only one predictable thing about pregnancy and childbirth, and that is that both are sometimes unpredictable. What should be normal for an individual woman could become, or may already be, a complication. Therefore, you need to learn to function within a flexible framework.

When complications arise, we as midwives must allow nature to correct them whenever possible. We have to be able to interfere when necessary, to wait when necessary, and to know when to do which. This is my motto for midwives:

> "When we do those things which complement the natural process by which God brings forth

mankind, then we are in accord with His plan for compassionate service."

Whether you intend to practice midwifery or not, all prudent individuals should build a home nursing file. The file should include practical home remedies that are built upon biological principles, not fads. I would also encourage everyone to learn as much as they can about physical therapies—massage and hydrotherapy, in particular—and to learn about preventive nutrition and exercise programs, in order to build and maintain good health. Be open-minded enough to learn from anyone, but be intelligent and discriminating enough to recognize fads, and be in tune enough to follow promptings. You cannot be deceived for long if you are being obedient to all the laws of God that you know you should be following.

A WORD TO MIDWIVES

Dr. Grantly Dick Read considered the hallmark of a good midwife to be her ability to instill confidence in labor.[1] A good midwife helps the mother to see success and to feel success in the way she is handling her labor. You teach and guide and praise her throughout labor. You help her to be confident that she can have this baby safely and without "dying!" This is your primary job.

A helpful and professional attitude begins the minute you receive a phone call from a mother who thinks she is in labor. You answer with enthusiasm and confidence: "Great! We'll check you and see."

When you enter your client's home, you enter with confidence, not impatience or dramatics. You are cheerful, quiet, reassuring, and calming as you set about your business. You ask questions you need to ask. Answer inquiries honestly, cheerfully.

If you are ASSISTING in a birth, don't take over or act bossy. Assist! Wait to be asked to do certain things even though you may know very well what to do. Each midwife develops her own way of handling things, and when it's your turn to assist, let the midwife in charge do it her way. No two midwives (or doctors, for that matter) will manage a birth exactly the same way. Be flexible and open--you'll learn more.

It is important to go to a birth in twos (or more) for several reasons:

1. To promote legality.

2. To have two people to witness techniques and outcomes.

3. To have another trained person present if the midwife in charge must deal with a crisis.

The assistant helps or assumes other responsibilities, or even other crises. For example, you may have a hemorrhaging mother and a baby that needs resuscitation. If you are the midwife in charge you may want to have a checklist of things for each assistant to do in order to lessen tension or confusion over duties.

As a midwife, it is important that you stay healthy yourself. It takes a lot of strength and energy and stamina to be on top of a situation for a long stretch at a time. If you do get tired and there's a lull in labor, don't crawl into the client's bed to sleep. A blanket on the couch or floor will do as your partner midwife spells you off, and vice versa.

Modesty is an essential feature of birthing. The considerate midwife dresses modestly, and she also helps the parturient preserve her modesty, especially during labor when often there are long periods of waiting. A drape should be close at hand, for convenient use. Birthing is a sacred process. The sensitive midwife will set and maintain a tone of modesty.

You should already have a feeling for the personalities and preferences of the couple you are serving before you come to help in the delivery, but you should nevertheless be sensitive to how the mother and father are reacting to labor when it actually begins. The father may be the awkward type—he doesn't know what to do but would like to help. Or he may be wholly terrified of the entire process. He may not want to be there at all, or he may want to be as involved as he possibly can be. You should learn to be sensitive to these different personalities and to deal with each kind appropriately, respecting wishes without judgmental remarks or attitudes.

In all my years of midwifery, I have seen only one father refuse to be there when his baby was born. Had I been there before he left, I feel certain I could have made him feel comfortable enough to stay in the house while his wife labored; then, as I would have needed his assistance to prepare for delivery, I would have taught him the measures we take to promote safety and I would have interested him in the tender aspects of seeing his own child come into the world. He would have stayed and been in on everything.

I believe that the husband should be with his wife in childbirth, if only he remains in the house. He needs to know what his wife goes through to give him children, and I know that he wants to give her support and assistance as he can. His gentleness and strength cannot be replaced by anyone else.

It is the midwife's job, however, to be sensitive to real or imagined tensions which would interfere with the success of the mother's labor. Tension alone will obstruct labor for a long period of time, to say nothing of the excruciating pain that will mount. Bad news, tension between two attendants, an impatient father, a worried grandmother or friend will render labor stressful. If the parturient is unable to handle stress and asks you to clear the air, you can do it without offending but with tact and firmness, for your client's welfare and safety.

WOMEN AND MIDWIFERY

I am convinced that midwifery is a woman's work. Nature has endowed women with an understanding about birth-giving. Dr. Beach, an M.D. from the Thompsonian era, made this statement after a number of years delivering babies:

> I have practiced this branch of medicine ever since I began my profession; but so fully convinced have I been that it is wrong, and belongs to the other sex, that I have abandoned it to its rightful owners, the female midwives: and I am therefore as anxious to bring about a reformation in this department as in other branches of medicine. I trust that I shall have at least the enlightened portion of the community to sustain me in a cause of such vital importance both to the moral and physical well being of the female sex. The tales that are told by designing physicians of the hair-breadth escapes of numerous women, to whom they have been called just in time to save life, and of the danger of trusting to females, have filled those over whom they have an influence with awful apprehension, and thereby secured to themselves a branch of medicine that reason, experience, and the finer feelings of the female sex loudly proclaim belong only to the females.[2]

12 POLLY'S BIRTH BOOK

I have infinite respect and appreciation for a number of fine men who have contributed much to obstetrics and to the cause of preserving birthing rights for birthing couples. I look with disdain upon others who place themselves much in the category spoken of by Dr. Beach.

Women offer a special tenderness and sensitivity in childbirth. The midwife has an excellent opportunity to help shape attitudes toward birth. Often physicians suggest that a woman should have her first baby in the hospital. If there are no overriding factors other than this being her first child, I believe home birth is preferable. A midwife can offer support and prevent the mother from having many unnecessary and unpleasant, routine hospital experiences (such as an episiotomy, for example: if a mother can deliver her first baby without one, it would be rare for her to need one with another birth).

A mother who can have her first baby with the assistance of a good midwife and without medication, forceps, or trauma will be ENCOURAGED to have the rest of her family. Low risk **gravidas** (pregnant women) are not made high risk simply because they are having home births.

It is interesting to know that 40 to 60% of the women who take my classes have intentions of becoming midwives. They give these reasons:

1. Most feel that the time will shortly come (or is already here) when they will need to be able to render this service. They consider this a vital part of emergency preparedness.

2. Many have felt a compelling urgency to learn to deliver babies. (Some are responding to spiritual pronouncements they have had.)

3. Others have always wanted to be able to assist those who suffer, rather than stand helplessly by.

4. Some view this preparation as potentially lifesaving, and therefore worth every effort.

5. Some are no longer of childbearing age, but they want to know how to successfully help their daughters, granddaughters, and friends during pregnancy and childbirth.

HOW TO CHOOSE A MIDWIFE

When you move into a new community, how do you choose a new family physician? Surely you would ask several people about their doctors and why they go (or no longer go) to them. You would be interested in finding out if the doctor is overanxious to prescribe drugs, perform surgery, run up large bills, and so on, or if he shows genuine concern and skill with his trade.

You would also consider candidates from among those who can fill your particular needs. For instance, when a member of the family has a visual problem, you don't go to an orthopedic surgeon. Likewise, when you need a dentist, you don't go to a urologist. And so it is with having babies. If screening with a midwife reveals complications which make you high risk, you need an obstetrician. If you are a well, normally healthy woman, you may simply need a qualified person(s) to assist you in pregnancy and childbirth. Unless and until you need the care of one who manages illness, dysfunction, or trauma, a midwife can meet your needs.

A midwife is investigated for qualifications and experience by visiting with those who recommend her, particularly those whom she has served. When you meet with her you have every right, as you should do with a doctor, to question her concerning her training and experience. Some of the questions you might consider asking are:

1. How long have you practiced (on a fairly regular basis)?

2. Have you ever lost a baby or a mother? What were the circumstances?

3. How many episiotomies have you performed?

4. What is your laceration percentage? How often do you suture?

5. What is your transporting percentage?

6. Do you give prenatal care?

7. Do you use herbs? drugs? medication of any sort?

8. Do you have a back-up doctor? (The midwife may also want to know if YOUR doctor will back you/her up.)

SELECTED REFERENCES

Listed below are a few books with information about pregnancy, childbirth, and other topics of special interest to women.

HOME BIRTH, CHILDBIRTH, RELATED TOPICS

Airola, Paavo. **Everywoman's Book.** Forward by Mary Ann Kibler, M.D. Introduction by Robert S. Mendelsohn, M.D. Phoenix: HEALTH PLUS Publishers, 1979.

Block, Polly. **A Superior Alternative: Childbirth at Home.** American Fork, Utah: By the Author, 1979.

Cohen, Nancy Wainer, and Estner, Lois J. **Silent Knife: Cesarean Prevention and Vaginal Birth After Cesarean.** South Hadley, Mass.: Bergin & Garvey Publishers, Inc., 1983.

Davis, Adelle. **Let's Have Healthy Children.** Completely revised and updated by Marshall Mandell, M.D. Bergenfield, N.J.: New American Library, Inc., Signet Books, 1981.

Eloesser, Leo; Galt, Edith J.; and Hemingway, Isabel. **Pregnancy, Childbirth and the Newborn: A Manual for Rural Midwives,** 4th English ed. Mexico, D.F.: Instituto Indigenista Interamericano, 1976.

Hazell, Lester D. **Common Sense Childbirth.** Seattle: International Childbirth Education Association, 1976.

Ingals, A. Joy and Salerno, M. Constance. **Maternal & Child Health Nursing,** 3rd ed. St. Louis: The C.V. Mosby Company, 1975.

Mendelsohn, Robert S., **Confessions of a Medical Heretic.** Chicago: Contemporary Books, Inc., 1979; (Warner Books Edition) New York: Warner Books, Inc., 1979.

_____. **How to Raise a Healthy Child . . . In Spite of Your Doctor.** Chicago: Contemporary Books, Inc., 1984.

_____. **Male Practice: How Doctors Manipulate Women.** Chicago: Contemporary Books, Inc., 1982.

Royal, Penny C. **Herbally Yours.** Completely updated ed. Payson, Utah: Sound Nutrition, 1982.

OBSTETRICAL TEXTS

Garrey, Matthew M.; Govan, A. D. T.; Hodge, C.; and Callander, R. **Obstetrics Illustrated,** 2nd ed. Edinburgh, London, and New York: Churchill Livingstone, 1974.

Hellman, Louis M., and Pritchard, Jack A. **Williams Obstetrics,** 14th ed. New York: Appleton-Century-Crofts, 1971. (Earlier editions are also useful reference books; later editions are more intervention-oriented.)

Myles, Margaret F. **Textbook for Midwives,** 8th ed. Edinburgh, London, and New York: Churchill Livingstone, 1975.

DRUG REFERENCE BOOKS

Long, James W., **The Essential Guide to Prescription Drugs,** 3rd ed. New York: Harper & Row, 1982.

Medical Economics Company. **Physicians' Desk Reference,** 34th ed. Oradell, N.J.: Medical Economics Co., 1980. (Consult current editions.)

NOTES

[1]Grantly Dick Read, **Childbirth Without Fear: The Principle and Practice of Natural Childbirth** (New York: Harper & Brothers Publishers, 1944), p. 159. This natural childbirth classic (in its original form) offers some superb instruction for midwives.

[2]Benjamin Colby, **The Guide to Health,** 4th ed. (Milford, New Hampshire: John Burns, 1946), p. 170. (Reprinted by Amtec, Spanish Fork, Utah.) Dr. Beach was President of the Reformed Medical College of New York.

CHAPTER 2

LEGISLATION REGARDING MIDWIFERY

Since the publication of my first book, **A Superior Alternative: Childbirth at Home,** a dramatic improvement in respect for the rights and desires of parenting couples during childbirth has taken place in Utah. In 1979, the state legislature passed a law stipulating that midwifery is not the practice of medicine, essentially giving midwives who are not licensed or registered freedom to practice within a certain framework.

It appears that health care people may be interested in providing consumers in the Intermountain area with alternative procedures in childbirth; at least, a stepped-up program to cater to the desires of some patrons has been initiated. Home birth activity in the Intermountain Area is second only to home birth activity in California, and a high level of competence is found among midwives all over the country. Even so, home birth supporters have to be on guard against unfavorable legislation.

It is my opinion that most laws enacted to control the practice of midwifery are too confining. This opinion is substantiated by many with a great deal of expertise and experience. We have found that midwifery training in this day broadens the potential for artful handling of births by women who have great sensitivity and intuitiveness, who by their maternal natures can become delicately precise in a lost art.

As with any kind of practitioner, there are midwives who perform their labors with deftness and expertise, and there are others who will never quite have the same knack. Unfortunately, some of the laws concerning midwifery currently in force are NOT designed to upgrade the standards of the less qualified, or to assist parents in their efforts to locate skilled childbirth attendants who will be responsive to their needs. Much to the discredit of certain states, they have enacted "harassment legislation": laws designed not to protect the welfare or well-being of parents or babies, but laws designed to eliminate the practice of midwifery, particularly lay midwifery. (Parents obviously wonder if there aren't individuals or groups whose REAL interest in support of this type of legislation is a FINANCIAL one; I don't believe that either couples who desire home births or midwives pose a MORAL threat to those seeking to squash the home birth movement.)

For example, some laws require TWICE-YEARLY qualifying examinations for midwives. (When did your doctor last have to requalify to continue practicing?) Other laws require that enormous amounts of minutely detailed records be kept. While some paperwork is obviously profitable to both midwife and client, compulsive piles of it (to be made available at any time--unlike medical records), demonstrate clearly the intent of such laws. Likewise, laws which prohibit the use by midwives of any kind of medication, and then define herbs as "medication," aim not at regulating the use of controlled substances, but at stifling those who assist with home births. Such laws are impractical and are bound to be as ineffective as Prohibition was. The truth is: many home birth patrons use herbs, like herbs, and want the benefits offered by herbs in childbearing.

In a similar vein, some laws in various states today make it impossible for midwives to take as a client a woman who is having her fifth or later child, or a woman who has had even one previous miscarriage, or a woman whose pregnancy indicates a malposition.

Midwives today are capable of screening for home births well enough that they know better than to try to deliver a grand multipara who has had bleeding problems from a placid or inert uterus. Mothers who have prevented possible inertia by maintaining good body tone may deliver several additional offspring safely. Limiting home births by law to the fourth birth is not only a form of unnecessary governmental intervention, but it is ridiculous.

Restricting midwives from delivering a woman who has had previous miscarriages but has been able to carry out a normal, unremarkable (without complications) pregnancy to term is also going a little far. Here again, as in other circumstances, screening is wise and a good midwife will consult and co-screen.

Malpresentations are not always "mal" (bad). Posterior, breech, or multiple births are to be avoided when other risk conditions enter into the question. Training and experience, not laws, should dictate many decisions. Breech, arm, transverse, and brow presentations, and other sticky situations, are successfully handled by experienced midwives.

The law should not be used as a political device to deny a couple a safe alternative in the setting of their choice. Parents are not seeking legislation which would require them to have within the walls of their own homes the same type of experience they would have had in a hospital. The medical approach, with little room for nonstandard procedure, is precisely what most people want to get away from in seeking out midwives who persist in using different means of assisting the pregnant and childbearing woman. Legislators contemplating passing laws requiring their constituents to conform their birthing experiences to the philosophies of organized medicine would do well to remember that parents do not want their midwives to manage a birth like a doctor would; that is what they are trying to avoid. (If they wanted such a birth, they would go to a doctor and not to a midwife.)

In addressing concerns about the safety of home birth, many things enter a given situation to dictate safety. Pregnancy and childbirth are so unpredictable in nature that legislation calling for black and white stipulations does not take reality into account. Training, experience, and cooperation seem to be the answer. Restriction and regulation should be replaced by responsibility. Informed parents are capable of screening their midwives (a responsibility not to be taken lightly) and of choosing the situation which is best for them, and midwives are capable of screening those desiring their services (likewise, a responsibility not to be taken lightly).

The home birth couple tends to have a greater level of consciousness and concern about preparing for birth in a manner which would ensure safety for both mother and baby. Home birth encourages mothers and fathers to be more responsible about the things they do during pregnancy. Also, midwives of today do a tremendous amount of preventive care not practiced by others. The home birth couple searches out birth attendants who will work with them and who will use methods they have confidence in, creating for them a better birthing experience.

Why legally deny them this alternative as long as they pursue their way of life without criminal intent or action? Generally, those in the home birth movement wish to maintain control of a sacred moment without compromising the rights or safety of EITHER mother or baby.

In 1981, a seasoned legislator was invited to speak with the Idaho Midwifery Council (IMC) concerning their fears about upcoming bills being prepared against them by members of the American Medical Association in Idaho. The IMC was of the opinion that they should write a defensive bill which would counteract the opposition stand.

The congressman suggested that the midwives might be better off without any legislation. He warned that once a bill is passed, amendments are more easily adopted to negatively reconstruct the provisions therein, and that this possibility was certainly to be considered. In order for the midwives to be able to practice without the proposed restrictions, all they needed to do was to prevent passage of the opposition bill.

He cited incidents of action taken by the home birth people in other states, particularly in Utah. For several years opposition bills, harassment bills, and shirt-tail bills (bills restricting midwifery practice tacked on to bills certain to pass into law, but totally unrelated to the subject of midwifery) were kept off the floors of the House and Senate by hundreds of telephone calls coming in within minutes after the appearance of these bills in committee. These calls were followed by hundreds of letters written with courtesy but firmness, conciseness but full explanation for displeasure with the bill. All letters urged their representatives to defeat any bill which would in any way prevent home births, home birth care by midwives, or home birth care by midwives using the preferred methods or approaches typically used in home birth settings (herbs, therapy, etc.).

The legislator reminded the Council that the current mood of legislative bodies was to stay out of the private lives of constituents. "Take advantage of this conservative mood," concluded the visiting legislator. "Make your wishes known by letters, especially, and telephone calls to your representatives and senators. Enough of a ground swell cry from you can pass or prevent passage of anything in congress."[1]

Bills in most states must be read several times (usually three) in committee before being presented on the floor for votes of passage or defeat. If the bill has been presented by one body (Senate or House of Representatives), it has to pass that body and also go to the floor of the other body and pass there before going to the governor to be signed into law.

Due to a network of home birth parents across the state of Utah, opposition bills at this writing have never come out of committee. Public opinion still is the biggest deterrent to or promoter of specific legislation. Interested parties who want their freedoms maintained need only to be loosely organized to make the difference. It is important to have a "spotter" in the legislative halls to catch the bills as they appear, in time to notify the consumer. So many times a large segment of lay citizenry feel for some reason that those halls are restricted, to all but legislators. This is not true. Those halls belong to the citizens of this country, and the laws being enacted there directly affect them. Legislators respond to the citizens who elect (and replace) them, but they need you to make your wishes on given subjects known, so they may adequately represent you. Appropriate arguments for the alternatives of home birth can be found in Chapter 1 of **A Superior Alternative.**

It is too bad that all of the time, energy, and money spent combatting undesirable midwifery legislation could not instead be invested in teaching and training midwives. Midwives are a valuable commodity in a community, even a life-saving resource. It seems quite absurd, in a society which encourages first aid knowledge and home nursing skills, as well as the development of livesaving and emergency preparedness resources (CPR, artificial respiration, disaster and crisis management, survival training, etc.), to make it difficult for lay persons to learn to skillfully assist with childbirth using natural methods and therapies.

A recent study concluded that home birth is here to stay, that no amount of persuasion or even legislation will stop it. The study recommended that doctors utilize midwives in their practices and back-up midwives in birth centers and home births, and it suggested that doctors encourage their colleagues to do the same.

The Instituto Indigenista Interamericano, an organization in Mexico City that trains midwives in three months of classroom learning and three months of clinical practice, is highly recommended by the World Health Organization for its ability to turn out very competent midwives in that amount of time. Women who have had no formal training in medical fields--some are even illiterate--are able to go into their remote communities and practice with great skill. It is their job to handle complications, for in most instances there are no doctors or hospitals within many miles.

I believe we in this country can quickly and competently train midwives, as well. We need good midwives.

NOTES

[1] Polly Block, notes.

CHAPTER 3

ABORTION

"From the moment of fertilization," says Dr. Hymie Gordon, chief geneticist at the Mayo Clinic, "the pattern of the individual's constitutional development is irrevocably determined. . . . Despite the small size and weight of this new being, it is, as the medical scientist Blechschmidt said, 'a unique individual--specifically human.'"[1]

In my opinion, to cut off this person from all possibility of development is murder. Dr. Gilbert W. Scharffs wrote, "The plight of unwanted children is one of the tragic problems of our society. Making it easier to empty life's chamber is not the solution. Efforts should be made to solve the problem of why children are unwanted."[2] I am an advocate for the unborn.

A middle-aged woman who was informed about abortion lived next door to a newly-wed couple. They often visited together. One day the young woman mentioned that she was pregnant, but she was going to get an abortion because she and her husband had not saved any money. Her husband was still in school and they thought it better to wait a few years to have children.

26 POLLY'S BIRTH BOOK

The older neighbor asked the young bride if she would do one thing before they made a final decision about the abortion. The young woman readily agreed to read a prolife pamphlet which explained that pregnancy provides the environment for a human being to live in and develop until it has matured enough to live outside the womb. It explained that abortion takes an innocent life.

The young woman took the pamphlet home so she and her husband could read it together. She returned the next day in tears to thank her neighbor for helping them to understand what they would have done had they carried out their plans. They were ignorant of what abortion really is and were grateful that an opportunity had been given them to understand the consequences of such action.

This story illustrates the point that a number of women choose abortion out of ignorance. With manipulation, ploy, and controversy about the subject common, it is no small wonder that young people are often confused. They simply do not know that from the moment of conception a unique individual is created, and its journey to become part of humanity has begun. We would do well to try to understand our friends who have chosen to have an abortion and to gently make sure they know what they are doing. The choice is still theirs, but it should be an informed choice.

Emotions run high about abortion, so sticking to a few facts can give a clearer perspective about what it really means to end the life of a fetus.

Spontaneous abortion is the medical term for a miscarriage. It is the natural expulsion of a fetus that for some reason the body cannot carry. **Induced abortion** (intentionally caused termination of pregnancy) was in the past known almost exclusively as **criminal abortion.** Now, the vast majority of induced abortions are termed **therapeutic abortions.** So subtly do words enable us to hide from unpleasant truth. Rarely is abortion therapeutic. (The life of the mother is, of course, paramount.)

Several methods are used to abort an embryo or fetus:

> Up to 10 weeks, the embryo is scraped out of the uterus with a curette or forceps or the physician's finger.
>
> Up to 13 weeks, the embryo is removed from the womb by vacuum aspiration with a metal suction curette and forceps. The risk of blood loss and of perforating the uterus or damaging the cervix is increased.
>
> After 13 weeks, an abdominal hysterotomy is sometimes performed. An incision is made in the mother's abdomen and the uterus is pulled out and scraped, then sutured and replaced. There is danger here that scar tissue on the uterus may rupture during succeeding pregnancies.
>
> After 14 weeks, a long needle is inserted into the bag of waters through the abdomen, some amniotic fluid removed, and a saline solution injected. Prostaglandins are sometimes given, either intravenously or injected into the amniotic cavity, to facilitate abortion. Abortion usually follows within 24 hours or, if there is any delay, labor is induced.

Complications from these methods include nausea and vomiting, incomplete evacuation requiring curettage (50 percent of the time), hemorrhage, and injury to the cervix.

In 1976, the national ratio of abortions to live births was 313 abortions per 1,000 live births. This figure rose in 1979 to 358 per 1,000. In Utah, the 1976 ratio was 67.5 per 1,000. This rose to 84.9 per 1,000 in 1979, and 94.7 per 1,000 in 1983.[3] (All of these figures refer ONLY to reported cases, and do not include Utah residents who had abortions in other states.)

Reasons for abortion cannot always be determined, particularly from public records. Nevertheless, the 1975 Utah statistics state that 2 percent of all reported abortions were performed for medical reasons and 6 percent for psychological reasons. That leaves 92 percent performed for other reasons, probably mostly reasons of convenience. The 1981 Utah statistics report that 93.5 percent of the abortions were performed for "therapeutic reasons."[4]

One of the cries from opponents of home birth is that midwives might perform abortions. It is impossible for me to condone the arts of midwifery being used in any way to abort a fetus for any reason. If there is a life-or-death situation for the mother and an abortion is needed, a physician must do it: under the right circumstances, after numerous evaluations and consultations. Taking a life is serious business.

The chapter on abortion in **A Superior Alternative** discusses in-depth this evil. Teach your daughters and clients so that they may never entertain the thought of having an abortion.

NOTES

[1] Polly Block, A Superior Alternative: Childbirth at Home (American Fork, Utah: By the Author, 1979), pp. 109-10, quoting Sean O'Reilly, M.D., "Physician Outlines Life After Conception" (pamphlet).

[2] Gilbert W. Scharffs, "The Case Against Easier Abortion Laws," Ensign, August 1972, p. 57.

[3] Utah Department of Health, Bureau of Health Statistics, statistical reports. (The 1983 Utah abortion ratio was obtained by telephone, prior to its publication.)

[4] Ibid. Abortions performed on behalf of the "emotional well-being" or the "emotional health" of the mother are among those classified as "therapeutic" abortions. Abortion can cause more psychoneurotic problems than it can cure. Dr. Victor Calef, of the Mt. Sinai Clinic in San Francisco, believes that "abortion itself is a potential source of psychiatric illness and a basis for mental breakdown. . . ." (Scharffs, p. 54)

CHAPTER 4

BETTER SIT DOWN FOR THIS ONE

MISUNDERSTANDING THE MARRIAGE ACT

Nope! Sewing up episiotomies tightly is not what marital intimacy is all about. The marriage act stems from something much more important than the physical pleasures that tend to promote it. I usually question the motives and the mind of the doctor who says to his patient's husband following the suturing of a large episiotomy, "She's better than new!" He certainly is not thinking of the mother and her childbearing responsibilities.

When hearts and minds are in the right place, a woman's physical make-up really doesn't matter that much when it comes to the marriage act. Becoming "one" is a marvelous expression of love. But becoming one on the physical level alone is only a part of what it's all about.

According to President Spencer W. Kimball, a religious leader, "The sexual drives which bind men and women together as one are good and necessary. They make it possible to leave one's parents and cleave unto one another."[1] We know how important bonding can be in a family to promote love, loyalty, faithfulness, and security. It is important for children to have deep, personal feelings within the family so they later can properly build loyalties to their own spouses and offspring.

One way this loyalty to spouse is nurtured is through intimacy. If husbands feel that their wives are not sexually responsive, it may possibly be that earlier in the day something went wrong—unintentionally.

Too few men realize that a woman needs to be approached on the mental level. When she is convinced that she is loved for her intelligence, her personality, her talents, and not her body alone, she readily feels the need to share her body and become one with her husband.

INTELLIGENCE? "Boy, honey, you sure handled the household funds nicely this month!" "My, you told that pressure salesman just the right thing." "How can you remember all those things about nutrition, dear? This is going to be a mighty healthy family!"

PERSONALITY? "You made me so proud of you tonight when that negative conversation came up with our friends. Your positive attitude turned the whole thing around." "I can always count on your looking at the bright side of things. Do you know what that means to me when I am trying so hard to make ends meet?"

TALENTS? "You made us shirts to match! How fun!" "Hon, when I hear our whole family singing while you play the piano so beautifully, it fills my heart." "You are a great little mother. I never worry that you will not know how to take care of our children." "I'm proud of you."

THIS, husbands, TURNS HER ON!

Controlled and exercised in love, the marriage act can be entered into upon all three levels: the physical, the mental, and the spiritual. Only when all those levels are involved does the union of a husband and wife reach its highest, most joyous consummation. It is meant to reach all three levels to be perfect. If one partner hurries to enjoy only the physical level, a rich and rewarding experience is forfeited for both partners.

In fact, the frequency with which the marriage act is participated in can either add to or diminish its specialness. Both husband and wife should practice restraint from ROUTINE intercourse, remembering that although begetting offspring is not the only reason, it is the major reason for this relationship.

A widespread misconception is the notion that when the husband has taken his wife to the altar, she is now his to do with as he pleases, when he pleases. Very soon after marriage many intimate and warm demonstrations of love between couples become routine and taken for granted. Some husbands expect this as submission to vows which were never meant to license such behavior.

It is true that sometimes it is the woman who makes demands upon her husband when he is less amorous. Indeed, at times it is when the woman is pregnant that her emotional-physical needs are highest. Perhaps this is hormone related or a subconscious freedom from conceiving that releases her feelings: the impulse differs with the individual.[2]

Because men are physically built the way they are, a woman has the obligation to be careful not to tempt by playing coy with her husband's affections during a time of planned restraint. If she expects him to be considerate of her, she must find warm and loving ways to express appreciation and regard for him and his efforts. A couple must come to an agreement on when and how to assist each other in their restraint.

Not even God asks a man or woman to stop having intercourse, for God instituted procreation and this manner of becoming one; but He does ask us to use purpose and wisdom and consideration. Changing for the better implies first a desire to change, then effort put forth, with prayer, to make the change effective. If a couple can do this together, blessings and rewards are inevitable.

I recall a friend who, at the death of his wife, stood back and looked at her body, and gently remarked, "My, how I've loved that body." Do you suppose for a moment that a man (or woman) who loved a spouse's body in such a way would ever abuse it? Certainly not! It would be treated with respect and care and loved with the tenderest of emotions. It would never be struck, handled roughly, or hurt just because the person inside the body may not have been amiable.

MARRIAGE COUNSELING

An excellent opportunity presents itself when young couples come to leaders, as well as to parents, for counseling prior to marriage. Why not counsel them to look forward to the three-level marriage experiences, instead of permitting couples to think that since they have abstained from intimacy before marriage, the reward is to be able to participate in "anything that is not offensive to the partner"? The idea that no holds are barred, all stops are pulled, and anything goes, is not going to build a permanent foundation of stability in marriage. Abusing the body with perversion is in no way considered restraining from appetites of the flesh and will not help in attaining righteous goals. Higher goals and concepts result in the rewarding, binding powers of heaven.

And for those couples who have been oriented in the less rewarding activities of marriage (or nonmarriage), now is the time to give them hope and help them set their sights and goals toward behavior that will give lasting joy and trust. Merely being "physical" is not all there is to a very happy union. There are those who would have us believe otherwise, but their sights are not set upon lasting relationships.

During my family counseling days a young friend told me that when she and her sweetheart were married, he cared enough about helping her make the transition from unmarried life to married life that they slept together for six weeks before they had intercourse. He offered her this time because he really cared for her, and she had been honest in her delay, wanting to feel fully prepared for intimacy. He, too, wanted to initiate their sexual relationship in a comfortable and purposeful frame of mind. I know of a number of couples who seem to have this eternal perspective and self-discipline, who are happily married and totally faithful to their spouses.

A WORD TO HUSBANDS

Because a woman gives herself to you, her husband, she sometimes conceives. After conception, something begins to happen to her: sexuality changes significantly, especially with succeeding pregnancies. She may not return to her preconception response to your advances until the full cycle from conception through lactation has been fulfilled. If husbands can understand this cycle, a new world will unfold to them. Interest will increase, not resentment.

Your wife does not become uninterested or "have headaches" because she does not love you or think you are any less a man. No. You, the love of her life, the only man in her life, have helped her maternal nature to be fulfilled. But because you—and perhaps your wife, also—have not recognized what is happening, you become confused. You want her to respond to your intimate feelings, but she cannot always respond as readily as before. What has happened? The two of you have set in motion her opportunity to fulfill a measure of her creation: to have a baby.

When a woman conceives she is becoming fulfilled, but the cycle is not done yet. Allow her and encourage her to finish that cycle. Her physiology has changed and reordered. And it will continue that way until the child is born and no longer needs the all-consuming sustenance she has within her to give him for the first few months of his life. When you place TOO MANY sexual demands upon her before this cycle is completed, frustration and tension and possibly a very natural lack of wholehearted cooperation on her part are the result. In other words, you have helped her to become fulfilled as a woman, but you didn't know it would take her 18 months to two years before she can respond to you as sexually as she did before she became pregnant.

If you want a happy, fulfilled wife, one who is ready to return to you with all the love and submission she once gave you, YOU MUST BE PART OF HER CYCLE. You can do this by being understanding and considerate of her feelings at this time in her life.

Every wife needs support, consideration, kindness, and approval while she performs her labor of love. She needs your help. When you come home from work to find the phone ringing, something burning on the stove, the baby in his highchair dumping food on the floor, Johnny crying because his bike is missing, and Mary Ann screaming because she's just mashed her fingers in the back door, don't push the panic button and then run away from the havoc.

Be the hero, the man of the hour. Tell your wife, "Go ahead, honey, get the phone," as you pull the burning food off the stove, clean up the baby's mess, and tell Johnny you'll help him look for his bike if he will play Red Cross and help you bandage Mary Ann's bleeding fingers.

Now, after being sensitive to what this day has done to your wife's tranquility, if you make no sexual demands on her, she, still grateful for your performance during the disaster and refreshed by a hot bath and some rest, may surprise you and ask for the intimate attention you desire. But if she doesn't at this time, your continuing to understand and protect and love her will surely bring greater rewards at a later time. This is worth waiting for.

When your wife is with child, and for the few months after childbirth, she needs much more assistance with the family and household. Fathers, I ask you to see to it that during your wife's pregnancies--which do take her extra strength and energy--she never has to perform exhausting labors or has to be excessively concerned with family problems. See to it that she has spare time for her quiet sitz bath and a leisurely walk each day.

If Mom can take a bath, read a book or do what she enjoys, go for a walk without the children (once a day), she can build the resources she needs to bear and nurture offspring and to be patient with the family while spending quality time as a loving companion to her husband. But this takes cooperation on the part of the whole family. One acquaintance had a rule that Mom, his sweetheart, was to do no work at all after the evening meal. Any chores or last-minute preparations for the morrow had to be taken care of by the children when they became old enough to do those things.

INTERCOURSE DURING PREGNANCY

In some cultures, past and present, womanhood and the procreative state was held in such reverence and awe that an expectant mother was "put away"; that is, no sexual demands on her were made. It was a cultural and social taboo to interfere with the childbearing or lactating mother. Her state of being was celestial. It was a holy thing which was going on within her, and to disturb or to violate her was unheard-of.

According to Elder Orson F. Whitney, also a religious leader, "During certain periods, those of gestation and lactation, the wife and mother should be comparatively free to give her strength to her offspring; and if this involves some self-denial on the part of the husband and father, so much the better for all concerned."[3]

Some physicians feel that intercourse is dangerous during the first and third trimesters. During the first trimester, the uterus is soft and still very low, sitting just behind the symphysis pubis and the bladder (see Chapter 6, Obstetrical Anatomy). It therefore is rather vulnerable to vigorous activity in that region; early spontaneous abortion can result. During the third trimester, the baby's head is low. Interference again becomes more likely at this time.

One midwife reported that one of the most moving experiences she had had with home birth came when she learned of a husband's behavior during his wife's pregnancy. He was a vegetarian, and he felt that this way of life had made him more sensitive to higher values. Throughout the entire pregnancy, he had voluntarily abstained from intercourse, and, upon discovering that the baby was coming breech, he had fasted the whole day of the birth for the infant's and mother's safety. They were delivered safely and there was much rejoicing, with the same quietness and simple joy that had been manifest during the whole gestational period.

FAMILY PLANNING AND BIRTH CONTROL

Pregnancy does not have to be and should not be a chore. A mother should be happy and healthy. She probably needs two years between the birth of one child and the conception of the next in order that: (1) her baby can be the baby for that time, (2) she can have at least one year or so to nurse the baby and give him a healthier beginning in life, and (3) she can have a rest and give her body a chance to rebuild.

One religious leader suggests nine months for pregnancy, nine months for nursing, and at least nine months for resting and rebuilding. This seems reasonable to thinking people. If a woman has not been able to nurse her baby for nine months to a year, she may not be taking proper care of herself, in which case she should not become pregnant until she feels better. (If mothers will make it their first priority to nurture and teach--not, to pick up after everyone--they will be better mothers.)

I know a mother of several children who found herself confronted with a problem well-known among married people: fertility! Though she felt strongly that motherhood is supremely important, she was concerned about having children in too close succession. She was worried that physically she was run down and couldn't handle another pregnancy right away.

This young mother decided to seek counsel about birth control from a respected and trusted church leader. He listened to her patiently and she tried to make sure he understood her motives. She explained that she was involved in church activities and also that she felt her priorities were properly set, but she still had a dilemma. "I truly want all the children the Lord would like me to have. I feel that I have not had all the children I want. But I need a rest! I cannot safely have another baby just yet. What can my husband and I do about it and still find favor with the Lord?"

Her wise friend--a man, no less--leaned forward in his chair and without flinching quietly asked, "Have you considered restraint?"

Whenever I have repeated this story to women, their inevitable response is, "Tell that to my husband."

I have not dared, until now, to tell it to husbands, but why shouldn't I? What surer way is there to prevent conception? By abstaining, you avoid the side effects of contraceptives. You also do not have to worry about using an IUD or the Pill: these do not prevent conception, but instead they cause the spontaneous abortion of a fertilized egg--a little, new baby.

Some may feel that restraint will cause tension and resentment between a couple. If, however, two people arrive at a decision to use this method of birth control and carry it out with loving intent, I believe abstaining from sexual relations at certain times can be a binding experience in their marriage.

When a woman needs a rest from childbearing, there are several ways of determining when she is fertile, and thus when to restrain from intercourse. The most constructive way to plan the arrival of newborns into your family is to use the **Billings Ovulation Method.** One health authority concludes that the Billings, calendar (or rhythm), sympto-thermal, and body temperature methods all coincide, and if they are used together to produce a "total fertility awareness," they are effective and far more safe than artificial means.[4]

It will take careful monitoring to discover the signs and symptoms which reveal your individual **fertility cycle.** Then, **fertility awareness** can help you plan your family.

While refraining from intercourse, observe and chart the quality and nature of vaginal mucus throughout an entire menstrual cycle (**Billings Method**). Intercourse stimulates secretions in the vagina and can confuse this determination of the normal changes in the mucus which occur. With an understanding of these changes, **ovulation**--the only time conception is possible--can be reliably anticipated each month.

The mucus comes from glands near the cervix. After menstruation, when the hormonal estrogen level is low, the vagina feels dry and mucus is scant, but opaque and sticky. As the body prepares for ovulation, estrogen levels increase and the amount of mucus increases. The mucus becomes progressively thinner and clearer, and quite slippery. About a day before ovulation, it will be slick, stretchy, and slippery, resembling egg white. (A thread of it will stretch, unbroken, between your thumb and forefinger.) OVULATION OCCURS AT THIS TIME OF GREATEST LUBRICATING SENSATION.

The increased slippery feeling facilitates intercourse at this particular period, so that conception and procreation will be more sure to take place. The alkaline mucus prolongs the life of the sperm cells as they are guided upward toward the ovum, protecting them against the acid pH condition of the vagina.

TO PREVENT CONCEPTION, YOU MUST ABSTAIN FROM INTERCOURSE FOR 4 TO 8 DAYS BEFORE OVULATION AND 3 DAYS AFTERWARD. The very fertile may wish to abstain an extra day or two before ovulation. Obviously, keeping good records is important.

Other indicators of ovulation can also be observed. On the day of ovulation, the wife's temperature (before she rises in the morning) will rise, up to one degree above normal. Irritability, pain, tender breasts, and edema are often apparent (**body temperature** and **sympto-thermal methods**).

Those with VERY regular cycles can predict quite well their **fertile days** (**calendar method**). An approximate chart follows, with the **first fertile day** counted from the first day of menstruation:

If your cycle is:	your first fertile day is:
22 days	4th day
24 days	6th day
26 days	8th day
28 days	10th day
30 days	12th day
32 days	14th day

TO PREVENT CONCEPTION USING THIS METHOD, YOU MUST ABSTAIN FROM INTERCOURSE FOR 7 TO 8 DAYS, BEGINNING WITH THE FIRST FERTILE DAY.

Nursing has been an effective contraceptive for many women. (I suspect that this benefit was by design, and that in a less degenerate physical state, lactation is the perfect birth control.) When a mother begins to feed her baby more and more from the table, however, her lactating processes begin to lessen and conception becomes more likely.

One mother told me that lactating, prayer, and the rhythm method had "planned" her eight children just the way she felt was warranted. I am sure this is the case with many. Several couples have told me they had recurring dreams about additional babies that were waiting to come to them; therefore, they knew it was time to conceive again. Prayer should play the utmost part in all family begetting.

THE ETERNAL PERSPECTIVE

It is assumed that most people would like to "lay up stores" of peace and enjoyment for the hereafter, and to accumulate experiences of integrity so that they may be still allowed to use talents and gifts to accomplish something besides playing a harp!

Better Sit Down For This One 43

If one is given dominions there, it stands to reason that powers like unto the model, or heavenly parent, would be unleashed for the good of mankind. Dominions are endowed, yet earned, through exercises of purpose, integrity, compassion, restraint, self-denial, and willingness to follow directions and to direct for the good of all.

It also stands to reason that the physical and emotional designs of the mortal being have pointed the way to primary roles in life, even Everlasting Life. The couple dreams and plans together. Then the man organizes, directs, provides, and protects with great love and tenderness. The woman stands beside her man, teaches, loves, and bears offspring with gentleness and compassion.

In this eternal perspective, perhaps men were meant to be more fulfilled, more quickly, in sexual intercourse than women, inasmuch as he must be about his particulars, and inasmuch as her long-range fulfillment is not consummated until she has brought forth the product of their union. Procreating takes time, and frustration might be her lot if she were adequately fulfilled in the moment, yet still had months ahead needed to finish her very special contribution. For her, gestation is a stewardship all its own, and is recognized as such in the anticipation of bearing her husband's child.

Only another woman can know the marvels and depths of joy of carrying a baby and giving it birth. Only another man can feel the wonder, the awe, the fatherhood of siring a son or a daughter. These are unmistakable roles, yet they are designed to create the need for gifts and talents that add variety and refreshing highs to everyday exercise of discipline. The counterfeit philosophy tells us to disregard the disciplines that make us accountable: "If it feels good, do it." I am convinced that only men and women who gain a certain amount of control over the appetites of the flesh (the desires and passions of the animal level alone) will ever have the privilege of claiming the joys and dominions longed for in everyday family life or in the eternities. Balance and order, timing, and the giving of time, and space, to each other are the essence of peopling and managing a world.

NOTES

[1] President Spencer W. Kimball, "Privileges and Responsibilities of Sisters," **Ensign**, November 1978, p. 102.

[2] Studies have shown that the degree of amativeness is, in part, correlated with the consumption of animal flesh. When people measured for amativeness are asked whether they are flesh eaters, those with low measurements (less responsive to purely sexual stimuli) invariably are vegetarians or persons who limit their animal protein.

[3] "Birth Control," **Relief Society Magazine**, June 1916, p. 367.

[4] See Dr. Paavo Airola, **Everywoman's Book** (Phoenix: HEALTH PLUS Publishers, 1979), pp. 339-44.

CHAPTER 5

MEDICATION AND THE MIDWIFE

This chapter discusses the use of drugs in pregnancy and childbirth, contrasting the approaches used by most doctors with those of the midwife. In general, the midwife enhances natural body processes with natural means, while the doctor frequently stimulates or depresses, hurries or slows these processes by introducing strong, potentially harmful substances. You need to be informed about these substances in case you must go to the hospital during labor or childbirth, and you will want to know alternative ways of dealing with problems that many doctors try to solve with drugs or other unnatural interventions.

DRUG USE IN PREGNANCY AND CHILDBIRTH

Because consumers have recently become more aware of the risks of drugs and are choosing natural childbirth more often, many hospitals have modified their routine use of drugs. They usually give painkilling drugs at the patient's request, and other kinds of drugs at the doctor's request. All too often, however, a mother in labor does not know about the potential effects of a drug on her soon-to-be-born child or on her; she asks for a painkiller without understanding either the harmful effects that the drug may have or the alternatives that are available. She may have some idea that a particular drug may not be good for her baby, but she is left to make such a decision at a very stressful time—a time when it can be difficult to think clearly or to reason effectively. All mothers, then, should know the facts about drugs BEFORE they are confronted with a decision about whether or not to use them.

During labor and delivery in the hospital, medications may be given for one or more of the following reasons:

1. To relax the patient.

2. To relieve pain.

3. To manipulate labor (slow it down or, more frequently, force or hurry it).

4. To make the doctor's work easier.

5. To deaden the senses prior to an obstetrical intervention (episiotomy, forceps, C-section, etc.).

6. To prevent or treat hemorrhage.

The first thing to remember about drugs is that they ALL pass through the placenta and the umbilical cord to the fetus. There are no exceptions. Furthermore, it is usually only a matter of seconds before something injected into the mother's blood stream also enters the fetal circulation. One doctor observed that when a local for an episiotomy is given before the head crowns, the baby will receive as much (or more) of the drug as the mother does. A drug's influence on the fetus begins almost immediately.

For example, some drugs cause **depression** (a slowing down or depressing of bodily functions). A depressed mother is groggy and lacks control; a depressed baby may lose its ability to breathe normally or its ability to fight for life.

If the baby is under any stress in the fetal environment or during delivery, a depressive drug such as **Demerol** or **morphine** (narcotics commonly used in childbirth; and yes, some doctors still use morphine) can substantially reduce the baby's chance for survival. Drugs to sedate the mother sedate the infant as well. If the mother has hallucinations or delirium as a result of the drugs used--and this DOES occur--what is happening to the infant? Not only does the baby have a much smaller system for the drug to be circulating in, but its liver and kidneys have not developed to a point where they can handle toxic chemicals.

In the hospital, a mother might receive several drugs during her antepartum hours and as she delivers: a tranquilizer, if she is apprehensive; a hypnotic, if she is tired; an analgesic and sedative or narcotic, if she is in pain; oxytocin (**Pitocin**), if her labor has slowed or stopped.

Several dangers are inherent in this use and multiplication of drugs, besides the possible side effects from each drug itself. First, if the laboring woman does not know her own capacities, she may ask for medication too soon, then be given further doses later when labor becomes harder and she "really" wants it.[1] The course of labor will be affected by any medication given, making it more likely that there will be additional drug intervention. By the time the baby is actually born, it may suffer severe depression.

Second, the administration of a second drug can expand the effects of the first. The risk of either drug producing side effects, as well as the strength of the toxic effect, is often multiplied severalfold.

Third, no two individuals will respond identically to a standard dose of a drug, nor will one person respond the same way to a drug administered alone as she will to the same drug administered in combination with another drug.

In general, the more drugs given, the harder it becomes for the baby to make its arrival safely. For the most part, drugs alleviate the mother's discomfort or hasten the doctor's work; they rarely enhance the natural work the body does by itself and they rarely help the baby at all.

Drugs affect childbirth in another way: an infant may be born with defects, malformations, or other problems with varying degrees of seriousness as a result of drugs taken by the mother during pregnancy. It has been estimated that pregnant women take an average of ten prescribed drugs. Jan Els, a pharmacologist, said at a midwifery conference for nurses at Idaho State University in July, 1977: "Drugs do not have any one effect in the body. There is no such thing as a drug affecting one area only--it affects all of the body." She further observed that "during pregnancy, pain relievers, diuretics, antihistamines, antibiotics, appetite depressants--ALL have effects, even up to neonatal and afterwards for months."[2]

Robert S. Mendelsohn, M.D., credits Eli Lilly, a pharmaceutical manufacturer, with having said that "a drug without toxic effects is no drug at all." Dr. Mendelsohn warns that EVERY drug, including aspirin, must be approached with suspicion, particularly during pregnancy. He states:

> . . . [I]f you're pregnant, you and your baby are better off if you stay away from all drugs **completely**. A drug that has minor side effects **on you** may do irreparable harm to a developing fetus. Hundreds of drugs are marketed long before their effects on the fetus are known. Unless you want to donate your baby's welfare to science and be one of the first to find out a drug's effects, don't take **any** drug unless your life is at stake.[3]

Surely there were mothers who expressed concern to their doctors about taking thalidomide, or DES (diethylstilbestrol), or bendectin, but were reassured that these drugs were "safe." After all, they were given for conditions directly associated with pregnancy. What mother whose baby was born with a defect due to her nausea medication would not have willingly foregone that means of dealing with morning sickness? Many women are finding out the hard way that drugs their doctors had said (or implied) were safe for their use were in reality harmful.

In addition to the immediate ill effects on both mother and baby from drugs used in pregnancy and/or childbirth, several studies show a marked, long-range effect from these drugs when in a few months or years dysfunctions become apparent. Physical impairment, mental retardation, or combinations of both can occur. Adverse reactions are not limited to the physical or the immediate: they may be emotional or behavioral and they may be separated in time from the administration of the drug(s). (Remember, it took a generation for problems with DES to surface, yet the time interval that had elapsed did not change the fact that this drug was responsible.)

Dr. Mendelsohn also cautions:

> ... Don't be mislead by risks that are expressed in small percentages. If you judge the danger of an iceberg by the size of the part that's above water, you're not going to stay afloat very long. Like a game of Russian Roulette, for the person who gets the loaded chamber, the risk is 100 percent. But unlike that game, for the person taking a drug no chamber is entirely empty. Every drug stresses and hurts your body in some way.[4]

You can read about the dangers of specific drugs in pharmacology books and the like (see Chapter 1, Selected References). Dr. Mendelsohn has written a very explicit chapter, "Fifty Drugs Every Woman Should Think Twice About Before Taking," in his book, **Male Practice: How Doctors Manipulate Women** (Chicago: Contemporary Books, Inc., 1982). He lists by trade and generic names the fifty drugs women most often ask him about, along with: (1) what the drugs are commonly prescribed for, (2) potential adverse effects, and (3) some personal comments.

You can also learn from the experience of others. In many of my classes a mother will begin to cry when we go through material on drug misuse. By the time we have finished, she will volunteer a painful, "THAT is exactly what happened to my son (or daughter)!" Then she will relate a heart-breaking tale of the damage suffered by her child due to drugs administered by a well-meaning practitioner during pregnancy and/or delivery, and of the sorrow caused the family by the death or defect of the child.

Instead of searching for ways to assist the laboring (or merely expectant) mother WITHOUT the use of drugs, the medical profession continues to search for what may be a myth: a drug or combination of drugs that will be "completely safe" for mother and baby. Until they find such a thing, both are vulnerable.

INDUCING LABOR

One of the most common uses of medications during childbirth is to induce labor. Dr. Anne Anderson, an obstetrician at the John Radcliffe Hospital at Oxford University, and Dr. Alec Turnbull, chairman of obstetrics there, together studied over 3,000 newborns. They found that the unborn baby knows better than anyone else, including the doctor, when it should be born. The study revealed that the baby triggers its own birth when it is ready. A hormone called **cortisol** (secreted from the baby's brain) stimulates the mother's uterine muscles and causes them to contract, beginning labor at the proper time.

> "When the unborn baby finds conditions in the womb deteriorating because of declining oxygen or reduced nutritional levels, he sends out this distress signal in the form of cortisol which triggers labor contractions. In the same way, overdue babies are often trying to tell us that they simply need more time to mature before they come out. We've found that in 80 percent of all births, the timing is strictly up to the baby himself. . . . In the past, doctors were prone to completely ignore these signals from the baby if they occurred before the expected date of delivery," said Dr. Anderson. The doctors prescribed bed rest and medication for the mother to suppress labor, . . . "but our research indicates that these distress signals should be taken seriously--it's better to let the unborn child have his way and come out early since he's the one who knows his environment best. On the other hand, doctors who induce labor take the risk that the baby's lungs or his disease-fighting mechanism may not be ready to cope with the outside world."[5]

For years midwives have noticed a tendency toward overdue babies or confused uterine functioning in mothers who have had their labors induced or controlled artificially (with Pitocin). When a uterus has been prevented from performing the task of expelling a baby on its own, it takes natural methods to encourage the uterus to function properly.

Inducing labor is always a dangerous interference. Midwives and mothers should be aware of the routine doctors use to induce labor so that they understand how steadfastly they should avoid it, except to save a life. A doctor who induces labor because he is relying too heavily on an approximated due date only--and ALL due dates are averaged and approximated--may not be using good judgment. Other factors, far more serious than labor setting in on its own a few days early or late, need consideration before induction of labor is begun. Certainly doctor convenience or impatience on the mother's part does not warrant induction.

The following routine is followed, with slight variations from doctor to doctor, for inducing labor in the hospital:

1. The amniotic membrane is ruptured. If this is done too soon--before the cervix has begun to retract or **efface** (thin and draw up to fit around the fetal head)--the parturient will go through a lot of pain for nothing because the inducement will not bring about the desired result: labor. Then the doctor may perform a C-section, since it is considered dangerous to let the gravida go more than 24 to 48 hours with the amnion ruptured.

2. For others, if contractions do not begin within two hours, **Pitocin** or **oxytocin** (a pituitary hormonal extract which triggers uterine contractions) is administered, usually intravenously. (It can be given orally or injected intramuscularly, as well.)

3. Because each individual's make-up is different, some women may respond to the Pitocin with unbearably painful contractions. If this

happens, and it frequently does, the woman is usually given Demerol to ease pain and calm her down. One of the problems with this is that sometimes the contractions slow down too much or stop altogether.

4. By this time everybody is tired, and if it is obvious that the mother isn't going to give birth in the next few hours, the doctor or nurse may say, "Let's give you something to help you get a good night's rest and we'll finish this up in the morning." So Demerol is again administered, but the mother gets only a little rest because contractions proceed right through the night, even though they don't accomplish much except to make the poor woman uncomfortable. She can't even go to the bathroom because of her IV. Her heart monitor beeps all night and may keep her awake.

5. The next morning, Pitocin is given again. This time doctors are going to stop fooling around and get that baby born, so a higher dose is given, and here we go! By now the woman is so tired and so discouraged that she is almost willing to go through anything to get the birth over with, and that's about what happens. She goes through more than she can bear. Pitocin forces contractions. They can be excruciating. No man can ever know how excruciating!

6. After a battle she'll not soon forget, the mother gives birth, much to everyone's relief.

If the above routine does not produce birth, doctors resort to the extraction birth (forceps or, in some places, a suctioning cup applied to the fetal head) or to cesarean delivery.

Because many women do not take care of themselves, their muscle tone becomes flabby. Interference with the natural birthing process then becomes routine. Who wants an overdue, hurting mom on their hands, a mom who will probably hemorrhage postpartum? Probably next to malpractice suits and hemorrhage, obstetricians fear most the bother of uterine inertia.

When a mother follows the dietary, hydrotherapy, exercise, and five-week formula program described in this volume, the above routine may be completely avoided.

NATURAL MANAGEMENT OF PREGNANCY

Rather than rely on drugs, many lay midwives stress the wise and regular use of herbs, massage, supplements (if needed), and other natural therapies throughout pregnancy, labor, and delivery. (It would be a rare thing to come across a Certified Nurse Midwife who can manage a birth successfully with the use of natural therapies and herbs. They simply are not trained in their use.)

Herbs and plant products include seeds, leaves, roots, or juice with medicinal value. Herbal preparations are a natural counterpart to drugs, without harmful side effects when used with prudence. Throughout the book I have included suggestions for using herbs to treat or prevent disorders that occur during pregnancy and childbirth (see especially Chapter 9, Herbs and Supplements).[6]

These natural products and therapies are superior to hospital-administered injections. They can prevent or treat specific problems associated with pregnancy, labor, and delivery. Herbal preventive therapy, a proper diet, exercise, sitz baths, and other procedures discussed in this work usually preclude the need for harmful medications.

NOTES

[1] One of the greatest advantages to birthing at home is not having the mother ever reach the point of wanting, needing, or asking for drugs. With constant, in-person attention and care, tension rarely reaches a point where this much discomfort is encountered. Without drug availability, the temptation to ask for drugs doesn't occur. If it ever did, there are other things that can help the mother, without side effects.

[2] Polly Block, notes.

[3] Robert S. Mendelsohn, M.D., **Confessions of a Medical Heretic** (Chicago: Contemporary Books, Inc., 1979), p. 39.

[4] Ibid., pp. 42-43.

[5] From a news article in the files of the author.

[6] The following account is of an earlier midwife who relied with promise upon the herbs:

> Ann Carling holds the unique position of having had the Prophet Joseph Smith lay his hands on her head and set her apart as a midwife. He told her that she would be successful if she used herbs exclusively in her work. Ann Carling then became known as the "Herb Doctor." She practiced her calling and brought hundreds of babies into the world and was blessed in this as the Prophet had promised her. She had her own herb garden and made her own teas and medicines. Most of the herbs grown in her garden had beautiful flowers. Her garden, therefore, was valuable not only as a producer of herbs for medicinal purposes, but was valuable as a garden of beauty.
>
> For many years she was the only midwife in Fillmore, Utah, and neighboring towns. Her fee was three dollars and she accepted it either in cash or merchandise. She was not only godmother to all the babies but doctor for all the ills of both young and old. Even the Indians came to her for aid. Without knowing the scientific reasons, she practiced most of the sanitary measures we now know are so necessary. [Kate B. Carter, comp., Heart Throbs **of the West**, vol. 3 (Salt Lake City: Daughters of Utah Pioneers, 1948), pp. 136-37; and Elda P. Mortenson, comp. and ed., Isaac V. Carling Family History, 2 vols. (n.p.: By the Author, [1964]), 1:8-9.]

UNIT II

Prenatal

CHAPTER 6

OBSTETRICAL ANATOMY

The purpose of this chapter is to acquaint you with the structure of the childbearing organs and the changes they undergo during pregnancy and labor. It is important that you learn the proper names for these organs and also their functions, not only for your own understanding, but so you can communicate well with your back-up doctor. If you need help fast, the more quickly you can express your needs, the more quickly you can be helped.

THE BIRTH CANAL

The **birth canal,** or the passageway the baby traverses in the process of leaving its mother's body, is shaped by the mother's pelvic structure and extends through the pelvis, vagina, and perineum.

The Pelvis

The **pelvis** (see Figure 1) is the muscle-covered, bony cage through which the fetus must pass. The baby enters the pelvic cavity through the **pelvic inlet,** and exits the cavity through the **pelvic outlet** (see Figure 2). The fetal head molds its shape and rotates to accommodate passage through this, the bony part of the birth canal. Thus, the size, shape, and relationship of the parts of the pelvis to each other are important.

The pelvis is made up of the **coccyx** (tailbone), the **sacrum** (the five, fused sacral vertebrae), and two "unnamed" or **innominate bones** (the hip bones). These innominate bones make up the greater part of the pelvis, and each consists of three bones fused together: the **ilium,** the **ischium,** and the **pubis bone.** The pubis bones meet each other and are joined by cartilage at the **symphysis pubis,** forming the **pubic arch.** (Because of the elasticity of the cartilage, this area "gives" some during childbirth.) The arch can easily be felt beneath the pubic hair. Internally palpating, it is the muscle-covered, hard ridge on the **anterior** side (toward the mother's front) as you reach into the vagina. The arch separates the pelvic inlet and pelvic outlet, anteriorly.

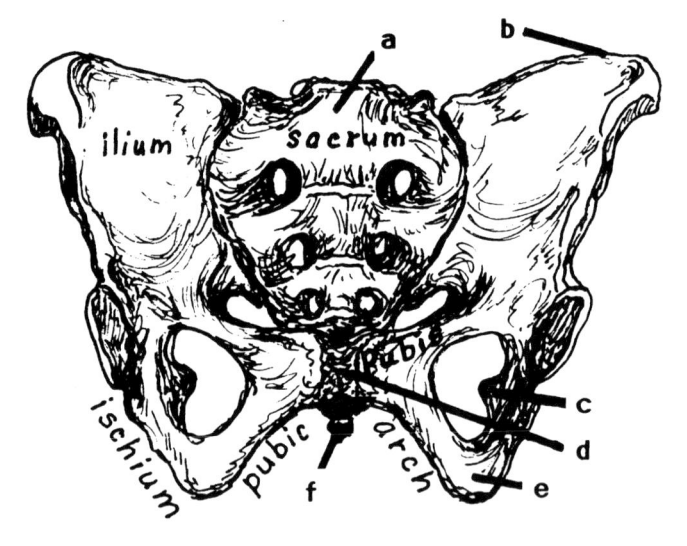

Figure 1. FEMALE PELVIS, FRONT VIEW. (**a**) sacral promontory, (**b**) iliac crest, (**c**) ischial spine, (**d**) symphysis pubis, (**e**) ischial tuberosity, (**f**) coccyx or tailbone.

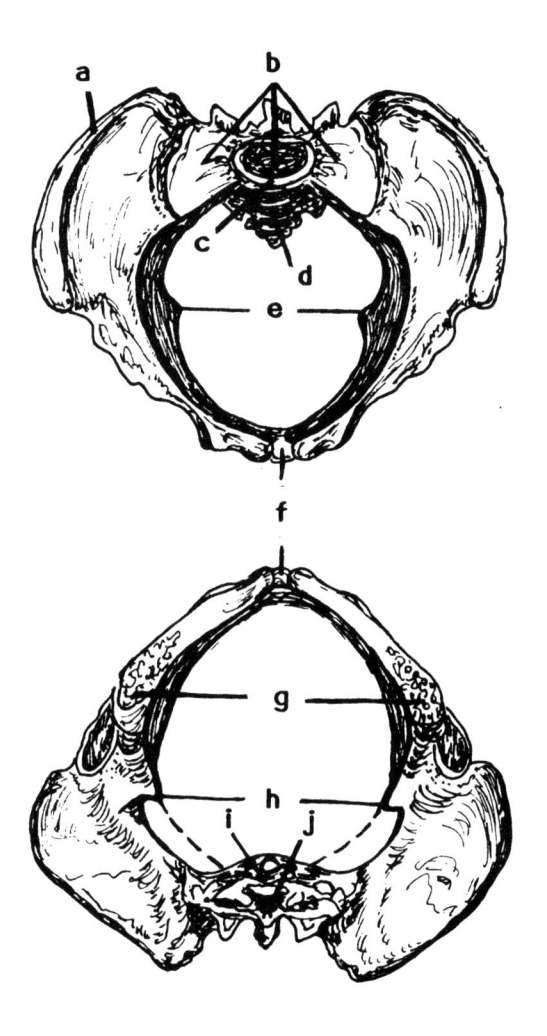

Figure 2. INLET AND OUTLET OF THE BONY BIRTH CANAL. **Pelvic inlet, seen from above:** (a) crest of the ilium (hip), (b) sacrum, (c) sacral promontory, (d) coccyx or tailbone, (e) ischial spines, (f) symphysis pubis. **Pelvic outlet, seen from below:** (g) ischial tuberosities ("buttbones"), (h) ischial spines, (i) coccyx, (j) sacrum.

The pelvic inlet leads down past the **sacral promontory** (the protruding part of the sacrum) and two bony protuberancies known as the **ischial spines.** The diameter between these spines is the narrowest diameter of the pelvic canal. Prominent ischial spines (ones that project into the pelvic cavity) can cause difficulty in labor. The progress of the baby's descent is usually measured by the baby's position in relation to the ischial spines.

In an upright position, the upper part of the pelvic canal is directed downward and backward; it curves and is directed downward and forward in the lower part (see Figure 3). The baby follows the curve of the sacrum, then moves between the **ischial tuberosities** ("sitting bones"; buttbones) and upward (past the symphysis pubis) to be born.

The Vagina

The **vagina** is the passageway between the uterus and the vaginal opening (see Figure 4). It varies in length and circumference according to a woman's build. It is muscular and expands during birth as the fetus moves through it. If it is healthy, it will not usually tear during childbirth, but if it has been plagued with yeast or other infections, it will usually have a soft and spongy or an old, tough texture from scar tissue. It may be ravaged with folds and irregularly shaped tissues from previous births, as well. If a woman stays healthy, this area will have good muscle tone and elasticity.

The Perineum

The muscles of the **pelvic floor** (base of the abdominal cavity) which surround the vagina, rectum, and urethra are part of the **perineum,** or

Obstetrical Anatomy 63

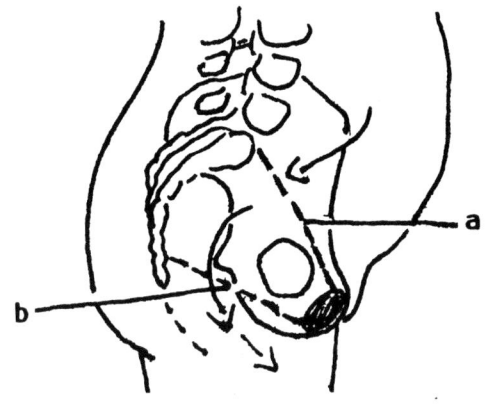

Figure 3. PELVIC CAVITY DIVISIONS. (**a**) plane of the pelvic inlet, (**b**) plane of the pelvic outlet. Arrows point the direction of the birth canal.

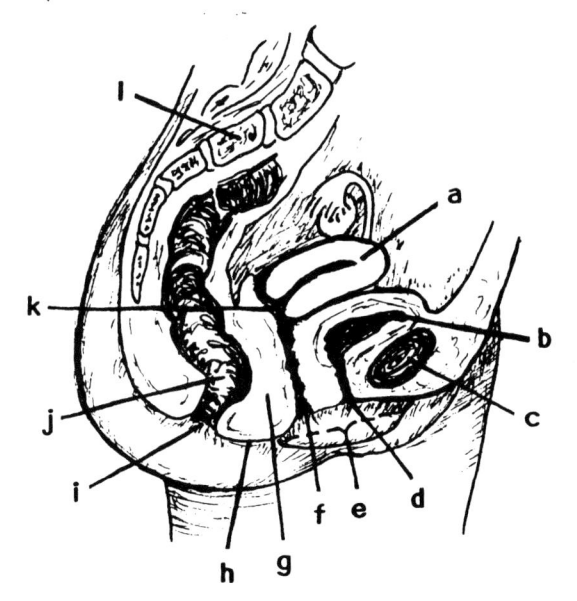

Figure 4. FEMALE REPRODUCTIVE ORGANS, SIDE VIEW. (**a**) uterus, (**b**) bladder, (**c**) symphysis pubis, (**d**) urethral opening, (**e**) vulva, (**f**) vagina, (**g**) perineal body, (**h**) perineum proper, (**i**) anus, (**j**) rectum, (**k**) cervix (external os), (**l**) sacrum (sacral vertebrae).

genital region of the body. Though the perineum includes all the area between the thighs, the term is used most frequently in childbirth to refer to the skin and muscle structure between the vaginal opening and anus--the **perineum proper,** or **"true" perineum.**

When the baby's head reaches the pelvic floor, it must "sweep" upward (along the internal perineum) to exit the mother's body. (Remember the direction and curve of the birth canal?) The fetal head compresses the **perineal body,** causing it to elongate and become very thin. This area is called upon to stretch the most; consequently, it is the area most frequently injured in childbirth. (Hospitals routinely resort to use of the **episiotomy,** an incision of the perineum; midwives utilize other techniques to avoid this trauma.)

THE VULVA

The **vulva** includes all of the external female **genitalia** (genitals): the **labia,** or lips (these stretch in childbirth), the **clitoris** (erectile organ), the **urethral** and **vaginal openings,** etc. (see Figure 5). The baby's head crowns through the **vulvar opening,** with more distension of the vulva at the perineal, or lower, margin than at the top and sides.

THE BLADDER

The small opening toward the top of the vulva is the opening to the **urethra,** through which the **bladder** empties. Bladder function can be impaired if the **parturient** (woman in labor) does not urinate fairly often. The uterus sits on, or leans over, the bladder. A full bladder may not just obstruct labor, but may become edematous (swollen) and occlude (close off) the urethra. An

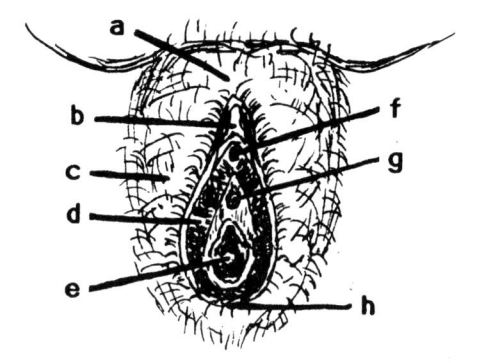

Figure 5. THE VULVA. (**a**) mons veneris (rounded, fatty pad over the symphysis pubis), (**b**) prepuce (fold of skin over the clitoris), (**c**) labium majus (larger, outer lip; pl. labia majora), (**d**) labium minus (small, inner lip; pl. labia minora), (**e**) vaginal orifice, (**f**) clitoris, (**g**) urethral opening, (**h**) fourchette (fold of tissue where the labia minora join below the vaginal opening).

extended bladder could rupture under the stress of strong contractions. Therefore, it may need to be **catheterized** if urine is trapped, obstructing labor. Catheterization is carried out by inserting a **catheter** (slender, flexible tube) into the urethra until it taps the contents of the bladder. It usually empties with some force, so be prepared to protect yourself.

THE UTERUS

The **uterus,** or womb, is found at the far end of the vaginal canal. It sits in the pelvic cavity, above and behind the bladder. In the nonpregnant state, it resembles a medium-sized pear. Composed of very elastic muscle tissue, after conception it becomes rounder and stretches to accommodate the growth of the fetus. It will rise quite high into the abdominal cavity, even displacing organs there when it needs more room.

The bottom portion of the uterus is secured in place, but the upper portion is free to move, responding to posture, gravity, and the contents of the uterus. The uterus normally leans forward, resting on the bladder, but sometimes it "tips" abnormally following childbirth. **Lochia** (drainage) can become trapped and infected (see Chapter 21, Anteflected Uterus). A tipped uterus can cause tenderness or pain in the abdomen or back, and often it causes menstrual cramping.

At the top right and left sides of the uterus are two armlike extremities, the **uterine (fallopian) tubes** (see Figure 6). These lead out to the **ovaries.** It is near the ovaries that conception takes place.

The uppermost portion of the uterus--above the uterine tubes--is the **fundus.** (Or, less precisely, the **fundus** is the entire upper portion of the uterus which is readily felt externally.) The height of the fundus is used as in indicator of fetal growth.

The uterus is divided into two main parts by the **isthmus:** the **corpus,** or body of the uterus (upper, somewhat triangular portion), and the **cervix,** or neck of the uterus (lower, cylindrical portion). The relative proportions of these parts change after the uterus has been stretched by pregnancy. Prior to carrying a fetus, the corpus and cervix are divided almost evenly by the isthmus. Following the birth of the first baby, the corpus is larger.

During pregnancy, the isthmus gradually thins and stretches to form the **lower uterine segment.** At term, the cervix **effaces** or thins and retracts into the lower uterine segment, and the **external os** (gateway between the vaginal canal and the cervix; also referred to as the cervix) **dilates,** or widens. The **upper uterine segment** (fundus/corpus) thickens and contracts to expel the baby, while the lower uterine segment and cervix thin and stretch and open to allow the fetus through. (See also Chapter 17, Figure 58.)

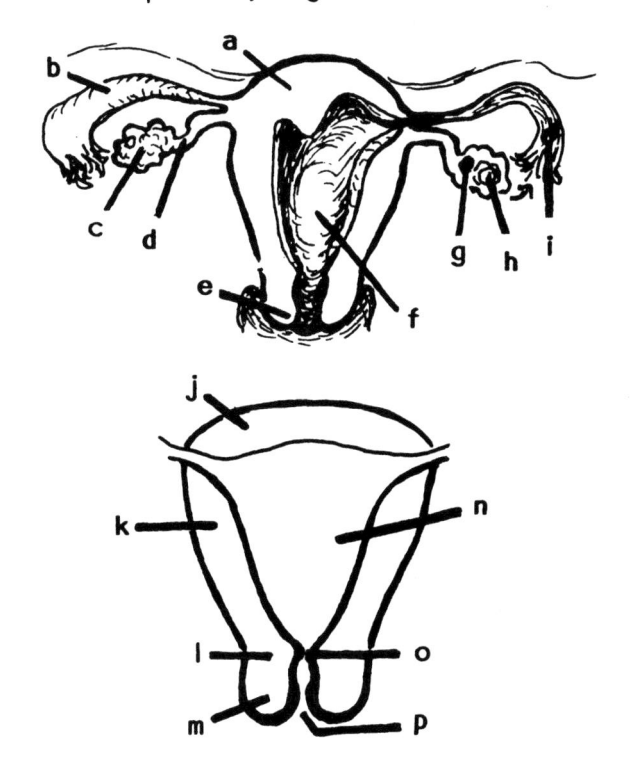

Figure 6. THE UTERUS. **Uterus, seen from behind:** (**a**) fundus, (**b**) uterine (fallopian) tube, (**c**) ovary, (**d**) ovarian ligament, (**e**) cervix, (**f**) uterine cavity, (**g**) follicle (protects the ovum as it matures), (**h**) corpus luteum (the follicle, now empty, changes in name, structure, and function after ovulation), (**i**) zygote (fertilized egg). **Uterus, inside view:** (**j**) fundus, (**k**) corpus, (**l**) isthmus, (**m**) cervix, (**n**) uterine cavity, (**o**) internal os, (**p**) external os.

68 POLLY'S BIRTH BOOK

The size and shape of the cervical opening differ between a woman who has given birth and one who has not. In a woman who has not given birth, the external os is usually a round, tight, pinhole opening resembling the anus (bowel opening). After a woman has given birth, the external os has an irregular shape resembling a slit (see Figure 7).

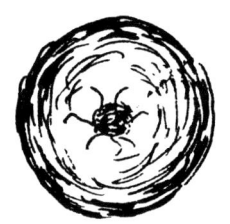

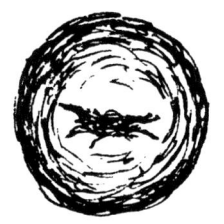

Figure 7. CERVICAL OS, BOTTOM VIEW. A nonparous external os (**left**) has never dilated to give birth to a fetus. A parous os (**right**) has been dilated by a fetus at least once.

THE CONCEPTUS

The term **conceptus** refers to ALL of the products of conception: baby, placenta, membranes, etc.

Each month the uterus prepares a bed, or **decidua**, for a fertilized ovum to implant within. After conception, the area of decidua at the base of where the fertilized ovum has implanted is called the **decidua basalis,** and that which lines the walls of the uterus is **decidua vera,** or **decidua parietalis**. **Decidua capsularis** lies over the developing ovum (see Figure 8). (By the fourth month, the baby has grown enough to fill the uterine cavity, and the decidua capsularis has fused with the decidua vera.)

The **amnion** (see Figure 9) is a membrane which encloses the fetus and amniotic fluid, encases the

Obstetrical Anatomy 69

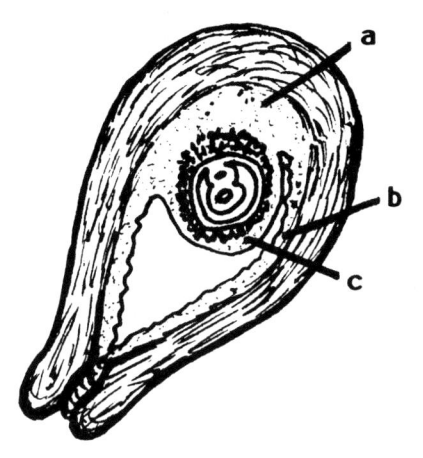

Figure 8. THE CONCEPTUS. The conceptus embeds in the uterine wall. (a) decidua basalis, (b) decidua vera, (c) decidua capsularis.

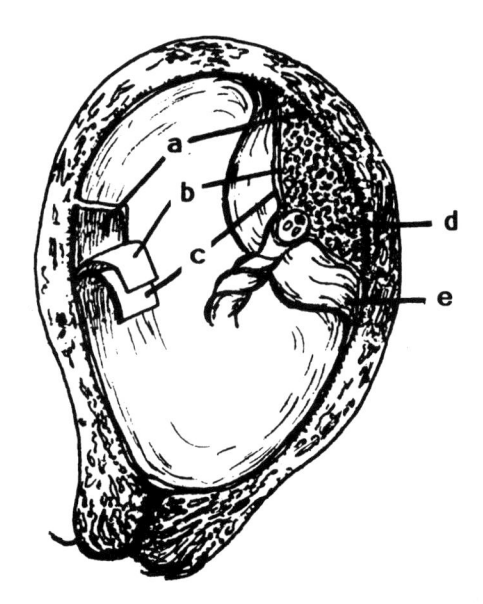

Figure 9. INTERNAL ANATOMY OF A PREGNANT UTERUS. (a) decidua, (b) chorion, (c) amnion, (d) maternal side of the placenta, (e) fetal side of the placenta.

umbilical cord, and covers the fetal side of the placenta. This membrane is backed by **chorion,** also a nutritive and protective layer. The baby draws support from the **placenta** through the **umbilical cord.** Amnion, chorion, placenta, cord, decidua, uterus—all change in size to accommodate the needs of the growing baby.

The Placenta

The **placenta** is the prime source of nourishment for the fetus. It has been stated that every enzyme known to exist in biology has been found in the placenta. While the mother and baby have two completely separate circulatory systems--the maternal blood does NOT circulate in the fetus-- the placenta allows those substances in the mother's blood stream to enter into the fetal blood stream. The mother's circulation provides oxygen and nutrients to the placenta; these are then absorbed, through the process of osmosis, into the fetus's blood stream. Within just a few hours after the mother eats (or drinks, or smokes, or ingests any other substance), the baby gets some of the very same supply. (Some substances affect the baby quite rapidly.)

Wastes from the fetus are delivered to the placenta, and the mother's system carries them off (along with her own) through her liver, kidneys, bowels, and lungs. Most of the time the placenta protects the baby from disease, although at certain stages it can allow some harmful viruses into the baby's body (rubella, for example).

Pregnancy is a state of elevated hormone levels. The placenta manufactures, in abundance, hormones vital to the mother, particularly **estrogen** and **progesterone.** After the first few weeks of pregnancy, the normal source of these hormones, the ovaries, becomes of little importance in hormone production and the placenta assumes this role. Estrogen levels increase throughout pregnancy, and at term estrogen production is stepped up to assist the cervix in parturition. Levels after delivery then drop abruptly. Progesterone is produced by the placenta in massive amounts (much more than estrogen). There is a gradual increase in these levels, which reach a plateau toward the end of pregnancy.

Hormones are important in uterine and fetal growth and in maintaining the pregnancy. They affect the baby, as well as the mother, and as a result the sex organs of the newborn are usually a little swollen. The hormone which stimulates milk production in the mother may sometimes cause the baby, male or female, to secrete a bit of milk from its breasts for a short time.

After the baby is born, the placenta voluntarily separates from the uterus as the fundus thickens and contractions push it downward. Still attached on the fetal side to the amniotic membrane, the weight of the placenta causes the amnioniotic and chorionic membranes (which are as one) to peel away from the walls of the uterus. Placenta and membranes--the **afterbirth**--are delivered shortly after the birth of the baby.

The Amniotic Sac and Fluid

The **amniotic sac** (**amnion** or **bag of waters**) is a balloonlike membrane that surrounds the fetus, encases the umbilical cord, and covers the fetal side of the placenta. It is a nest of fluid that is constantly renewed--about 35 percent of the fluid is replaced every hour.

The **amniotic fluid** is alkaline. About 98 percent of it is water. The remaining 2 percent consists of solids--organic and inorganic materials. Some of the substances found in the amniotic fluid are proteins, fatty acids, enzymes, hormones, electrolytes, glucose, fructose, nitrogen, calcium, phosphorus, lecithin, cholesterol, urea, uric acid, and miscellaneous fetal cells.

The amniotic fluid serves several important functions: (1) it keeps the baby at an even temperature, (2) it cushions the baby against injury, and (3) it provides a safe way for the baby to move around easily. The baby drinks and inhales the fluid. Some of it is absorbed by the fetus. The combination of amnion and fluid serves to protect the spongy, fibrous placenta from the movements of the fetus.

During labor, the amniotic sac usually breaks because of the pressure exerted by contractions. You may have to rupture a tough membrane to encourage delivery or to prevent the baby from being born with the membrane over its face. Occasionally, the membrane will rupture high on its surface (more toward the fundus) and will emit fluid in dribbles, perhaps weeks prior to or during early labor. Rupture of the membrane nearer the external os usually produces a flush of water.

The Umbilical Cord

The placenta is attached to the baby by the **umbilical cord (funis)**, which is wrapped in a sheath of the amnion. This cord consists of a large vein, which carries blood to the baby, and two smaller arteries, which take wastes from the baby back to the placenta. Inside the cord, **Wharton's jelly** suspends these three blood vessels traveling from the placenta to the baby (see

Figure 10). The cord, which is attached at the baby's **umbilicus** (navel), must be severed carefully shortly after birth. This creates an **umbilical stump** at the navel which requires special attention until it atrophies and falls off.

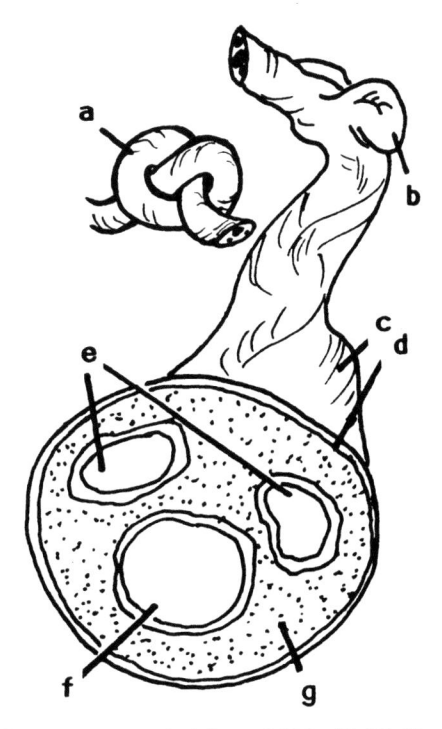

Figure 10. THE UMBILICAL CORD (FUNIS). (a) true knot, (b) false knot. Encased in an amniotic/chorionic sheath (c, d), the funis has two small arteries (e) and a larger vein (f). They are supported by a substance called Wharton's Jelly (g). The cord has no nerves or feeling in it; therefore, it does not hurt when cut.

Development of the Embryo

Fertilized ovum, embryo, fetus, infant—all these terms refer to a baby in earlier or later stages of development, but to a baby, nevertheless. Within the first three weeks of gestation, the spinal cord, brain, and heart have begun to develop. The spinal cord is complete by the twentieth week, the brain by the twenty-eighth week, and the heart by the sixth week. The face, limbs, and genital system are complete by the thirtieth week. Imagine the jawbone moving by the seventh week, and the hands and fingers moving between the ninth and sixteenth weeks, as well as the legs and vertebrae!

By the sixteenth week the mother can be feeling movement: the fundus is nearing the mother's navel, the baby's skin is less transparent, and the heartbeat can be heard with the fetalscope. There may be some hair on its head and a fine **lanugo** (covering of hair) will be found all over the body.

By the twenty-fourth week, the fetus CAN live if born prematurely, but is unlikely to do so. By now, the first fat is being deposited under the skin, which is still quite wrinkled.

At the twenty-eighth week the baby is about thirty-seven centimeters (fourteen and one-half inches) long and weighs about 1,000 grams (a little over two pounds). From this point on, the chance of survival with good care increases. (However, a premature birth in the planned home setting is not advisable if the premature period extends earlier than two weeks.) Deliveries of premature babies at home have been successful, but the reality of the risks must be realized. I weighed four and one-half pounds (and was born at home when there was no other alternative) and made it fine, as did many others in those days, but there were many who did not make it under the same circumstances.

We should realize that all these changes, all these intricate processes that take place during pregnancy in both the mother and the baby, are part of the great procreative program of Diety. If our Heavenly Father had not been the architect of this delicate process, the mother's body would reject the baby in her womb, just as human and animal bodies reject organ transplants and foreign materials that are incompatible with their own physiological make-ups. (At this point in time, a person's natural protection against disease must be impaired in order for him to not reject the incompatible, transplanted tissue.) But the baby, though an entity all its own, grows and lies within its mother's body. The Lord has provided all the proper balances to secure a grand environment and safe fulfillment for this marvelous phase of earth life for His children.

CHAPTER 7

DETERMINING HOME BIRTH FEASIBILITY

ASCERTAINING PREGNANCY

Many physical indicators and tests are used to assist with the determination of pregnancy; however, most of them are not by themselves conclusive evidence of pregnancy, particularly in the early stages. Other conditions may be accompanied by similar physical symptoms, and test results are not always reliable.

Amenorrhea is by no means conclusive evidence of pregnancy: some women miss periods when they are not pregnant, and a few women continue to have one or more periods following conception (some never stop!). The **ballottement test** (see Figure 11) is a little surer, but in my opinion it is a risky thing to be doing too early for several reasons, including: (1) possible introduction of infection, and (2) interference that could bring about miscarriage. **Uterine palpation** (holding the fundus and palpating internally with the other hand) is useless to determine pregnancy if done prior to the second to third months, since other conditions may imitate the feel of pregnancy. By the third month, a more accurate assessment can be made (enlargement and presence of the conceptus). Palpation of cervical and uterine tissue earlier than about the tenth week of pregnancy may disturb delicate growth progression to the point of causing the fetus to abort. **X-ray examinations** are not safe in pregnancy, according to most

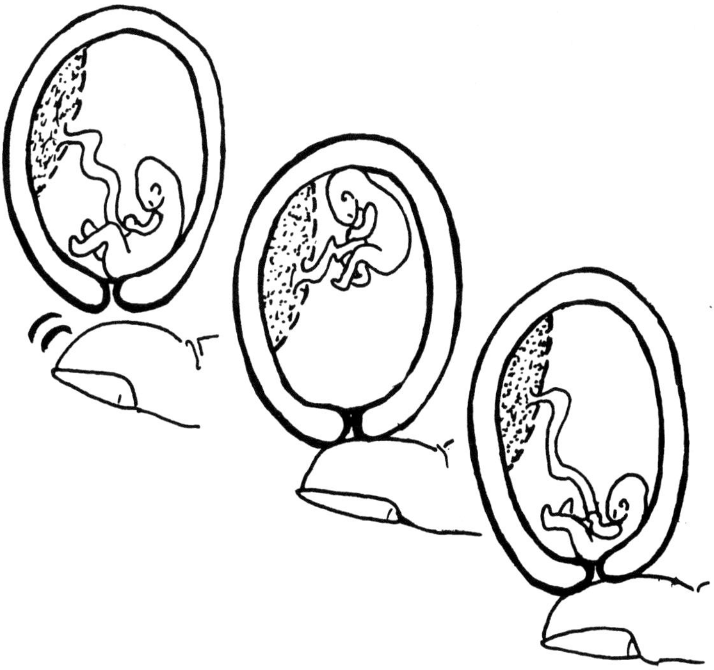

Figure 11. INTERNAL BALLOTTEMENT. Internal ballottement during the fourth and fifth months of pregnancy can be done by GENTLY tapping ONCE on the cervix, then leaving the finger tip against the cervix while the embryo travels up in the amniotic fluid. The embryo, if present, will return with a soft bounce. Extreme caution and gentleness must be exercised if ballottement is used. (External ballottement can be done from one side of the abdomen to the other at 24 weeks, with palms of the hands placed on abdominal sides.)

doctors. **Ultrasonograms** should not be given, especially in early pregnancy, just to ascertain pregnancy. They have not proven safe or completely reliable (see Chapter 8, Ultrasound). And, with the **endocrine test** for pregnancy, I have had more than one mother in class say that she was six months along with each of her several children and laboratory endocrine tests were still showing negative.

Most women seem to want a confirmation of pregnancy at an early date, since special attention to nutrition and to other preparations is wise, and perhaps also because of impatience or prospective changes in work or lifestyle. One of the many rewards of pregnancy is the joy of anticipation, of preparing materially and emotionally for the birth of a new little one. A woman's intuition at this point is probably as valuable as any test, if she does not allow wishful thinking to confuse her.

There is something exciting and special about the DISCOVERY of the more sure signs that come along, those that attest to the very life and undeniable presence of a baby: hearing the heartbeat, feeling unmistakable fetal movement, watching the body change to accommodate growth, and feeling the outline of the baby's shape through the abdomen.

Many of the interferences done to detemine pregnancy need not be done at all unless there is a cause for concern about a problem that might affect pregnancy, or vice versa. When fundal growth, fetal heart tones, fetal movement, etc., occur, it is time enough to KNOW a baby is on the way. If a mother SUSPECTS she is pregnant, she can and should pay extra special attention to her nutrition, as these first weeks are an extremely important period of fetal development.

The positive, probable, and presumptive signs of pregnancy are listed below:

POSITIVE SIGNS OF PREGNANCY

1. FETAL HEART TONES (can be picked up by the 20th to 22nd week with fetalscopes, later by ear to the abdomen, and much earlier with Doppler equipment).

2. SPONTANEOUS MOVEMENTS OF THE FETUS detected by the midwife (discernable after about the 5th lunar month[1]). These movements are felt by placing a hand over the appropriate place on the mother's abdomen. They vary in intensity from a faint flutter in early months to brisk (even visible) movement in later months.

3. RECOGNITION OF THE FETUS THROUGH X-RAY EXAMINATION (the presence of the fetus can be picked up by the 5th lunar month about one third of the time, by the 6th lunar month half of the time) OR ULTRSONOGRAPHIC EXAMINATION (usually reveals the fetus by the 5th to 6th week). Neither of these methods are considered entirely safe, especially in early gestation. Sober consideration should be given to resorting to these methods of determining pregnancy.

PROBABLE SIGNS OF PREGNANCY

1. ENLARGEMENT OF THE ABDOMEN.

2. CHANGES IN SIZE, SHAPE, AND CONSISTENCY OF THE UTERUS. Vaginal examinations should not be attempted until at least the 2nd or 3rd months of pregnancy.

3. CHANGES IN THE CERVIX (softening).

4. BALLOTTEMENT (tapping on the bottom of the uterus at the 4th to 5th month of pregnancy to feel the fetus rise in the amniotic fluid and rebound against the finger tip). This is unnecessary and could upset the pregnancy with infection or miscarriage.

5. OUTLINING THE FETUS (feeling body parts through the abdomen in the second half of pregnancy).

6. POSITIVE HORMONAL (ENDOCRINE) TESTS (standard pregnancy tests; these measure levels of chorionic gonadotrophin).

PRESUMPTIVE SIGNS OF PREGNANCY

1. CESSATION OF MENSES (periods cease).

2. CHANGES IN BREASTS (firmer, enlarged, more color at the nipples).

3. NAUSEA AND VOMITING (anytime during the day or night).

4. QUICKENING (first perception of fetal movement).

5. DISCOLORATION OF MUCOSA (TISSUE) OF THE VAGINA AND SKIN OF THE VULVA (to dark, blue red tones).

6. STRETCH MARKS (and some pigmentation of the skin).

7. URINARY DISTURBANCES (frequent urination).

8. FATIGUE (and extreme sleepiness for a few weeks).

DETERMINING A DUE DATE

Never expect to arrive at an EXACT due date for delivery. There is no way to accurately calculate this. Less than 5% of all babies are delivered on the estimated dates. Due dates are approximations based solely upon averages. EXACT PERIODS FOR GESTATION VARY ACCORDING TO THE INDIVIDUAL FETUS. This is the key, but it nevertheless remains an unknown. There is just no way to tell, so we must be content with approximations.

The AVERAGE length of gestation is approximately 280 days or 40 weeks (10 lunar months) COUNTING FROM THE FIRST DAY OF THE LAST MENSTRUAL PERIOD. About two-thirds of the babies are born within ten days of their due dates. Some feel that mothers who have longer or shorter than average (28-day) menstrual cycles will have longer or shorter gestational periods accordingly (because the actual dates of ovulation and consequently conception will be earlier or later than the estimated date of ovulation used in the formula for determining the due date). The thing to remember is that the maturation needs of the individual fetus are of primary importance, and each situation is different.

Due dates are commonly figured according to **Naegele's rule:** COUNT BACK 3 CALENDAR MONTHS (or add 9 months) FROM THE FIRST DAY OF THE LAST MENSTRUAL PERIOD AND ADD 7 DAYS. This date for a normal, full-term pregnancy is a good estimate. MOST babies are born within two weeks (before or after) of an accurately calculated due date.

Menstrual irregularities may interfere with the determination of a due date. Sometimes it is difficult to determine even an approximate due date. The point **quickening** occurs (first perception of life; said to happen between the 16th and 19th weeks), fundal height measurements, and **lightening** (when the baby drops into the pelvic cavity near term) can provide clues to a due date, but even these will vary with different individuals.

INITIAL SCREENING

A successful outcome for all concerned may depend largely upon a midwife's ability to screen the expectant mother for a safe home delivery. The initial screening is carried out with both parents present, if possible. If the gravida proves to be low risk, a refinement of screening is continued throughout pregnancy.

Cooperation between husband and wife at this time usually engenders in the couple a joyful anticipation of carrying out suggested ideas for: (1) improving health, (2) preventing problems along the way, and (3) making needful preparations for delivery and postpartum.

Information gathered from the mother will assist you in judging outcome trends for her current pregnancy. These trends will indicate which corrective measures may need to be taken to promote a safer pregnancy and birth. From this initial screening you will have an estimation of the gravida's physical build, the risks revealed by her past obstetrical history (previous birth outcomes), and the risks posed by her current health and diet habits. The advisability of pursuing plans for home birth will become clearer when you take into account the overall picture drawn by: (1) your interview with the mother (and father), including the answers given to the prenatal questionnaire, and (2) your assessment of the condition of the mother's pelvis and vagina for giving birth.

Prenatal Questionnaire

In addition to certain autobiographical (or personal) information (name, address, husband, phone numbers, etc.), you should ask other questions which will help you determine whether the gravida can be considered a candidate for home birth or if risk factors rule this out.

In all instances, use common sense and careful evaluation of the entire situation to determine whether home birth is advisable.

1. How old are you?

2. What is your past history of pregnancies?

   Number of previous pregnancies:
   Number of full-term babies:
   Number of live births:
   Number of stillbirths:
       Reasons given for death(s):
   Number of miscarriages: (give approximate dates)
       How far along in pregnancy?
       What caused each miscarriage?
       Did you have a D & C afterward?

3. Information about each birth:

   Date:
   Was your labor induced?
       Why?
   Duration of labor:
       From loss of mucous plug to delivery?
       From first regular contractions to delivery?
       Did your contractions ever stop during midlabor or mid-delivery?

Drugs used: (general or local anesthesia, narcotics or painkillers, "Pit drip," "blocks," etc.)
Type of delivery: (vaginal or cesarean)
    If vaginal:
        What was the presentation of the baby? (vertex, breech, posterior, face, etc.)
        Were extraction tools (forceps, etc.) used?
        Were there tears or incisions requiring extensive suturing?
        Did you have an episiotomy?
    If cesarean:
        What kind? (classical incision or "bikini"/lower uterine segment incision)
        What reasons were you given for needing a C-section?
Did you hemorrhage?
When?
Size of baby:
    Weight:
    Length:
    Head measurement:
Baby's condition at birth: (stillborn, died neonatally, had birth injuries or defects, needed resuscitating, was drug-depressed, Apgar was excellent/good/fair/poor, everything was fine, etc.)
Were there any complications with the labor or delivery?

4. What is your blood type?

    Are you Rh-negative?
        If Rh-negative, have you ever had RhoGAM?
        Are you "sensitized"?

5. What is your nonpregnant weight?

6. Are you going to breast-feed your baby?
7. Do you really want this baby?
8. Have you ever had an induced (performed by a doctor) abortion?

>How many? (give approximate dates)
>Was there any:
>Excessive bleeding?
>Elevated temperature? (give length of time)
>Other complications? (specify)

9. Have you ever had a D & C (dilation of the cervix and curettage of the uterus)?

>When? (give dates)
>Why?

10. Have you ever had an IUD (intrauterine device)?

>Was it removed? lost?
>Do you have one now?

11. Were you on birth control pills when you conceived?

>How long had/have you been on contraceptive pills?

12. List the medications and drugs that you currently use, and for what reason:

Were you using any kind of drug (including marijuana) when you conceived? (list)
Was your husband using any kind of drug (including marijuana) when you conceived? (list)

Do you consume alcohol?
Do you smoke?
Does your husband smoke and/or are you exposed to secondhand smoke at home, work, etc.?

13. To your knowledge, do you now have or have you ever had any venereal disease?

    What is/was it?

14. Have you ever broken your back, coccyx, pelvis, or hip?

15. Have you ever had:

    A heart disorder (rheumatic fever, murmur, etc.)?
    Hypertension?
    Kidney disease?
    Emotional disorders?
    Diabetes? (Has any member of your family had diabetes?)
    Gestational diabetes (diabetes present only during pregnancy)?
    Lung disease?
    Cancer? (Where?)
    Polio?
    Rickets?
    Varicose veins or other varicosities? (How serious?)
    Allergies (asthma, hay fever, etc.)? (How serious?)
    Epilepsy?

    Most of the above disorders will preclude home birth.

16. Are you in good general health?

    Do you tend to be anemic?

Do you have hemorrhoids?
Do you have at least one bowel evacuation per day?
What percentage of the time do you eat the "great American diet" (commercially processed, refined, and packaged foods, short-order fare, junk food, etc.)?

17. Do congenital defects appear regularly in:

    Your family? (name any)
    Your husband's family? (name any)

18. Do multiple births appear in:

    Your family?
    Your husband's family?
    Have you been taking fertility pills?

19. How long are your menstrual cycles (beginning to beginning)?

    How long do your periods last and what kind of flow (normal, heavy, light) do you have?

20. What was the date of the FIRST day of your last menstrual period?

    What is the expected due date (using Naegele's rule)?

Commentary on Prenatal Questionnaire

1. **Age of the mother.** Those under 16 and those over 40 pose higher risks because of possible incomplete maturational development (younger women) and possible lack of muscle tone and elasticity (older women).

2. **Past pregnancy history:**

   Neonatal death. A history of neonatal deaths or stillbirths probably indicates problems a midwife may not be equipped to handle. If the death(s) was unexplained (not due to drug depression, premature separation of the placenta, cord stress, toxemia, mongoloidism, fetal brain hemorrhage, etc.), consider the possibility that it may have been caused by diabetes. Whether you should accept for home birth someone who has had a stillbirth or neonatal death would depend upon the cause of death.

   Miscarriage. Some causes of miscarriage are either preventable or handled just as well at home. A woman who seems to have a problem with miscarriage may have to take extra precautions. If miscarriages have occurred more than once, consider the cause and possible corrections before dispelling the idea of home birth. Also consider a trend to miscarry at a particular stage of pregnancy. Miscarriages that happen in early pregnancy pose less problems than those occuring in the second or third trimesters, which may involve a viable fetus. (See also Chapter 11, Unexplained Spontaneous Abortion.)

   A spontaneous abortion may be the result of:

   A DEFECTIVE FETUS.

   A HORMONAL IMBALANCE. May be corrected.

   BLOOD VESSELS THAT ARE NOT ELASTIC ENOUGH. May be corrected; additional vitamin C and hesperidin complex are needed.

Determining Home Birth Feasibility

SMOKING BY MOTHER OR FATHER OR THE USE OF PRESCRIPTION OR NONPRESCRIPTION DRUGS. A year of nonsmoking, without drugs and with a good systemic cleanse will lessen the chances of damage to a future placenta and fetus.

TRAUMA, AN ACCIDENT, EMOTIONAL STRESS, OVERWORK, EXHAUSTION.

COITUS (intercourse) during the first trimester.

DIABETES. Treatment outcome is unpredictable; VERY high risk for home birth.

NEPHRITIS OR OTHER KIDNEY DISORDERS.

HYPOTHYROIDISM.

UTERINE ABNORMALITY, including uterine immaturity. Dilatations, carefully done, will sometimes correct uterine immaturity.

TUMORS. Usually high risk, depending upon where and how removable or operable they are, and whether they are malignant.

CERVICAL EROSION. This is not usually inflammatory, but the breakdown of cervical tissue can interfere with effacement and dilation. High risk.

UTERINE INCOMPETENCE (incapable of natural function: the cervix is without sufficient tension or elasticity to give needed support to the growing conceptus). Without correction, the weight of the fetus, fluid, cord, and placenta creates stress and the conceptus displaces or separates and is lost. In some cases, this can be remedied by the physician after the 12th week with a purse-string suture. This is removed before labor--38th week--to prevent destruction of the cervix as it dilates. Risk is too high for home birth.

INFECTION OR ILLNESS. Infection of the vagina or uterus or infectious diseases such as measles, typhoid fever, hepatitis, scarlet fever, etc., can disrupt and abort a pregnancy.

Children close together (several pregnancies less than 2 years apart). This invites uterine inertia unless a serious program is undertaken between pregnancies to keep the body tone good.

3. **Information about previous birthing experiences:**

    Induced labor. A uterus sometimes won't function well on its own when Pitocin has never allowed it to follow through with a normal delivery; the sooner it learns to function on its own, with natural aids, the better. (See also Chapter 5, Inducing Labor; Chapter 15, Uterine Inertia.)

    Duration of labor. It would hardly preclude home birth if labors have been long in the past, unless there is a very narrow and long "tunnel" canal through the pelvis. While long labors are normally cut in half when the gravida is on the Good Program and takes the Five-Week Antenatal Formula, the tunnel canal does take a longer labor and a longer, more persistent, bearing-down stage to deliver. Normally, if such a mother does not seem to be overdue and she does not have a history of large babies, this narrow canal does not pose much of a problem.

Previous uterine inertia. If found previously in a young woman (22 to 28 years old), inertia can usually be prevented by a strict pre-pregnancy exercise program, by building confidence through good care, and by teaching the gravida about birth. Fear CAN stop labor or prevent labor from progressing. Inertia due strictly to lack of muscle tone is high risk in home birth.

Drugs used in labor and delivery. Drugs used in previous births to hurry labor or delivery often strip the uterus from experiencing its own trials and successes. The uterus needs an opportunity to perform correctly. If drugs were given for pain, it usually means there was either a lack of REAL understanding of the mechanism of labor (fear of the unknown) or a lack of the kind of care offered on a one-to-one basis in the home (fear from past experiences). This person has been cheated out of a normal, joyful, birth experience and should have that opportunity with the right kind of help.

If drugs were given because a gravida "never" goes into labor, work needs to be done to build this uterus that is apparently not "receiving instructions" from the readiness signals (hormones) of the baby. This "hormonal disharmony" can be safely remedied with herbal formulas begun between pregnancies and continued throughout the current pregnancy. While longer-term efforts give better results, sometimes this correction can be made during pregnancy alone if a good program and the herbal formulas are strictly adhered to.

Extraction delivery, previous suturing. Was the mother told that major suturing was needed following her extraction birth? Did she have a "blowout" or lacerate through several layers of tissue? Did she have a bladder repair? At times this suturing following heavy lacerations (or incisions) creates an imbalance in the walls and floor of the vagina which curbs mobility and stretching. This means there is a possibility of tearing at the site again during a birth. If tears or incisions were extensive originally and vaginal tissue is NOT YET HEALTHY, home birth would be inadvisable. However, excellent results can come from a very strict regime for repair and rebuilding of such tissue, especially if it is begun a few months prior to conception.

Previous episiotomies. Heavy scar tissue does not stretch easily, so a program of softening the tissue surrounding the vaginal opening will have to be undertaken. Too much scarring of the perineum will eliminate the benefit during labor of foot therapy.

Cesarean delivery. Whether you have had one or three previous cesarean deliveries, vaginal delivery is entirely possible. If abdominal and uterine incisions were "bikini" (horizontal in the lower segment), home deliveries are possible provided the mother is in good condition. Excellent material on the subject can be found in **Silent Knife: Cesarean Prevention and Vaginal Birth after Cesarean,** by Nancy Wainer Cohen and Lois J. Estner (South Hadley, Mass.: Bergin & Garvey Publishers,

Inc., 1983). Statistics are being reported which demonstrate very high rates of successful vaginal births after cesarean sections. (See also Chapter 22, Cesarean Sections.)

Previous hemorrhage. The gravida should be able to correct and control this problem through prenatal diet and supplements. There are also extra precautions the midwife may wish to take during delivery (see Chapter 17, Hemorrhage).

Size of previous babies. A trend toward large babies (10+ pounds) may be a genetic factor, a weight problem of the mother, or an indication of diabetes; small babies may indicate the presence of a trend toward premature births or short gestational periods, a smoking mother, etc.

Condition of previous babies. Was each baby born in a healthy condition? Was its color good at birth or did it need resuscitation? Did any grunt and grimace with each breath? Were any stillborn, injured, or defected in any way? Only if these conditions in previous births present a trend are we concerned. This might indicate a predisposition toward poor prenatal care, or it might reflect previous poor labor and delivery care.

Previous complications. Complications that would impose hazards on this pregnancy would include a history of:

1. Excessive hemorrhage.

2. Repeated malpositioning.

3. Very large or very small babies.

4. Premature or postmature babies.

5. Uterine inertia.

6. Deformations, stillbirths, or unexplained neonatal deaths.

7. Chronic or acute **intrapartum** (during childbirth) response to a physical condition (asthma, heart disorder, epilepsy, toxemia, etc.). (The mother may have believed her condition to be of no particular consequence.)

4. **Rh-negative.** The fact that a woman is Rh-negative does not of itself preclude home birth (see Chapter 12, Rh Factor and Hemolytic Disease).

5. **Weight of the mother.** If the woman is 40 pounds or more overweight at the beginning of pregnancy, risks increase for premature delivery, hypertension, uterine inertia, overweight baby, and hard delivery.

6. **Breast-feeding.** It would be uncommon to have a gravida ask for home birth who has not planned to nurse her baby. This must be encouraged for two major reasons: (1) the baby's welfare (long-range and also at birth), and (2) to help prevent postpartum hemorrhage, as well as to help all reproductive organs resume their proper positions in good condition. There is not usually a good reason why a mother cannot breast-feed her babies, unless she does not have breasts. Even inverted nipples can usually be dealt with successfully.

Determining Home Birth Feasibility 95

7. **Does the mother WANT this baby?** If the mother does not, the REASON would prevent a midwife from being judgmental. If the reasons are emotional ones--such as hate of the father, rape, inconvenience, just plain does not want children--the probability of the gravida's being totally dissatisfied with any part of her care (and thus holding the attendants liable for her displeasure) is too great. High risk.

8. **Abortion.** The chances of having had the uterus damaged and scarred from almost any kind of manual abortive technique increases the risk for home birth. Co-screening with a physician is advisable.

9. **D & C.** The complications from a D & C depend on the competence of the physician who performed it and whether the procedure was done in conjunction with an induced abortion. Risk of uterine damage increases with the number of D & C's that have been done.

10. **IUD.** With an IUD that is currently in place (including one that has been lost in the uterus), there is a high risk that: (1) tearing of the uterine tissue will occur, and (2) the growing conceptus will become involved with the IUD. Also, tearing and scarring of the uterine tissue may have already taken place with use of an IUD.

11. **Birth control pills.** Dr. Robert S. Mendelsohn, an M.D., reported in 1979 that women who take "the Pill" have a six times greater risk of high blood pressure, four times greater risk of stroke, and five times greater risk of thromboembolism (blockage of a blood vessel by a blood clot). They run the risk of

cardiovascular disease, liver tumors, headaches, depression, and cancer. The risk of dying from a heart attack is multiplied by a factor of three for women from age 30 to 40, and by a factor of five for women over age 40.[2] Such women may have incurred health problems from use of the Pill which make them too high risk for home birth, though sometimes it takes years for some of these results to show up. If contraceptive pills have been used for only a short period of time, the mother may be low enough risk for home birth.

12. **Harmful substances:**

   Drug use. The use of any medication in any amount needs evaluation. If the potential harm from the medication itself does not veto home birth, the reason for which it is being given may. Women under medication for chronic diseases or illnesses must be screened out because prolonged use of medication places such a high risk on the fetus. With drug use by wife or husband, risk increases for malformations, fetal addiction, etc.

   Marijuana. See Chapter 9, Avoid Harmful Substances (Marijuana).

   Alcohol and Smoking. There has been a movement underway to publicize the dangers to the unborn of using alcohol. Pregnant women should abstain from its use entirely, as well as from the use of tobacco. Tobacco and alcohol increase the risk of placental insufficiency, retarded fetal growth, mental retardation, etc. Secondhand smoke poses the same hazards as does personal use. The pregnant woman who stops smoking is better off than if she continues; however, it takes about a year

Determining Home Birth Feasibility 97

to rid the body of the effects of smoking. If she stops, but her husband continues to smoke in her presence, risks are still present. If the mother abstains during pregnancy (from alcohol AND tobacco), home birth may be a possibility as long as there is medical back-up available and the higher risks are understood. Pregnancy and childbirth will have to be closely monitored.

13. **Venereal disease.** Venereal diseases can lie dormant for periods of time, yet still affect the fetus either in utero or as it passes through the birth canal. V.D. can cause blindness and can infect those who give prenatal, parturition, and postpartum care. VERY high risk. (See also Chapter 12, Venereal Disease.)

14. **Broken pelvic bones.** If the pelvis, etc., has been broken and not healed correctly, or vertebrae have fused in the lower back, risks are obvious. Specific pelvimetry screening must be done if the bones of the birth canal have been affected. If tailbones have broken previously, breakage may occur again (though the parturient may not feel this breakage).

15. **Various disorders:**

    Heart disorders. Risk depends on the kind, severity, and present status of the heart condition. Of cardiac patients with very limited activity who become pregnant, about one-third suffer heart failure before the reproductive process is completed. (Heart disease is never an indication for C-section. It is, rather, a contraindication. Mothers with heart disease often cannot take the operation.) Careful screening of those with minor ailments, who are on an active program and are in excellent health otherwise, would determine the wisdom of home birth.

Hypertension, kidney disease. Both high risk; no home birth. Kidney disease is the most commonly known cause of hypertension (high blood pressure). The kidneys need to be able to function normally so that toxins can be eliminated freely. If they cannot do this, uremia or renal failure will cause edema in the mother and child and can cause death of the fetus. In early stages, the symptoms are not noticed. Later signs are fever, high blood pressure, back pain, edema all over the body, etc. Any chronic malfunction or impairment of the kidneys predisposes toxemia, infection, and possible heart failure to the gravida.

Emotional disorders. Most severe emotional disorders require ongoing medication, which is very high risk to the fetus. The gravida may vacilate in her ability to handle stress. Home birth is high risk to her and a liability to the attendants.

Diabetes. A midwife must NEVER accept the responsibility of a diabetic gravida in a home birth. You should be cautious if other family members are diabetic (even in previous generations). A thorough medical checkup is required to determine whether diabetes exists. (See Chapter 12, Diabetes Mellitus.)

Gestational diabetes. Prenatal tests will reveal signs of gestational diabetes. A change of diet may bring this under control. If it persists, the gravida will be too high risk for home birth.

Lung disease. Lung diseases affect the pregnancy, and pregnancy almost always disturbs the disease, causing reduced oxygen supply to fetus and mother, etc.

Cancer. If there has been cancer, regardless of where it was in the system, careful scrutiny and present status have to be considered. If cancer is found at the cervix only and in an early stage, sometimes one or possibly two children can be borne before penetration occurs. In the meantime, early cervical cancer can be treated even during gestation without harm to the fetus if methods other than chemotherapy, radiation, or surgery are used. Cancer is found to be a hard knot or lump in the tissue on the cervix. Advanced stages must receive immediate attention, whether pregnancy exists or not.

Polio, Rickets. Specific pelvimetry screening must be done if there have been diseases or accidents affecting the birth canal.

Varicose veins. When varicosities exist, particular prenatal measures (diet and therapy) must be taken to reinforce and support the liver and circulatory system. The presence of varicosities indicates a deficiency in the tone of vascular tissue. The weight of pregnancy in the third trimester also increases the risk of rupture and discomfort of vulva and leg varicosities. (See Chapter 10, Hemorrhoids, Other Varicosities.)

Allergies, Asthma. Risk for home birth depends on the kind and severity of the allergy, the medications used, etc. Patients with mild asthma usually can go through a pregnancy and labor without much difficulty.

Chronic and severe cases are high risk for home birth. Emotional stresses during gestation and labor can intensify asthmatic attacks and even bring on anaphylactic shock.

Epilepsy. Home birth can be planned only if cleared by the doctor, and his decisions will be influenced by the kind of seizures and the medication required for regulation. (Some anticonvulsant drugs cause birth defects.) A seizure during childbirth could cause trauma in that the lungs are usually partially paralyzed and this would inhibit oxygen supply. Seizures could expel the fetus by propulsion or could injure the fetus by restriction.

16. **General health of the mother:**

    Anemia. Red blood cells carry oxygen and nutrition to the fetus, so they have to be full and strong. If iron-deficiency anemia is present at term, the hemorrhage risk is increased. (See Chapter 10, Anemia, Other Deficiencies.)

    Hemorrhoids. If this condition is severe (hemorrhoids protruding and bleeding) and not corrected prior to delivery, ruptures can be expected during bearing-down contractions. This can lead to heavy hemorrhaging.

    Bowel regularity. Less than three bowel movements a day constitutes constipation. Particular attention to promoting regular evacuations lessens the chances of developing toxemia, as well as the discomforts of headache, nausea, and fever that sometimes accompany this condition. Care must be taken to increase exercise and water and bulk in the diet. Normal progression of pregnancy often hinders regularity. Hypertension can be a major cause of constipation in any person. Often the sitz bath and B vitamins help to maintain a more calm nature. Chronic constipation does not necessarily rule out home birth; it does give the gravida something she immediately should set about to correct in order to enjoy her pregnancy and labor.

Diet. See Chapter 9, THE GOOD PROGRAM.

17. **Congenital defects.** Whether home delivery is indicated will depend upon the kind and cause of defects that may occur. Some defects are accompanied with specific labor and delivery problems. Defects such as web feet, missing limbs, and extra fingers would present no problem. (See Chapter 21, Birth Defects.)

18. **Multiple births.** Particular prenatal, antenatal, and delivery care plans have to be developed in anticipation of multiple births. Twins have been delivered safely at home. (See Chapter 8, Diagnosis of Multiple Pregnancy; Chapter 20, Multiple Births.) The gravida on fertility pills must realize the possibility of her delivering several offspring at once. In this case, she definitely needs the problem-preventing care a good midwife can offer during pregnancy. She needs a superior, well-monitored diet to assure proper balance between adequate nutrition for "the family" she is carrying and her weight. She needs special care to help her carry the babies as close to term as possible, in reasonable comfort. Other plans for delivery—whether in the hospital or at home—need to be carefully made. Good back-up personnel should be present and in readiness for any eventuality during labor or postpartum.

19. **Menstrual irregularities.** Heavy menstrual flows, strong cramps (that have posed physical and emotional problems prior to conception) sometimes indicate lack of uterine efficiency. At other times, pregnancy seems to remedy the malady and menstrual periods improve between pregnancies.

20. **Due date.** See this Chapter, Determining a Due Date.

Pelvic and Vaginal Assessment

An important part of screening for home birth consists of evaluating the structural capacity of the pelvis and the condition of the vagina for giving birth.

If a woman has given birth to infants six pounds or heavier and her labors have been 18 hours or less, with about two hours or less of bearing down, her pelvis is probably adequate. If this is her first baby and her growth and development are normal, her pelvis is probably fine. Even if her pelvic measurements are a little small early in pregnancy, they will be somewhat larger by the end of the pregnancy, especially if she has exercised and taken her sitz baths. If you can fit your fist comfortably between the "sitting bones," or **ischial tuberosities** (see Figure 12), then probably all is well.

INTERNAL PALPATION (VAGINAL EXAMINATION)

To make a thorough assessment of the pelvis in order to determine whether a mother has an adequate build for vaginal delivery, you will need to palpate internally (see Figure 13). Before you do so, make sure the mother has emptied her bladder

Determining Home Birth Feasibility   103

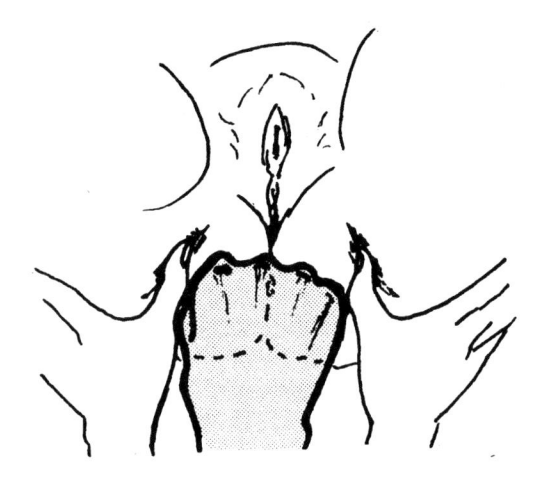

Figure 12. EXTERNAL PELVIMETRY. The pelvic outlet measurements are found between the ischial tuberosities or "buttocks bones." A general assessment can be made by placing the closed fist between the bones indicated by the thumbs. This will approximate 11 cm, but remember to deduct 1 to 2 cm for the fat and tissue. This can also be measured when the gravida is on her side.

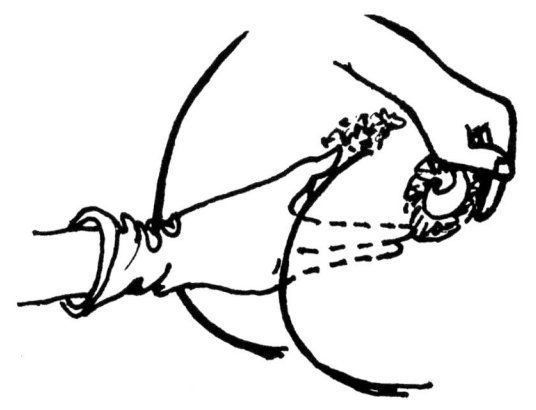

Figure 13. FIRST VAGINAL EXAMINATION. This is carried out at 2 1/2 to 3 months of pregnancy by palpating internally with one hand while cupping the other hand down behind the uterus, externally.

and is comfortable and well-draped. If you are doing this in your own home, use fresh linens to cover your bed and to drape her.

A caution or two should be inserted here. VAGINAL EXAMINATIONS TOO EARLY IN PREGNANCY CAN DISRUPT THE DELICATE FETAL ENVIRONMENT TO THE POINT OF CAUSING THE FETUS TO ABORT. Consequently, many midwifes have adopted as a rule of thumb that they do not conduct vaginal examinations until about the third month. Cervical and uterine tissue should not be palpated earlier than about the tenth week. Also, LEARN HOW TO BE AS CLEAN AND AS SANITARY AS POSSIBLE, AND DON'T DO VAGINAL EXAMINATIONS INDISCRIMINATELY. ANYTHING ENTERING THE VAGINA BRINGS WITH IT THE POSSIBILITY OF INFECTION.

After hand scrubs (see Appendix A, Aseptic Technique) and application of a lubricant to the palpating fingers, point the index and middle fingers of the left hand down and part the vulva. Insert the index and middle fingers of the right hand very slowly and gently while following the vaginal canal in a slight downward direction. It will be less uncomfortable for the gravida if gentle right and left rotations are made along the way. Examinations are made by sweeping the fingers across the inferior side of the canal, then turning the palm upward and sweeping across the superior sides.

Experience with many examinations over a period of time will help you to be able to make judgments accurately. The midwife should develop a skillful sense of observation with her fingertips. She needs to be able to assess the birth canal quickly and systematically in order not to forget any point. She should leave the area knowing all she needs to know, without having caused discomfort.

Determining Home Birth Feasibility 105

1. Note the overall shape and size of the canal, including the placement and dimensions of the points through which the baby's head must pass in birth: the sacral promontory, the floor, the ischial spines, and the pubic arch. Palpate to the lower right and left to see if the ischial spines (the two bony protuberances) are particularly prominent or just normally protruding (see Figure 14).

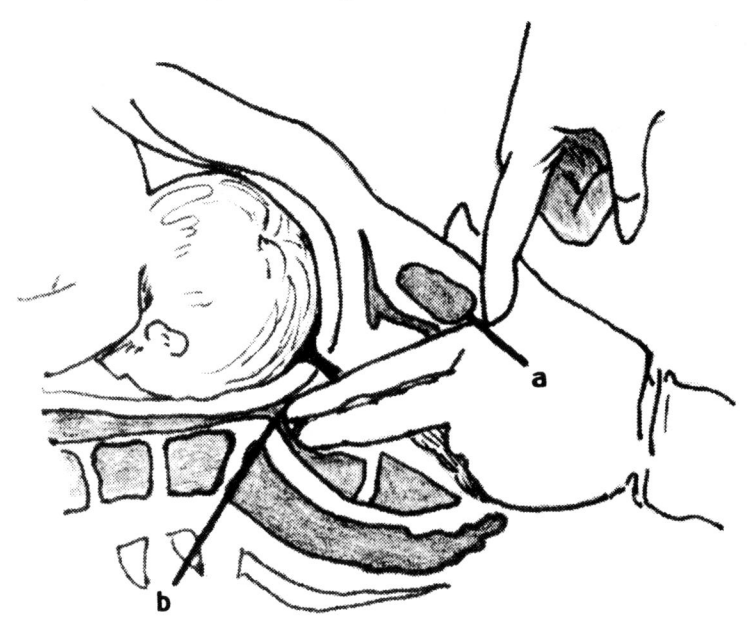

Figure 14. INTERNAL PELVIMETRY. (a) inferior edge of the symphysis pubis, (b) sacral promontory (prominence upward from the coccyx). Know your own index finger-to-thumb length to measure the **diagonal conjugate** (distance from the sacral promontory to the lower margin of the symphysis pubis). Subtract about 2 cm (to allow for the depth of the pubic bones) and find the space across the pelvic inlet to be about 12 to 13 cm for average, safe passage.

2. Is the tailbone (coccyx) moveable? It should be. If it rises sharply from the vaginal floor, it may break during birth. (The mother may or may not feel the breakage; following childbirth, breakage discomfort can be relieved by sitting in a sitz tub on a plastic "donut.")

3. Check the condition of the vaginal floor. The muscles should be smooth and firm. The floor should have a normal curve, not be wide and flat. A mother with a sacral hollow that is flat and wide will need additional attention during late first stage and second stage labor (see Chapter 16, Transverse Head Arrest). If you find that the mother has a narrow canal, tell her, "You have a rather small canal, but it is not abnormal. It just means that you may have to push longer and harder than most women to give birth." This prepares her emotionally and intellectually for a longer labor (see Chapter 16, Narrow Build, Therapies for Birth Canal Expansion).

4. Are there any irregularities: scar tissue, warts, hard knots, cysts, varicosities, excessive vaginal discharge (leukorrhea), excessive tenderness, etc.?

   Most abnormalities should be referred to a doctor. If there is a discharge that is irritating, green, and frothy, or bloodstained or profuse, the mother should be seen by a physician. Internal edema, vulva warts, or lesions indicate there may be venereal disease. This demands IMMEDIATE medical attention. Simply tell the mother what conditions you have found (not what you think it may be) and that this must be taken care of before you can consider her for home birth.

PAP SMEAR

This procedure is done in order to determine if the gravida is free of cervical cancer; it should be done with each pregnancy, particularly if the gravida is past 30. Prior to palpating at the first vaginal exam, a closed speculum should be inserted carefully, so that matter adhering to and around the external os is not disturbed. Open the speculum and secure it in an open position so you can insert the wooden spatula through it. With this you will gather a sample for a **Pap smear** from the external rim of the cervix. To obtain another smear from the os itself, you will enter the point of the irregular end of the stick into the cervical opening, make a complete turn, and withdraw the sample. The samples will be "smeared" on glass culture slides, covered or mixed with fixative (which dries quickly), and examined for cancer cells. This you can do yourself if you are trained and have the equipment; otherwise, the samples, packaged according to directions in the kit, are sent to a lab for results.

NOTES

[1] A lunar month is a four-week (28-day) period. **Gestational age** of the baby--in weeks or lunar months--is based on the **menstrual age**, or time elapsed since the first day of the last menstrual period before conception (about 9 1/3 calendar months, or 40 weeks, altogether). This time frame is about two weeks before ovulation and conception, and about three weeks before implantation of the fertilized egg. Embryologists and those concerned with the specifics of development of the baby use the **ovulation age** or conception age, the time (in days or weeks) since ovulation or conception.

[2] Mendelsohn, **Confessions of a Medical Heretic**, p. 29. Of interest also is Dr. Mendelsohn's chapter on the Pill in **Male Practice: How Doctors Manipulate Women**, "'It's Safer Than Pregnancy.'" (Chicago: Contempory Books, Inc., 1982), pp. 119-29.

CHAPTER 8

PRENATAL TESTS AND VISITS

NATURE OF PRENATAL CARE

If you find that the mother who wants your services is low risk and appropriate for home birth, you should help her prepare for the birth with good prenatal care. This care includes:

1. Regular prenatal exams.

2. Thorough instruction in nutrition.

3. Instruction about exercises, therapies, and herbs that prepare the gravida's body for childbirth.

4. Instruction about what normal body changes occur as pregnancy progresses and labor begins.

5. Instruction about danger signals she should watch for during pregnancy and when she should call you for delivery.

6. Instruction about which items the mother should have ready for the birth.

7. Instruction about what is expected of the mother and what she can expect from you.

PRENATAL TESTS

Laboratory Tests

It is recommended that you run standard blood tests early in pregnancy in order to determine some factors that screen for high risk mothers and other factors that will help you know how to best deal with the gravida throughout her pregnancy and delivery. You can run these tests yourself if you have the facilities, training, and desire to do so.[1] If you don't, you should have your clients also visit a doctor or clinic or lab at the time of their initial prenatal visit. Most states and counties have Public Health facilities which will run these tests for you at minimal or no cost. Whenever borderline high risks prevail or questionable conditions exist, it is advisable that a physician also be seen.

A single blood sample can be tested to disclose:

1. Whether the mother has an adequate white blood cell count (so her system can fight disease and infection).

2. Whether the mother's red blood cells are rich enough in iron and other minerals and components to sustain a pregnancy well. Hematocrit testing should be repeated late in pregnancy and whenever there is concern about the sufficiency of the mother's iron level.

3. The mother's blood grouping, or blood type (in case a transfusion is needed), and Rh status (negative or positive). If the mother is Rh-negative, you need to find out if she is "sensitized." Also, if a sensitized, Rh-negative mother is pregnant, usually with her second child or more, a periodic antibody

screening may be called for. (See also Chapter 12, Rh Factor and Hemolytic Disease.)

4. The mother's immunity to rubella (see Chapter 12, Rubella).

5. Whether the mother has an active venereal disease (see Chapter 12, Venereal Disease). A prenatal serology test is required by most states.

Tests can be costly. Only the above are considered essential, unless present health conditions warrant further laboratory investigation. Tests should also be run, if conditions warrant, to discover:

1. Sickle cell anemia. (Since intermarriage has become more common, the number of nonblack and non-Mediterranean cases of sickle cell anemia is increasing.)

2. A blood disorder or infection (such as leukemia or hepatitis).

3. Tuberculosis.

4. Cancer.

5. Any other condition which would interfere with a safe pregnancy and delivery.

Ultrasound

Along about the fifth month, many women notice a jump in weight gain. They suddenly have a lapful! At this, some doctors wonder about twins. (I begin to wonder about the doctor, about this time.) Too many of them suggest an ultrasonogram to determine multiple birth when this sudden jump is a normal development at the fifth month.

The ultrasonic diagnostic machine transmits a beam of sound waves far above the range of human hearing. When this beam strikes objects of different densities--fetal limbs, fluid, skull, or placenta--the returning echoes are amplified and displayed as dots of light that can be recorded with a camera. The image produced is an **ultrasonogram,** or "echo picture."

Some practitioners decline to use ultrasonic equipment because they feel it disturbs the fetus. Indeed, excessive fetal activity, indicating stress, has frequently been recorded during and after the use of ultrasonic equipment. My own daughter's baby was excessively active for 1 1/2 days beginning with an ultrasound test at her fifth month of pregnancy.

Another problem with ultrasonographic diagnosis is its unreliability. Many times disorders appear in the ultrasonogram which, in reality, do not exist.

I remember delivering a mother who had attended a prenatal class that was taken on a tour through the hospital in anticipation of their deliveries there. To demonstrate the effectiveness and wonder of the ultrasonogram, the nurse offered to have one of the expectant mothers jump upon the table to see her baby in utero via the equipment. The class and the mother saw the outline of her baby--with two heads and one or two of the extremities missing! The nurse got excited but said there was nothing to worry about, they would have a doctor make the test again. The doctor found the same thing. This mother went through great trauma expecting that her baby would be thusly affected, but when the baby was born it was formed perfectly.

Another woman from Arizona came to me to deliver her expected twins. They had just moved to our valley and the babies were due in three weeks. An ultrasonogram had positively diagnosed twins. Besides, she was a twin, as I recall, her mother was a twin, and "Why wouldn't this be a very normal thing to be happening to her?" Her labor produced a single, normal-size, healthy baby. The stories could go on and on.

It now appears that even babies who seem to be normal and healthy at birth may suffer disorders later on as a result of the use of ultrasound equipment. The routine use of ultrasound has been a relatively recent development, so the jury is still out while more long-term results are being surveyed. But it looks as if the verdict is going to go against ultrasound.

There are books now available which give us clues to the damage that may be occurring due to diagnostic ultrasound. One book I recently read reported that studies done using ultrasound on laboratory animals found genetic alterations in chromosomes, decreased blood clotting ability, liver cell damage, brain enzyme damage, and corneal damage. In some animals the EEG activity was altered (brain messages were confused) and reflexes were impaired (delayed). A study of human infants disclosed disruption of the spleen's ability to produce antibodies with which to fight disease.[2] These are among the many problems being recognized.

Doris Haire (Director, Association of Maternal Child Health in New York) has called ultrasound "the DES of tomorrow."[3]

Dopplers. The small, hand-sized detectors rubbed over the abdomen (after petroleum jelly has been applied to enhance the acoustics) transduce the fetal heart tones by utilizing ultrasound and the Doppler effect. These are ultrasound "mini-units": they operate in the same way, by bouncing sound waves off fetal parts. It is likely that they, too, have some of the same effects upon the newborn.

External Fetal Heart Monitors. The external fetal heart monitors used in hospitals also utilize ultrasound. Almost any variation on the monitor which is not understood or is not interpreted correctly can alter the labor outcome drastically. MANY C-SECTIONS ARE PERFORMED UNNECESSARILY because such things as the mother's apprehension, slow fetal heart recovery after contractions (which can sometimes be corrected by changing the mother's position), excessive activity of the fetus (BECAUSE he is hooked up to the monitor), etc., cause the needle on the monitor to change its course for a while. Even the supine (lying down) position used with the monitor can contribute to fetal stress and failure of labor to progress. Those supervising labor become concerned, and a cesarean delivery results.

Confusion in interpreting the monitor results can stem not only from insufficient training, but from questions as to whether the monitor is working properly. Many mothers are hooked up to unreliable--but available--monitors. Hospital policy or the doctor may require that monitors be used with each laboring mother. One researcher concluded that monitor information is inadequate "as much as two-thirds of the time," and that it "shows an entirely false sense of precision."[4]

Serious concerns are raised with the use of fetal heart monitors, not only because of the increased rates of C-sections that accompany their use, but also because of the potential harm from the use of ultrasound.

It really doesn't matter that Doppler or fetal heart monitoring or ultrasound equipment is expensive, because this equipment probably would be worth having IF IT WERE SAFE AND GOOD FOR THE BABY. But these items have not proven safe; in fact, there is much evidence to suspect real harm from them.

In some situations, using ultrasound might be the lesser of two evils. Then, you would have to simply hope that the results are portrayed and interpreted accurately. ANY kind of interference (ultrasound, amniocentesis, or whatever the latest procedure might be) should be used with extreme caution and NEVER at the drop of an inquisitive hat. There may be times when it is important to ultrasonically determine where the placenta is, or whether there is an ectopic or a multiple pregnancy, etc., but most of the time ultrasound isn't ABSOLUTELY ESSENTIAL. It is easy enough to wait or find a more acceptable alternative, rather than expose the fetus to the risks of ultrasound.

Amniocentesis

Amniocentesis is a process used to determine whether the fetus has Down's syndrome, a congenital abnormality, hemolytic disease, etc. The process consists of inserting a very long needle through the abdominal wall, through the uterus, and into the amniotic sac. Then some of the amniotic fluid, which contains cells discarded by the fetus, is withdrawn.

The risks for both mother and child are considerable, according to Dr. Robert S. Mendelsohn:

> ... [Amniocentesis] doubles the rate of spontaneous miscarriage and of fetal abnormalities such as respiratory distress syndrome, pneumothorax (air in the baby's chest) from multiple puncture wounds, orthopedic problems, and gangrene of a limb. The mother may experience infection, bleeding, possible mixing of her own and the baby's incompatible blood types, premature rupture of the membranes during pregnancy, and postpartum hemorrhage. There is also sufficient incidence of false positive findings to cause a significant number of abortions of normal babies.

Dr. Mendelsohn adds:

> Although most doctors will deny it, there is considerable evidence that many parents seek amniocentesis not to determine fetal abnormalities, but to determine sex. Their intention, of course, is to abort the baby if it is not of the sex they prefer, and there isn't much chance that the aborted baby will be a boy. In fact, qualified medical observers tell me that in abortions performed after amniocentesis, girls are aborted in four cases out of five."[5]

The possibility of a malformation—resulting from a freak of nature, drug use, poor health habits, aging, etc.—can cause stress and demand major decisions. A couple can decide to let nature work things out, allowing a natural outcome (whether it be good health or retardation, death, deformation, or miscarriage—in other words, let nature dictate the results), or they can call for an amniocentesis, accepting the risks it poses (including the possibility of damaging or losing the baby, healthy or otherwise). Still, some defects can be discovered, and at times limited corrections can be made that may or may not bring the desired results. Many infants have been helped through amniocentesis. Many have not, and occasionally tragedies result from the interference.

PRENATAL VISITS

I am thoroughly convinced that prenatal exams are crucial to a safer pregnancy, labor, and delivery. They may seem unnecessary to the mother when things are going along fine, but panic and delay in catching and solving problems can usually be avoided through regular, careful exams.[6] Detecting protein in the urine early is especially important. Becoming familiar with individual maternal and fetal heart rates, monitoring maternal blood pressure, and knowing about any varicosities (especially in the vulva) are also important.

Prenatal visits allow you to keep abreast of changes occurring in the mother and to be on the lookout for anything unusual or abnormal, and for anything which might indicate a potential problem or a high risk situation developing which would preclude home birth. These visits give you an opportunity to instruct the mother about caring for her body and about preparing for childbirth. They allow you to appraise how the mother is doing with her prenatal preparations (diet, exercises, sitz baths, supplements, birth supplies, etc.).

You should teach mothers to take much of the responsibility for prenatal care themselves, but unless the mother is experienced in midwifery, you are more qualified to make many of the judgments that need to be made. You should also understand, however, that a mother's intuition can be invaluable to you. She often knows intuitively when things are wrong.

For example, one day a grand multipara (older mother of several children) I was working with came to me in tears and said she no longer felt pregnant, even though she was in her third month.

I looked her in the eye and said, "I believe you. If you don't feel pregnant, you probably are not anymore."

She quieted and asked, "What will happen?"

I answered, "The baby's life has probably terminated already and nature will take care of it. Just go about your business. In a short while you will begin to have symptoms of labor and the deceased fetus will pass. Call me when this happens and we will watch for any extra bleeding and take care of everything. Don't worry or fret. Everything will be fine." It was less than 24 hours before she called me and said she had had cramps and some bleeding all morning, and that when she went to the bathroom, she had passed everything. The conceptus was intact, but the embryo had embedded in the decidua basalis OUTSIDE the unruptured bag of waters. The pregnancy was not normal and the fetus could not live. This mother sensed the death of her child intuitively.

Prenatal visits should be made monthly during the first seven months of pregnancy, then every two weeks between the 32nd and 36th weeks, then each week until delivery. The more frequent visits later in pregnancy are important to check for signs of anemia or toxemia.

At each prenatal exam, do the following (be sure to carefully record the results):

1. Take the mother's blood pressure.

2. Do a urinalysis.

3. Weigh your client and look for signs of edema (swelling).

4. Measure the fundal height.

5. Listen to the fetal heart tones.

6. Answer any questions.

Keep track of your client's red blood count, as it should be adequate during the course of pregnancy. Hemoglobinometers are available and this test can easily be done anytime you suspect that her iron level is low. Early in the last month, do another blood count to check the mother's iron level. If it is borderline, check it weekly. If your client is anemic, it is imperative that you determine whether the anemia is caused by a nutritional deficiency (see Chapter 10, Anemia, Other Deficiencies) or by an undetected blood loss. An increase in blood pressure and pulse rate, if sharp, will likely indicate obscured bleeding. TIME IS OF THE ESSENCE in correcting the problem and building the blood, PARTICULARLY IF A BLOOD LOSS IS CAUSING THE PROBLEM. A physician should be seen if this determination is not clear.

Blood Pressure

To determine blood pressure, follow the instructions that come with the sphygmomanometer and stethoscope. Some general principles about taking blood pressure follow. (See also Appendix B, Blood Pressure.)

The upper number of a blood pressure reading is called the **systolic pressure;** it measures the ventricular contractions in the heart that force blood through the arteries. The lower number of the reading is called the **diastolic pressure;** it measures the force of blood pressure during ventricular resting or relaxation.

Prenatal Tests and Visits 119

A "resting" person is more likely to give you the average norm for an individual. Have the mother sit down for a few minutes before taking her blood pressure. Wrap the cuff snugly around the upper arm or biceps. The arm should not be any higher than her heart. Do not allow any parts of the equipment to touch while you are checking the pressure, because the stethoscope is very sensitive and this can distort or hide the "thump" of the heartbeats you are listening for.

Position the bell of the stethoscope directly over the vein inside the elbow. Bell and cuff should not touch each other and the arm should have been bared to minimize sound distortion. Remember to have the arrow on the cuff point to this vein. Study the gauge to become familiar with its measurements.

Close the screw, or the gauge valve, so air can be pumped into the cuff to about 180 to 200 mm Hg (millimeters of mercury—units of pressure). Open the valve just enough to allow the needle on the gauge to fall slowly and steadily. When you hear the first thump of the heartbeat through the stethoscope, make a mental note of the reading on the gauge at that point, BUT ALLOW THE NEEDLE TO CONTINUE TO GO DOWN. When you hear the last clear thump before all becomes silent, make a mental note of that point on the gauge. The first thump occurred at the systolic or highest pressure, and the last occurred on the lesser or diastolic pressure. For example, the needle may have read 120 on the first thump and 90 on the last. That person's blood pressure would be 120 (systolic) over 90 (diastolic), or 120/90.

Each person has his or her own norm. The average American's blood pressure (male and female) is probably too high. A good average for a woman of childbearing age is 113/72 to 125/80. As pregnancy progresses, a slight elevation in blood pressure is not uncommon. Chronic hypertension is indicated by persistent blood pressure above normal, and may or may not be accompanied by pre-eclampsic symptoms. Hypertension is high risk and not advisable for home birth.

Urinalysis

You can do your client's urinalysis routinely during each prenatal visit. Purchase a bottle of Uristix (or a similar product). These are clear plastic strips ("dipsticks") with patches of various chemicals on them which enable you to monitor the presence of protein, sugar, casts (blood particles), and other substances in the urine. The patches are dipped into the urine sample, then matched with scaled color patches on the bottle label. (Complete instructions appear on the label.)

Protein in the urine (**proteinuria**) is one of the signs of pre-eclampsia; when a trace of protein appears, begin therapy to avert this problem. Higher levels of glucose in the urine (**glucosuria**) indicate the mother should be more careful with her sugar/carbohydrate intake; she may even be developing gestational diabetes (which usually can be corrected with diet and rest). The gravida may need to have her BLOOD sugar checked for hypoglycemia or diabetes if the problem continues. In this case, co-screening with a physician is advisable.

To collect a urine sample, the gravida should void for just a few seconds, catch the "midstream" urine in a sterile container, then remove the container before the last of the urine passes.

Catching midstream urine lessens the possibility of contaminating the specimen.

Should Uristix or labs be unavailable and you wish to do your best without them, hold a fresh, early morning sample of urine (in a clear container) up to the light. Since bacteria build rapidly in urine, you should do this within a few minutes after obtaining the sample. After it has settled, evaluate its transparency, color, and odor:

TRANSPARENCY

>**cloudy:** Suggests the presence of protein, bacteria, and/or infection; may be caused by urinary tract infection, excessive diarrhea, vomiting; may be symptomatic of pre-eclampsia. (Protein may be present in crystal-clear urine, as well.)
>
>**clear:** Suggests good alkaline/acid balance (urine itself is usually acid).

COLOR

>**straw to amber:** Normal.
>
>**red to dark brown:** Indicates the presence of blood (dried or fresh--the darker the color, the older the blood), most often from vaginal bleeding; may be dark brownish red (or chocolate) in cases of eclampsia.
>
>**other colors:** Deep orange, green, methylene blue, brown may be due to the presence of chemicals, drugs, or medication in the mother's system; the presence of bile results in a greenish gold or a greenish brown color; also, different foods, vitamins, and minerals may affect the color of the urine (for

example, vitamins B and E make it more yellow; beets, more red; asparagus, more green).

ODOR

ammonia scent: Usually results from the ingestion of certain foods (for example, asparagus).

fruity odor ("Juicy Fruit Gum"): Suggests a diabetic or metabolic disorder.

other odors: Residual (retained) urine causes several odors (rancid, pus, ammonia, infection); inadequate water intake will result in a strong smell. (Odors are manifest through all the eliminative systems, including the skin.)

Any IRREGULARITY in urine transparency, color, or odor indicates that you must immediately start the mother on a stringent diet.

These techniques for evaluating may seem primitive; nevertheless, they are reasonable standbys that can be used in the absence of more precise methods. A midwife must use the resources she has available to discover potential problems, and then either initiate measures to correct them or refer her client to the back-up doctor.

Weight

RAPID weight gain of 3 to 5 pounds in any one week calls for examination to determine if there is edema due to lack of proper kidney function or if edema associated with toxemia is present (see this chapter, Diagnosis of Pre-eclampsia).

Fundal Height

Fundal height is used to measure fetal growth and can therefore indicate abnormally slow or fast growth. It can fail in accuracy, but at least it is an aid to monitoring a pregnancy. With a metal tape measure--inch/centimeter ones are available--measure the distance in centimeters from the upper edge of the symphysis pubis to the point where the top of the uterus (**fundus**) rounds off and turns inward. Fundal height charts (see Figure 15) approximate gestation time, in weeks, according to fundal height. After **lightening** occurs (the baby drops into the pelvic cavity, at about 38 weeks), the height of the fundus is lower and the contour of the abdomen is more round than oval. The gravida generally goes into labor between the 38th and 41st weeks.

Fetal Heart Rate

The fetal heartbeat can be heard at various times with different mothers. It can usually be heard about the 16th week with the fetalscope. When the abdominal wall is quite thick, the room is noisy, or there is an excessive amount of amniotic fluid, it may be some time before the sounds are audible enough and the baby remains in one place long enough to get a good heart count. If a doppler (ultrasound device) is used, a heart tone can be picked up by about the 12th to 14th week (see this chapter, Ultrasound). Oftentimes, the fetal heart can even be heard with the naked ear.

The fetus will have a **fetal heart rate (FHR)** of about 135 to 165 beats per minute. Little girls TEND to have faster heart rates than little boys do. When taking the fetal heart tone, do not mistake other rhythmic sounds for the fetal heart. The **maternal heart rate** and the **uterine souffle** (a

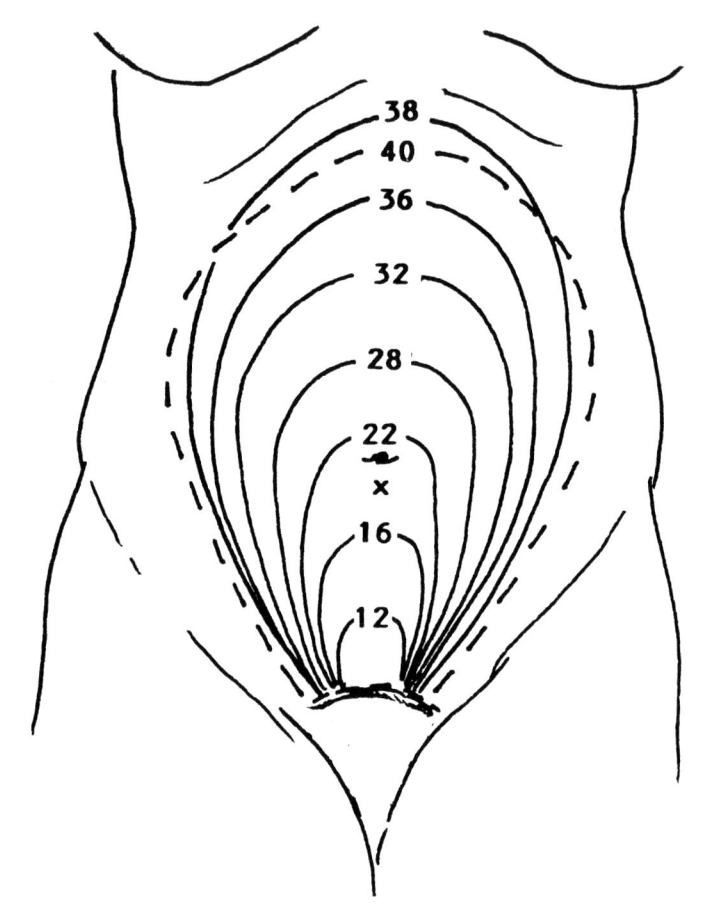

Twelfth week: The uterus, the size of a small grapefruit, fills the pelvic cavity and the fundus reaches just above the symphysis pubis.
Sixteenth week: 7 1/2 centimeters
Twentieth week: 15 centimeters
Twenty-fourth week: 20 centimeters
Thirtieth week: 24 centimeters
Thirty-sixth week: 30 centimeters (highest point)
Thirty-eighth week: 28 centimeters (32nd to 34th week level)

Figure 15. FUNDAL HEIGHT MEASUREMENT (shown in APPROXIMATE weeks of gestation). Listen for fetal heart tones (FHT) just under the navel (x).

blowing sound) will have identical beats and will be much slower than the baby's heartbeat. The **cord tone** (a swishing sound) and the fetal heart rate will be the same; both can be picked up at various times and places along the abdominal sphere.

Vaginal Exams

Vaginal examinations (beyond the initial examination to determine pregnancy, pelvic proportions, and the condition of the vaginal tract for delivery) are seldom called for in midpregnancy, unless some problem arises that needs to be investigated or monitored. Late in pregnancy, vaginal examination to determine fetal lie, cervical readiness, and dilation will give clues for delivery preparations and can be safely done if there has been no spotting. Cleanliness of mother and examining hands is always important. (See also Chapter 7, Pelvic and Vaginal Assessment; Chapter 14, Determining Engagement; Chapter 15, Dilation and Effacement; Appendix A, ASEPTIC TECHNIQUE.)

DIAGNOSIS OF MULTIPLE PREGNANCY

Suspect a multiple pregnancy if an unusually large uterus develops throughout the third trimester. Actual fundal height will be higher than normal for the weeks/months of gestation and the uterus becomes globular in shape earlier in the pregnancy. (Beware of a mistaken due date, though.)

Without ultrasonograms, a 50% correct diagnosis rate is made by doctors when infants weigh less than about 5 1/2 pounds; they have a 70% rate when the larger twin is 5 1/2 pounds or more. Some twin pregnancies are not diagnosed until the birth of the first baby.

To determine multiple pregnancy, include abdominal palpation, auscultation (listening for fetal heart sounds), and vaginal examination.

If a lot of small parts (elbows, knees, heels, toes) are palpated, twin pregnancy should be suspected. When two heads are palpated, two breeches, or two backs, or perhaps one back but four opposite ends of the body, then at least twins are known to be gestating. With many gravidas it is easiest to feel the body parts early in the third trimester. On very rare occasions, a tumor may be mistaken for a little round head.

Auscultation is probably a better source of information. When two fetal heart tones are heard from parts fairly well removed from each other, and especially when the heart tones are at least 10 beats per minute different from each other, then you know there are two babies.

Palpating at the cervix sometimes reveals the presence of a breech (especially a foot), and this should also cause suspicion of a twin pregnancy if the uterus is exceptionally large.

DIAGNOSIS OF DEATH IN UTERO

There may be those rare times when a question arises as to the vital conditon of the fetus in utero. In determining whether the fetus has died, look for a combination of the following signs:

1. The uterus has remained the same size for a number of weeks.

2. Repeated endocrine tests for pregnancy are negative.

3. Fetal movement ceases over a number of weeks.

4. The mother's breasts become softer and flabby instead of firm.

5. The fetal heartbeat ceases. (Don't mistake cessation of FHT for your inability to find heart tones for a few days.)

6. Palpation of the baby's skull through the cervix reveals a loose skull, as if it were in a flabby bag.

7. X-ray shows the bones of the fetal skull overlapping at the sutures (sign of shrinkage of skull contents).

If a fetus has died in utero, there is usually no need to get the baby out right away. Nature will almost always trigger birth when it is ready, and the mother is not usually in any danger. Labor need not be induced, as a rule. Herbal remedies probably will not bring on labor, but a small amount of lobelia, false unicorn, or squawvine will not hurt. The five-week herbal formula should be followed so that bleeding, which is sometimes a little excessive under these circumstances, is curbed when birth does occur. An early conceptus will sometimes reabsorb into the system.

DIAGNOSIS OF PRE-ECLAMPSIA (TOXEMIA)

In my opinion, the stressful condition commonly referred to as **toxemia of pregnancy (pre-eclampsia or eclampsia)** is brought about primarily by an unhealthy system. One may or may not realize the extent of this unhealthy condition at the beginning of pregnancy.

An unhealthy body that is slow to eliminate toxins may be asking too much when it becomes pregnant and asks its kidneys and bowels to take on the added resonsibility of eliminating wastes for another body (to say nothing of trying to build and maintain that other body).

If pregnancy occurs in a very unhealthy body, sooner or later vital signs will begin to show the degree of stress the parent and fetal bodies are really under. Protein (albumin) will appear in the urine, the kidneys, unable to function well enough, will leave too much water in body tissues (edema), causing sudden weight gains, and the overtaxed condition of the body will put stress on the heart to push impure blood through a clogged vascular system (elevated blood pressure). At any point along the way maternal and fetal bodies are in peril. Eclampsia (severe toxemia) can indeed bring about convulsive revolts to the impositions placed upon the maternal and fetal systems, and at times it even brings about death.

Pre-eclampsia is the early stage of toxemia. Physicians cannot predict when this condition may progress into **eclampsia,** which is the later stage and an extremely serious, convulsive (and possibly comatose) condition. One person may go into convulsions (eclampsia) more quickly than another who shows more signs of trouble.

Pre-eclampsia is most often seen in young primigravidas, especially those whose diet has been poor. You will want to watch these mothers especially closely, particularly during the last few weeks before due date.

Signs of toxemia may have been negative all during pregnancy, then begin to show up the last week or two. (If toxemia is going to show up at all, it will usually show up in the third trimester. If it shows up before then, the woman probably had problems before she was pregnant.) Frequently signs will not show up until the days between the last prenatal checkup and delivery, especially if the due date has passed or if a particularly stressful event has occurred in the mother's life.

Toxemia is a serious condition, posing threats for both mother and child. Home birth is definitely not safe if the condition is advanced or is rapidly advancing. Experience and intuitiveness will help make the decision about home birth if the mother shows MILD symptoms at term.

Pre-eclampsia too serious for home births occurs when any two or three of the following symptoms are present (one symptom alone is not conclusive):

1. A rise in blood pressure of 30 mm or more above usual in the systolic measurement, or a rise of 15 mm above normal in the diastolic measurement.

2. Significant protein in the urine (proteinuria) of 3+ (or 300+).

3. Edema (swelling) of the hands and face.

To check these signs out further, do the following:

1. If the blood pressure shows above normal, there may be a superficial reason. The mother may be hurried, worried, or excited. You should check the pressure again in 6 to 12 hours. If it remains high, you should suspect pre-eclampsia and begin corrective measures. (This may also be indicative of hypertension alone.)

2. Obtain a fresh, early-morning urine specimen. A 2 or 3+ reading in the antenatal period, in conjunction with any other of these three symptoms, would prove too high a risk for home birth.

3. A SUDDEN weight gain, of three or more pounds in any one week, is probably due to edema and is cause for concern that toxemia may be present (see also Chapter 11, Edema).

Outside a prenatal visit setting, some physical indicators, if positive, would indicate that a prenatal visit should be set up without delay:

1. Have the mother cross her knees. Tap just under the lower edge of the kneecap. If she responds with a sharp, quick, high kick she should be checked for pre-eclampsia.

2. Have the mother point her toe away from her body, and then bring her toe back up toward her knee. If the toe jerks three to five times as it is pulled back, suspect toxemia and test for elevated blood pressure, proteinuria, and excessive weight gain (edema).

WHAT TO DO:

When TRACES of pre-eclampsic symptoms appear, bed rest and a change in diet are called for immediately. The gravida should eliminate all soda pop, fried foods, meat, sweets, and breads from her diet. She should eat raw fruits and vegetables. One or two servings of steamed vegetables per day is permissible. She should also drink one tablespoon of lemon juice in a tall glass of water in the morning before eating. Vitamin E (600 IU per day) is very helpful. An average intake of water is fine. Kidney-herb teas should be taken: parsley, uva ursi, juniper berries, shave grass, watermelon seeds, etc. (See page 81 of **A Superior Alternative** for further details.)

Notify your back-up doctor so that he is aware of the mother's pre-eclampsic condition and can help you determine if hospitalization is needed or if he can be available to help you treat the gravida.

If severe pre-eclampsia does not improve in one to two days, termination of the pregnancy is usually advised for the safety of both mother and baby. If the cervix is ready (retracted), labor may be induced. If not, a cesarean delivery may be necessary. These procedures are NOT undertaken by midwives.

It behooves every expectant mother to faithfully play the role of a happy guardian in preparing a healthy body for her child by carefully monitoring her diet and exercise program. Both she and the baby can have a wonderful experience in childbirth if care and caution and discipline are the watchwords throughout pregnancy.

NOTES

[1] During my midwifery classes, I have found a number of class members who worked in labs or clinics and were trained to make blood tests. Some were interested in providing this service to midwives and parents. It seems that this need is being fulfilled by very competent technicians. Back-up doctors, as well, are coming out of the woodwork, so to speak, because of the increasing interest in out-of-hospital care for healthy people.

[2] Nancy Wainer Cohen and Lois J. Estner, **Silent Knife: Cesarean Prevention** and **Vaginal Birth After Cesarean** (South Hadley, Mass.: Bergin & Garvey Publishers, Inc., 1983), p. 142. Ultrasound is discussed in Chapter 8, "Diagnostic Time Bombs?," pp. 140-45.

[3] Ibid., p. 141.

[4] Ibid., p. 181. Chapter 9, "Birth Interventions and their Consequences," discusses both internal and external fetal heart monitoring on pages 180-83. Though I do not discuss here the INTERNAL fetal heart monitors (electrode attached to the fetal scalp) used in hospitals, they have some very serious risks associated with their use.

[5] Robert S. Mendelsohn, M.D., Male Practice: How Doctors Manipulate Women (Chicago: Contemporary Books, Inc., 1982) p. 186.

[6] See page 80 of A Superior Alternative for an anecdote about a fetal rate that went down with each prenatal visit, signaling a problem early.

CHAPTER 9

THE GOOD PROGRAM

I frequently refer in this book to the Good Program. This chapter includes information about foods, water, the use of herbs for nutritional and medicinal aids, exercise, and sitz baths, all specifically designed to assist the childbearing woman and her family. The avoidance of harmful elements is also discussed.

NUTRITION

A woman's primary biological contribution to the human race is childbearing. In order for her to make this contribution and still enjoy life and be a bright spot in the lives of her family and associates, she must enjoy good health. It is each woman's obligation to make every effort to be healthy. One mother put it to her daughters this way: "You have no right to eat 'any way you like,' if it will tear down your health and reflect in the health of your offspring."

Certainly, a long-term poor diet can leave the alimentary canal so stressed that it, in turn, leaves the eliminative systems hardput to function properly.

As an example, look at the dependency one set of physiological systems has upon another. The eliminative systems (I include the lymphatic system, lungs, skin, kidneys, and bowels) must be functioning adequately to maintain life. The body will tolerate a great deal of abuse, but even then it will tolerate just so much. Sooner or later accumulated wastes set in motion life-threatening putrefaction and decay. This makes the body vulnerable to all kinds of disease and to malfunctioning of the endocrine system (which balances and controls body growth and activity).

A body laden with undigested protein, unremoved fecal matter, and impure blood needs to rid itself of such. To do this, it needs adequate, balanced nutritional intake and body motion.

The lymphatic system must have a body in motion, and the body must have enough clean water and roughage present to help move waste through the blood stream, liver, kidneys, and bowels, or else decay and infection set in and large, painful lumps appear in the lymph nodes. Headaches, stomach cramps, pimples, and skin disorders appear, bladder infections become frequent, and temperature, blood pressure, pulse, and respiration begin sending out distress signals. When the kidneys are overloaded, bacteria multiply rapidly and the infection is manifested in numerous ways: it shows up in the urine, in pain, in fever, etc. Bacteria are seldom isolated for long. They penetrate through tissue after tissue and, unchecked, eventually will involve the whole body to bring about death.

It makes sense that these conditions can be avoided if the clean-up of the body and maintenance of good health is undertaken with regularity.

Most of us assume that we are healthy if we can get out of bed each day, take a pill to hide nature's warning signals, and not suffer constantly. Seldom do we recognize the adverse conditions we are courting by the way we live until it is a little late. Pregnancy comes along and suddenly we are made aware of the dangers we have imposed upon self and body.

Pregnancy should be prepared for more conscientiously than any other project we undertake.

A pregnant woman need not change her diet if she already has a good one. Most women, however, have less than the ideal diet. For those of us who are feeling the consequences of a generation or two of malnutrition—and too much and too rich is malnutrition—the answer is to work out a balanced diet and stick with it.

Furthermore, we must not get discouraged when reversals seem to come along in the pursuit of a good program, for often when you begin to eat properly and to exercise, you give nature such a boost that all of a sudden you are thrown into a body cleanse. One health authority makes this observation: If the bowels are constipated the body may be fighting a disease. If the bowels are in good shape (three stools a day) the discomfort may be due to a body cleanse (simulation of a "cold" or disease). Instead of finding fault with my efforts to find solutions and to make health repairs after a personal crisis, one man said, "Look what might have happened had you not been on your good program!" A good program is essential for childbearing women. It may possibly take a woman in poor health one to three years to get into shape to bear offspring without physical distress and complications. Then again, by launching on the Good Program, she may breeze through her pregnancy feeling better than she has ever felt in her life. Certainly her pregnancy will go much better and the outcome will be more rewarding than if she had never refined her efforts to feel good, to look good, and to produce a fine and healthy baby.

Implementing a good program leaves her with one additional responsibility, that of feeding her family correctly henceforth so their habits will build a better generation to follow. I suppose the whole motive for this chapter is to encourage people to prepare for and to have offspring more safely than ever before.

It goes without saying that health and nutrition experts are trying to help us allay future problems by admonishing us to READ LABELS on all foodstuffs. They tell us that the "insignificant amounts" of additives, etc., have climbed to rates so high as to be very significant, because virtually everything we purchase contains them. Let us say here that the more foods we can grow for our own families, the better off they will be nutritionally. Clean food would suggest to us that pure foods are to be free of contaminants. There are several ways to preserve foods without contaminating them. This volume is not meant to replace other volumes that are elaborate, eloquent resources for this kind of help. The message is simply to eat good, clean foods, and many raw foods, with a minimum of animal protein. No flesh-eater will tell you to do without meat, because he has been taught that there are values to be found there. A vegetarian will tell you there is more harm done to the body by eating flesh than can be compensated for by those few values. Each person must work out his own regimen; however, an exceptional feeling of well-being comes from eating fruits and vegetables, accompanied by sufficient quantities of higher proteins to balance out the growing and maintaining that must be done in the body.

Vegetarianism

Plants are a valuable, complete source of food. Although Dr. John A. Widtsoe, scientist and nutritionist, seemed to favor an overall diet of plant, animal, and dairy foods, he made the following comments about vegetarianism:

> The protein of fresh eggs and clean milk have the highest value . . . ; meat and animal products are also good protein foods, though meat has certain drawbacks. Modern research has shown . . . that all the necessary food constituents are found in plants. From that point of view vegetarianism should be practicable. The legumes, (peas, beans and lentils) and nuts are the richest vegetable protein foods and their protein compares favorably with those of meats. The proteins of nuts are more nearly complete protein than those of legumes, but soybeans, peanuts and peas have protein which may safely be relied upon for growth and maintenance throughout maturity if eaten in the right proportion. Therefore when meat is not eaten both nuts and legumes are indispensable in the diet, . . . Some form of good protein must be eaten every day. . . . In fairness, it must be said that many vegetarians have lived well and happily to a ripe old age.
>
> . . . Man may live entirely upon the products of the soil, and do an effective work and attain a high age--if he understands and uses well the facts of complete nutrition. Indeed, many find that their health is improved when meat is excluded entirely from their diet. But such a diet may be unwise, especially for growing children and adults also, unless the vegetable proteins are chosen most wisely, and with full understanding of the laws of human nutrition . . . .[1]

If one uses meat, it must be used sparingly and in winter or famine only, as stated in a wise law of health, the Word of Wisdom.

It may well be said, as Dr. Widtsoe said of vegetarianism, that any man could live, do effective work, and attain a high age if he understood the facts of complete nutrition. Who of us--whether vegetarian or not--understands the facts of complete nutrition and abides by all he knows to do? Follow your heart and continue to learn.

Diet

The program for eating found in this volume was built around recommendations of two vegetarian medical doctors, Drs. Paul and Charles Smith, two of the most energetic, accomplishing, soft-spoken, and composed persons I have known. Their research into nutrition has brought out the fact that Americans usually eat many more grams of protein than are actually needed for growth and maintenance of good health. Between 25 and 40 grams daily are adequate for even the pregnant woman. Each individual has certain body and energy requirements. The quantities needed to fulfill these requirements may have been assumed, until one has been on a vegetarian diet for a few months. When the body begins to regulate to real--not assumed--needs, it becomes easier to meet those requirements adequately. Heavier proteins are recommended for the earlier part of the day, before 2:00 p.m.

A general menu-graph of your plate is shown in Figures 16 and 17. Follow this outline for successful eating without excessive weight gain. In fact, you are likely to lose weight on this program, but if you are getting a variety and not overdoing the nuts and sweets, you will be getting good nutrition for your own strength and energy, plus ample quality nutrition for Baby Dear. (Some ideas for utilizing good foods are found in Appendix C, SAMPLE RECIPES FOR THE GOOD PROGRAM.)

The Good Program 139

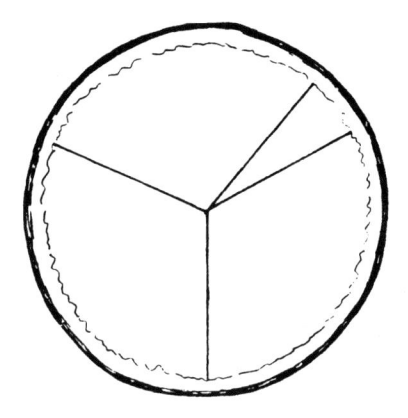

Figure 16. BREAKFAST PLATE VOLUME. **Going clockwise, the first large area at the top:** cereals, bread, milk; **smallest section:** nuts, peanut butter, margarine, avocado, olives, etc.; **two bottom sections:** fruit (one portion citrus if you live where it grows).

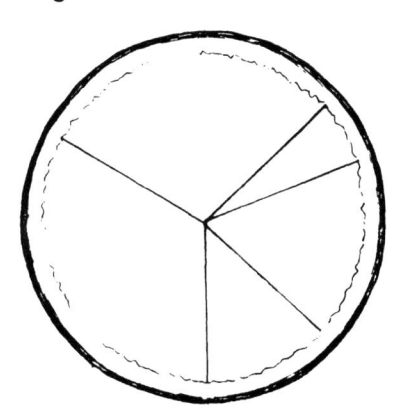

Figure 17. DINNER PLATE VOLUME. **Going clockwise from the top:** salads; **smallest section:** nuts, honey, raisins, dates, margarine; **third section:** fat, 20% (in food and food preparation); **next section:** protein, 10 to 12%; **last section:** green vegetables. Hypoglycemics may want to divide these portions into six SMALL meals a day.

Basically, I refer here to groups of foods that are grown from the soil (as opposed to "nonfood" or packaged foods): vegetables, fruits, nuts, and grains. We are reminded that the soil should be properly prepared--as naturally as possible. I cannot argue with those who have successfully recycled nutrition by using mulches and composts. If they can do it, we can. Mass production of huge crops has demanded, it seems, that the growing of foods be handled in different ways, using chemical fertilizers and sprays. But on a smaller scale, such as the individual family garden, we should take another good look at what the small-scale experts are saying.

Once the soil has been properly maintained over the years, and rested when appropriate, we can expect good, balanced nutrition from our home-grown foods. Probably the utilization of the VARIETY, as well as the kind, of foods needs closer attention. The WHOLE FOOD in many instances--the potato peel, the apple peel and seeds, the whole grain, etc.--provides most of what is needed to digest and utilize the product.

Any changes we make in the original food perhaps should only change the form, not necessarily the make-up or content of the product itself. We may slice, dry, grate, juice, chill, warm, arrange, and have taste in variety and abundance.

Fruit intake is unlimited, except for bananas, raisins, and dates. You may choose not to use nuts with fruits. Remember to use at least three fruits at a fruit meal time. Bottled fruits prepared with not more than 2 T. honey, and perhaps 1/4 teaspoon vitamin C to prevent discoloration, are acceptable (see Appendix C, Canning Recipes).

In the GREEN VEGETABLE group we find, for example:

artichokes	cabbage	parsley
asparagus	cauliflower	spinach
beet greens	celery	summer squash
bean sprouts	cucumbers	sweet peppers
broccoli	green beans	watercress
Brussels sprouts	lettuce	other leafy greens

In the WHOLE GRAIN and BEAN food groups, we find:

barley	rye	great Northern beans
oats	wheat	lima beans
buckwheat	mung beans	soy beans
corn	navy beans	peas
millet	pinto beans	lentils
rice	garbanzo beans	

Eat from these two groups daily for a balanced quality and amount of proteins. Whole grains are delicious for breakfast and can also take the place of breads. They can be soaked overnight to release full value in their use as cereals. Beans must be sprouted or cooked thoroughly to release a usable protein.

To supplement fat and protein needs, eat small amounts of NUTS and SEEDS:

almonds	caraway seeds	sunflower seeds
peanuts	cashews	pumpkin seeds
poppy seeds	pecans	walnuts
sesame seeds	filberts	

Beets, carrots, potatoes (sweet or Irish), winter squash, and pumpkin, steamed until tender, can be eaten in smaller quantities. Beets, carrots, and either kind of potato are nutritious and delicious raw.

SEASON with garlic, onions, herbs, mushrooms, and vegetable powders (which taste salty when dried and then powdered, but have very small, if any, amounts of salt). Use lemon juice also for seasoning.

It is indeed possible to add variety and still maintain original nutritive values in our foods. So you want a little spicier taste today! Dried forms of vegetables give interesting and delightful salty tastes without additional salt. (Watch labels: some products on the market do contain mineral or sea salts.) One such preparation took the fancy of my fifteen-year old son. You couldn't get him to put gravy or sour cream on his baked potato anymore. He likes the taste of Jensen's Broth or Seasoning Powder, a dried preparation of uncooked barley, alfalfa, onion, tomato, celery stalk and leaves, pimento, orange, parsley, spinach, watercress, and carrot, spiced with chili, garlic, celery seed, and yeast. Anyone on a low sodium diet will enjoy this. Other preparations are good too. Two teaspoons of Jensen's Broth and Seasoning Powder in hot water with a pinch of cayenne give energy in sickness.

The Lord didn't forget anything! We do get much natural salt in foods themselves, probably as much as we need under normal circumstances. Two or three grams of salt come in normal amounts of food per day. This is plenty. You get seven or eight and up to thirty grams of salt per day if you salt things during cooking and at the table, or if you use salt tablets. Essential salts and potassium are already in the body. Potassium is a great regulator for the heart, is needful for alertness of mind, and has other benefits.

According to Dr. Paul Smith, M.D., there are 10,000 chemical reactions possible in a cell. Microscopic bodies within the cells of our bodies contain enzymes responsible for the conversion of food into energy. A membrane encloses each cell and keeps some elements (such as potassium) in the cell and some elements (such as sodium) out of it. Hormones, for example, can be likened to "keys" which unlock areas of the cellular membrane and activate the cell to produce the substances it needs. "Medicines, in general," says Dr. Paul Smith, "are 'blocking' or 'poisoning' agents to our cells." They don't allow the cell to function normally. Good foods enhance cell activity and are better medicines for us.[2]

Seasons Point The Way

We might take a hint from the example nature gives us when we think of what to eat and when to eat it. For instance, those heavier roots and thick-skinned vegetables have built-in preservatives that help them to last for months for our use. Potatoes, carrots, squash, and beans (with such a variety!), seeds and grains and nuts all have nature's own preserving qualities. These foods are harvested in the fall and can be stored for use during the time of the year our bodies need what these foods contain for extra warmth.

As the growing season begins, we find fresh greens and blossoms on the trees to herald the coming of foods designed to build and "house-clean" our bodies and to prepare them for different activities in warmer temperatures: foods such as strawberries, rhubarb, asparagus, dandelions, greens, and fruits of the cleansing varieties.

It is said that fruits cleanse and vegetables build, primarily. Since a variety provides the essential nutrients, the whole summer is filled with an abundance and a variety.

While raw foods not only provide bulk, they also provide nutrients, alive and ready, as it were, to fulfill their missions of contributing to our well-being. Overcooked foods are destroyed foods.

Steamed foods and some baked foods for variety (squash, potatoes, etc.) are also wholesome.

We know that individual body chemistry differs, and so certain foods needed by one person may cause stress to another. Therefore, it is wise to learn which foods benefit your body best as you cleanse and build better health. Some find it helpful to take pulse rates before eating a particular food, then take the pulse rate again 20 minutes afterwards. An increase of up to 10 beats can be normal. A rate increase of 16 beats or more indicates that food has imposed some digestive stress upon the body.

Avoid Harmful Substances

Harmful substances are sometimes called food, when they are not. Some manufacturers are honest enough to label some of their products as "nonfood." We thank them. Popular forms of adverse materials taken into the body are refined foods, carbonated drinks, chocolate, alcohol, tranquilizers, and tobacco. It is easy to see that childbearing women are risking much when they partake regularly of these elements.

Dyes in foods are typically coal-tar products, perhaps carcinogenic. I became indignant when I discovered that maple sugar tree growers were putting formaldehyde tablets in the cuts of their trees to hasten the flow of maple sap. Great care must be taken to refuse harmful substances that hurt not only the mother but the baby as well. Generally, avoid the use of:

> **Refined foods,** especially sugars and white flour products. Americans consume over ten million tons of sugar each year. Refined sugar has empty calories and no nourishment.

"One piece of apple pie puts 50% of your white blood cells to sleep," says Dr. Paul Smith, M.D., "so they aren't active to fight disease." Sugar clogs the system. It causes a stasis in the blood supply to the tooth, so the tooth cannot be fed properly.[3] A person becomes addicted to sweets just as surely as he becomes addicted to other harmful agents. Natural sweets are sweets enough. Fruits, fresh or dried, are an excellent source. Dates, figs, raisins, honey, dried apricots, bananas, and other sweet fruits are fine if eaten sparingly.

Excessive dairy products. Buttermilk and plain yogurt are best; others are more mucus-forming. (Over the years midwives have repeatedly found that when the gravida drinks more than small amounts of milk during either gestational periods or lactating periods, the baby has heavy mucus accumulations that make breathing more difficult. Some babies have to be suctioned at birth numerous times; blessings and constant care are given to prevent choking for weeks because of milk-drinking on the mother's part.)

Carbonated drinks, which contain salts, sugars, caffeine, and other additives. Carbonation itself lowers the nitrogen level of the body so that it cannot easily digest protein, according to one nutritionist.

Chocolate, in any form. Theobromine in chocolate operates similarly to caffeine in coffee and cola drinks. The pickup obscures a detrimental effect upon the nervous system. This addictive substance "shorts out" the normal transmission of electrical impulses in the nerves which naturally jump from one synapse to another. Malfunctions then occur in the system. Chocolate prevents calcium absorption from our foods, therefore negates the calcium in foods, such as milk, used with chocolate. Carob, a healthier product than chocolate, is a taste-alike and contains 40% natural sugars, as much vitamin B_1 (thiamine) as asparagus or strawberries, as much niacin as lima beans, lentils, or peas, and more vitamin A than eggplant, asparagus, or beets. It is also high in B_2, calcium, magnesium, and iron. (Carob, a long, brown bean from the honey locust tree, is said to be what John the Baptist lived on while he was in the wilderness preparing for his mission.)

Stimulants or depressants, such as coffee, alcohol, tannic acid teas, tranquilizers, aspirin, etc. Both alcohol and tranquilizers are depressants of inner function. Depression starts at the top in the highest center of the brain and goes down. The conscience is affected during the time an individual is depressed from drugs. The alertness of the mind is affected; the motor areas of the brain and the autonomic nerve responses are disturbed.

All drugs and medications, if at all possible (see Chapter 5, Drug Use in Pregnancy and Childbirth).

Tobacco affects the potency of the husband, the size and condition of the placenta and infant, and imposes adversities upon the whole family. Nicotine in tobacco paralyzes the cilia that line the bronchial tree. Cilia were meant to cleanse the air that goes into the lungs; smoke changes cells into atypical cells and then into cancer. (Atypical cells become normal in a year if smoking is stopped; however, the rate for cancer cure is small, since there is a direct diminishing of the blood vessels all the while smoking occurs.)

Marijuana. Since a wide number of people in the world have been convinced that marijuana is neither a drug nor harmful, I would like to persuade them that marijuana is definitely harmful; not just by an emotional plea from someone who has suspected all along that it was not to be trusted as a totally pleasurable euphoric, but because now there has been time for science to make objective tests. The results of current tests are frightening and the story has just begun.

Smokers of marijuana on a regular basis have cooperated in tests—some apparently to prove that marijuana is harmless, even beneficial, and some who have been "burned out" on it and are facing the hard facts they know are attributable to smoking the plant. They testify to the severe lack of memory recall they once had. Certain periods of time and activity are totally gone from their memories. This observation and current findings now fall into perspective and become part of the many startling discoveries being made. Under a microscope, portions of brain and nerve cells look as if they have been tarred, and are literally unrecoverable (truly "burned out") in those people who have smoked five joints of marijuana daily over a period of a few years.

The thoughts of having marijuana parties during parturition, or of smoking marijuana during pregnancy, alarms anyone who realizes that a small body and small brain will be getting massive doses compared to those the mother gets. It is perfectly safe to fill the lungs with good, fresh air. It can usually be trusted to be safe and wholesome. We know fresh air can help build bright, healthy children with minds to recall, evaluate, and make decisions through processes of associational memory. Fresh air will also help mothers to have a sense of well-being.

If one is troubled with nervous tension, there are several excellent remedies—besides walking in fresh air and sleeping with windows open at night (although city dwellers sometimes have a real air pollution problem). There are good herbal formulas for NOURISHING and calming the nerves).

Water

Water is essential to our lives. It cannot be omitted from one's daily intake for long without causing damage to his system. Clean water is vital. Unfortunately, much of our drinking water has become polluted in one way or another, and an efficient water purification system is useful. Most health authorities recommend drinking six to ten glasses of water each day.

Water also carries into our system trace minerals which support life and mental well-being. Without water our circulatory systems could neither provide oxygen to our cells, nor provide nutrition, nor return wastes to our eliminative systems. Water helps us to have the bowel evacuations we should have (30 to 45 minutes following each meal) to keep poisons from building up in our bodies. Without water in our bodies we would not have tears, perspiration, or urine, and we could not salivate in anticipation of food.

We must have adequate clean water daily. In pregnancy the demand for water is as great as at any other time. Drinking water does not cause one to "hold water" in the system. That is caused by other upsets, including the intake of too much salt.

Ingesting the nutritional herbal teas helps to fulfill the need for a plentiful supply of water. Drink the teas at least forty minutes before eating solids, and do not drink liquids immediately after eating--instead, wait at least an hour. Allow digestive juices to have a chance to do their job without being diluted. Most foods have enough liquid content to aid mastication of foods.

HERBS AND SUPPLEMENTS

If you are not acquainted with herbs, you need a good herbalist to take you, and others who are interested, into the field to teach you to identify herbs. Collect them, dry them, and learn to use them by attending classes or by reading books on the subject.

These same sources (knowledgeable people, classes, books) will teach you how to make teas (usually 1 teaspoon of herb to 1 cup of boiling water; steep and strain and cool), tinctures, salves, tonics, etc. (NOTE: Never make teas in aluminum pans.)

A number of herbal preparations are described throughout this volume as they pertain to pregnancy and childbirth. The herbs I have recommended are typically available in North America. If you live elsewhere, use those herbs from your area which are particularly adapted for the same use.

During pregnancy the mother's body requires extra doses of certain vitamins and minerals. For example, vitamin E is essential to growth and to the assimilation of vitamins A, C, and K; it also carries oxygen to all parts of the body. Herbs useful to the expectant mother because they contain these essential elements (and many others we will not mention here) are these:

>**Red raspberry, comfrey,** and **alfalfa,** combined, provide a balanced combination of vitamins and minerals needed during pregnancy. They build uterine tone, help control nausea and hemmorrhage, and help provide good maintenance of pregnancy. RED RASPBERRY leaves contain vitamins A, B, and E, and also calcium, phosphorus, iron, and an acid neutralizer. ALFALFA contains vitamins A and B_{12} (found in all sprouted seeds), D, and E; also calcium and phosphorus. COMFREY contains assimilable calcium, vitamin K, and potassium, and has its own pain-relieving and penicillinlike properties. These herbs can be taken as follows:

>>LAVAY'S PREGNANCY TEA
>>
>>Combine two parts red raspberry leaf, one part alfalfa, and one part comfrey (the root is stronger than the leaf). Mix herbs well and add 4 rounded teaspoonfuls to one quart of water and steep as a tea.
>>
>>One quart of this mixture daily adds substantially to the mother's health throughout pregnancy, and helps to prevent bleeding and discomfort during parturition.
>
>**Dandelion** contains vitamins A, B, and E, as well as calcium, iron, and potassium; great for the liver. Use fresh in salads.

Cayenne contains vitamins A and C, and has numerous other vital properties; gives a lift during those days of tiredness. Add it to bayberry bark tea and bleeding from the uterus stops immediately.

Mistletoe contains calcium, magnesium, potassium, and sodium; a natural nervine, tonic, antispasmodic, and narcotic; has been used with very good results in parturition to contract the uterus and control bleeding.

Lobelia is a marvelous catalyst, enhancing the effect of other herbs; is excellent for discomfort when taken in small doses with a stimulant herb.

Peppermint, spearmint, catnip, etc., enhance the effectiveness of other herbs, add to the taste of teas, and aid digestion.

Fennel, mullein, nettle, parsley, and **peppermint** are all high in potassium; fennel seeds are also high in sodium.

Shepherd's-purse is high in sulphur and helps to purify the blood.

Preventive Supplementation

When the following substances have been faithfully ingested during pregnancy, many problems do not find their place in the home birth: repeated spontaneous abortive trends; hyaline membrane disease; malformations (if drugs or the strong genetic influences are absent); poor teeth and poor eyesight; and "blue babies" (the cyanotic newborns that have come through a long or very hard labor or that have experienced cord stress). These and other morbidities have an extremely low appearance in home births.

Additional daily intake of the following, either by food or supplements, is suggested for most gravidas:

1. LAVAY'S PREGNANCY TEA, 3 to 4 cups daily. Red raspberry leaves, comfrey, and alfalfa provide good procreative support, along with extra calcium and vitamins with vitamin K-like properties (for bleeding).

2. 1,500 units of VITAMIN C for vascular elasticity, infection, assimilation of folic acid, and as a diuretic. According to Richard A. Passwater, Ph.D., "Calcium ascorbate is a natural form of Vitamin C . . . . [It] is not acid, therefore, more people can take larger amounts without 'acid upset' or diarrhea. . . . calcium ascorbate replenishes the calcium that is excreted in the urine due to the chelating properties of Vitamin C."[4]

3. 350 mcg FOLIC ACID. Use extra folic acid (up to 1000 mcg) for mothers who are past age 40.

4. 400 to 600 units of VITAMIN E WITH LECITHIN (the oil form is preferable), for good pregnancy maintenance; provides the lecithin ratio needed to help prevent hyaline membrane disease, and assists the oxygenation of the blood.

5. 60 mg VITAMIN B COMPLEX, provides sufficient strength and energy; especially good for the nerves.

6. CALCIUM , as needed, for leg or muscle cramps, building strong bones, teeth, and muscles, restful nights, and calming the nerves.

7. 15 mg IRON per day, if needed. Persistent fatigue usually is an indication for more iron. (An excellent preparation by KAL, iron orotate, replaces iron without the offensive side effects of ferrous sulphate that few people can tolerate.)

Ample amounts according to the individual needs may be taken daily. I might say here that I recommend supplements only in certain circumstances. The ideal thing is to learn to use vital food sources. It does take time—not only to learn, but usually to make transition in our current habits. In order to help us make that transition not at the expense of the unborn fetus, I recommend supplements to assist in providing more adequately for the baby.

Hesitation is made to recommend more specific amounts of each supplemental item, inasmuch as individual requirements vary. This may be a problem with many who are trying to be helpful and recommend "average doses" for everyone. We are not all alike and since our needs are so different it is recommended that each person work to discover his own. List symptoms and their apparent degrees of effect upon your systems. Learn by reading and experimenting—as your physician does when he says, "Let's try this, and if it doesn't work, we'll try something else"—to discover how much will be adequate for you. A word of caution: Be sure your resource material is not based on trends of fad or fiction. Reliable sources are available.

Hormone Helpers

During pregnancy, labor, and childbirth, a woman's body secretes hormones to aid it in caring for, nourshing, and finally parting from the new person within her. A description of some of these hormones and how they work follows:

1. **Progesterone** maintains the pregnancy, calming early or false contractions of the smooth muscles. Sarsaparilla, ginseng, spikenard, and wild yam are herbs that either produce or aid the body in producing this hormone; they are not foreign materials which slow or stop any body process.

2. **Estrogen** is essential for conception, but too much may prevent the fertilized egg from implanting in the uterus. (This is the hormone from which the Pill is made.) Estrogen levels normally rise at the time for delivery. Since pennyroyal and black cohosh increase estrogen levels, their use at this time may encourage excessive bleeding. Blessed thistle and wild yam are preferable sources of estrogen.

3. **Adrenalin** and **cortin** help bring up low blood pressure and prevent or help correct hypoglycemia and sugar/insulin imbalances. Herbs that aid in the production of this hormone include valerian, hops, wild yam, Brigham tea, and licorice.

4. **Oxytocin** helps to produce strong contractions during labor, stimulates milk production, and encourages uterine contractions after the baby is born (to prevent hemorrhage). It aids in the let-down reflex of breast-feeding as well. Herbs that aid the production of oxytocin are blue cohosh, blessed thistle, and mistletoe.

Polly-Jean Five-Week Antenatal Formula

We have found the Polly-Jean Formula--an herbal combination that gravidas begin taking five weeks prior to anticipated date of delivery--to be a boon to the home birth movement. It assists in the following ways:

Much easier labor and delivery.

Longer and easier labors for women who tend to have precipitous births.

Shorter and easier labors for women who tend to have long labors.

Bigger dilation before discomfort arises.

Minimization of postpartum bleeding when taken in conjunction with the Good Program.

Shorter periods before lochia stops.

Other formulas on the market have helped many mothers, but over the years midwives have found that these formulas did not assist enough in preventing hemorrhage in women with borderline anemia, the Rh-negative factor, and other conditions. We found that when pennyroyal was included in the formula, bleeding continued to be heavier than it should be. We also found that black cohosh seemed to increase the normally stepped up production of estrogen, adding to the hemorrhage problem. Jeanne Johnson and I elimated both these herbs when we developed our formula.

Midwives who recommend this formula for use have frequently reported only 1 teaspoon to 2 tablespoons of bleeding with the placenta separation in normal deliveries. Even in problem deliveries, only 1/2 to 3/4 cup blood loss (considered normal) was reported. If these assessments are correct, the results of the Formula are phenomenal.

POLLY-JEAN FIVE-WEEK ANTENATAL FORMULA

If measurements of cups are used, 1/2 part would call for 1/2 cup, and 1 part would call for 1 cup of the following powdered herbs. Mix thoroughly and encapsulate. Six to nine capsules a day are recommended. It is recommended that dosages begin the FIRST week (five weeks before due date) with two capsules in the morning and two nightly, before meals. Increase the SECOND week (four weeks antenatally) to two capsules, three times a day. Increase the THIRD and FOURTH weeks up to about three or four capsules, three times a day, according to individual tolerance levels. Maintain this dosage until delivery. The formula can also be used a week to ten days postpartum advantageously.

    1/2 part motherwort
    1/2 part wild ginger
    1/2 part lobelia
      1 part squawvine
      1 part blue cohosh
      1 part blessed thistle
      1 part red raspberry leaves
      1 part false unicorn
    1/2 part wild yam
    1/2 part bayberry root bark

WHY DO WE CHOOSE THIS PARTICULAR COMBINATION?

Here is the breakdown:

  Motherwort: Nervine, hepatic (for liver problems); good for suppressed urine; excellent pregnancy herb.

Wild ginger (Canada snakeroot): Enhances other herbs in their action upon the system; good for diarrhea which sometimes precedes labor; prevents griping; especially good for action in lower parts of the body.

Lobelia: Antispasmodic, nervine; excellent in enemas with catnip; improves oxygenation of blood; has great influence upon regulatory systems and restores interaction between the functions of the organs.

Squawvine: Diuretic; helps to make childbirth wonderfully easy--especially when used with red raspberry leaves; good for uterine troubles, female complaints; excellent for sore nipples when combined with olive oil; astringent and tonic.

Blue cohosh: Regulates menstrual flow; brings on effective labor contractions; for chronic uterine trouble, leukorrhea (a discharge, sometimes profuse, of whitish or yellowish mucus from the vagina), inflammation of the vagina; good for high blood pressure; has potassium, magnesium, calcium, iron, silicon, phosphorus; helps alkalinize the blood and urine.

Holy or blessed thistle: Great power in purifying and circulating of the blood; strengthens the heart; soothing to headaches; good for memory; lifts spirits; excellent in puberty; aids in the production of quality mother's milk.

Red raspberry leaves: Antacid; decreases menstrual flow; soothes—doesn't excite; mild laxative; assists in parturition; removes cankers; allays nausea as an anti-emetic;

astringent;[5] used as a tonic and alterative to restore health and vigor.

False unicorn: Female herbal director: balances the direction of female changes, puts functions of reproductive organs in right perspective. If fetus is malformed, or an uncorrectable problem exists, false unicorn will encourage spontaneous abortion; if all is well and some other cause has threatened miscarriage, false unicorn will change directions to retain fetus in utero to successful conclusion of pregnancy. (Begin use with first symptoms.) Assists in the discharge of retained placenta and membrane fragments.

Wild yam: Good to combine with squawvine; in frequent, small doses allays nausea; relaxing and soothing to nerves; one of best herbs for pain in childbirth; good for discomfort in late pregnancy; combine with ginger to prevent miscarriage.

Bayberry root bark: Astringent properties suppress bleeding; aids in the separation of the placenta; increases flow of urine; excellent for dispelling fermentation in stomach and bowels; for relief of cramps when uterus is contracting; stimulates the uterus to function properly.

As one can see, many of these virtues are to be used postpartum.

EXERCISE

Exercise is good for the pregnant woman, but she must be cautious. Activities or exercise that jar or jolt or cause her to overexert herself or to become exhausted should not be engaged in. (See Figure 18.)

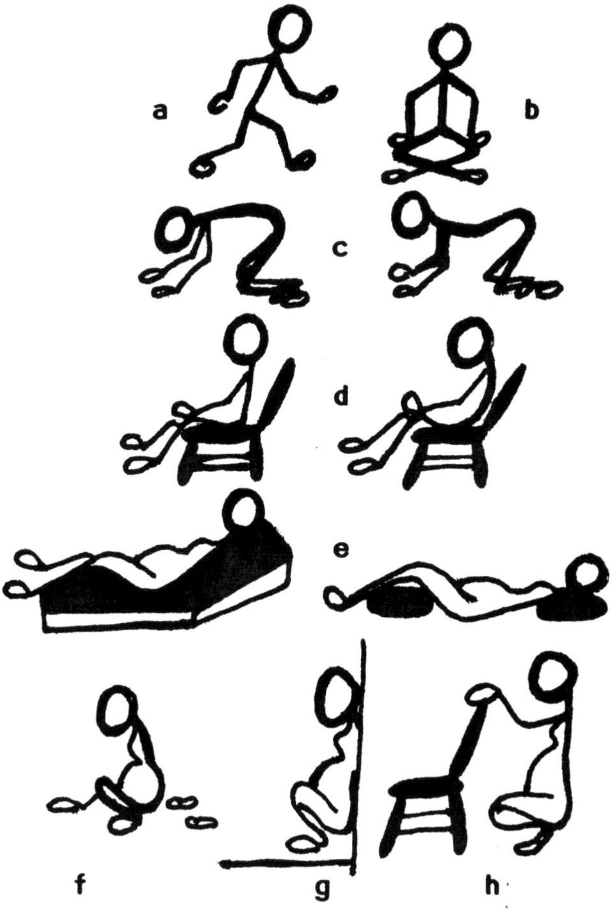

Figure 18. PRENATAL EXERCISES. Begin slowly and increase slowly. Adjust to needs in very late pregnancy. (a) walk, (b) sit cross-legged on the floor often, (c) pelvic rock, (d) arching exercise: sit straight on chair away from the back, arch and straighten, (e) abdominal breathing: support head, shoulders, and knees while practicing abdominal breathing, (f) duck walk, (g) squat with back support, (h) knee bends for sacral adjustments.

Walking

Walking is by far the best exercise for pregnant women because it is not apt to do the harm some exercise might and because it accomplishes a variety of good things for the expectant mother. It:

> Stimulates good circulation throughout her system.
>
> Slims and trims the body.
>
> Increases fresh air intake.
>
> Aids in good elimination.
>
> Provides a change of scenery.
>
> Gives a sense of well-being.
>
> Diverts away from routine and demands.
>
> Promotes sound sleep.
>
> Strengthens leg muscles for carrying the extra load.

Walking a mile or two a day during the hours of the day when it is not too hot and when the air is not filled with hurried, noisy sounds is ideal if it can be managed. Cold weather, if not severe, is no problem if the gravida dresses warmly. As she becomes heavy with child, exercise will naturally decrease somewhat. Care must be taken not to fall. Wear comfortable walking shoes. After the walk, skin-brush, shower (hot, then cold water), and nap (out-of-doors, if possible).

Pelvic Floor Exercise

This exercise is also known to the pregnant woman as "doing her **kegels.**" It is very effective in building perineal muscle tone. It can be practiced while waiting for a red light to turn green, while sitting in the bathroom, while in the tub, or while watching TV.

To learn the principle of this exercise, try squeezing off urination during midstream. Then release the urine for three seconds and squeeze it off again. If you are able to do this successfully, you have good muscle tone. If you are not able to terminate urination at will, you have some work to do.

Practice 100 kegels a day as follows: Squeeze those perineal muscles; hold tight for 10 seconds. Relax completely for 5 seconds, squeeze again. You may not be able to hold the squeeze for more than 2 to 3 seconds at first, but work on it until you can hold the squeeze for a full 10 seconds, 100 times a day.

This exercise also promotes good bladder control and tones the vaginal floor muscles. It pays every female to keep tone in this area, because as age comes upon us all, postchildbearing years can leave us with something to be desired in bladder control. If this simple exercise is engaged in regularly throughout life, bladder control will remain stong.

Abdominal Breathing Exercise

Abdominal breathing strengthens abdominal muscles, and also teaches a person how to cooperate with contractions in first stage. The greatest rewards come when total relaxation is accomplished with this breathing exercise.

Find a quiet place and do the following:

1. Lie on your back, with knees, head, and shoulders supported.

2. Completely relax.

3. Inhale. Let the air "fill the abdomen" instead of the chest. Pretend your lungs are in your abdomen. Extend abdomen as high as comfortably possible.

4. Hold to a slow count of 5.

5. Exhale completely to a slow count of 3.

6. Repeat until you are breathing FROM THE ABDOMEN AS NATURALLY AS YOU BREATHE FROM THE LUNGS AND CHEST WHILE WALKING.

7. Twenty minutes of this exercise, two or three times a day, will pay real dividends when you are in labor.

Stomach and Back Exercises

1. Sit in a straight chair with hips and shoulders against the back of the chair.

2. Place your feet on the floor directly below your knees.

3. Keep head erect.

4. Press hip, hollow of back, and shoulders hard against back of the chair.

5. Hold this position to the count of 5, relax; repeat 6 times.

Another exercise to strengthen back and stomach muscles is to sit out from the back of the chair, arch the back, then straighten; repeat several times.

Pelvic Rocks

Pelvic rocks also strengthen back muscles; they should be done regularly from the beginning of pregnancy. They are done as follows:

Get down on all fours. SLOWLY roll the buttocks down (by slightly arching the spine) and back up again (by relaxing the abdomen); repeat over and over again, in a rocking motion. Injury to the back may come with fast rocks. It is important to get as much of the rocking as possible coming with the hips, NOT THE BACK OR SPINE.

Begin with perhaps 10, then increase to 20 rocks a day (see Figure 19).

Sitting and Squatting

SIT ON THE FLOOR often—to read, to fold socks, to darn, to read to the children. Getting up and down will keep you limber and more agile. Sit with legs crossed, Indian style. If a pillow is used, make it rather thin and soft. SQUATTING OR DUCK-WALKING daily will tone muscles in preparation for squatting after full dilation in labor. Do this as you weed the flowers, pick the garden produce, etc. TO RELAX THE BACK and regain circulation, stand and "stretch for a star" with one hand and then with the other. TO STRENGTHEN THE SACRAL AREA, especially when it seems to be "out," hold to the doorknobs of an open door, place feet about six inches apart (a few inches from the door), toes pointed slightly out, back straight. Let yourself down almost to a squatting position,

164 POLLY'S BIRTH BOOK

then rise to a standing position again while supporting yourself by holding to the doorknobs. This can also be done using a chair for support.

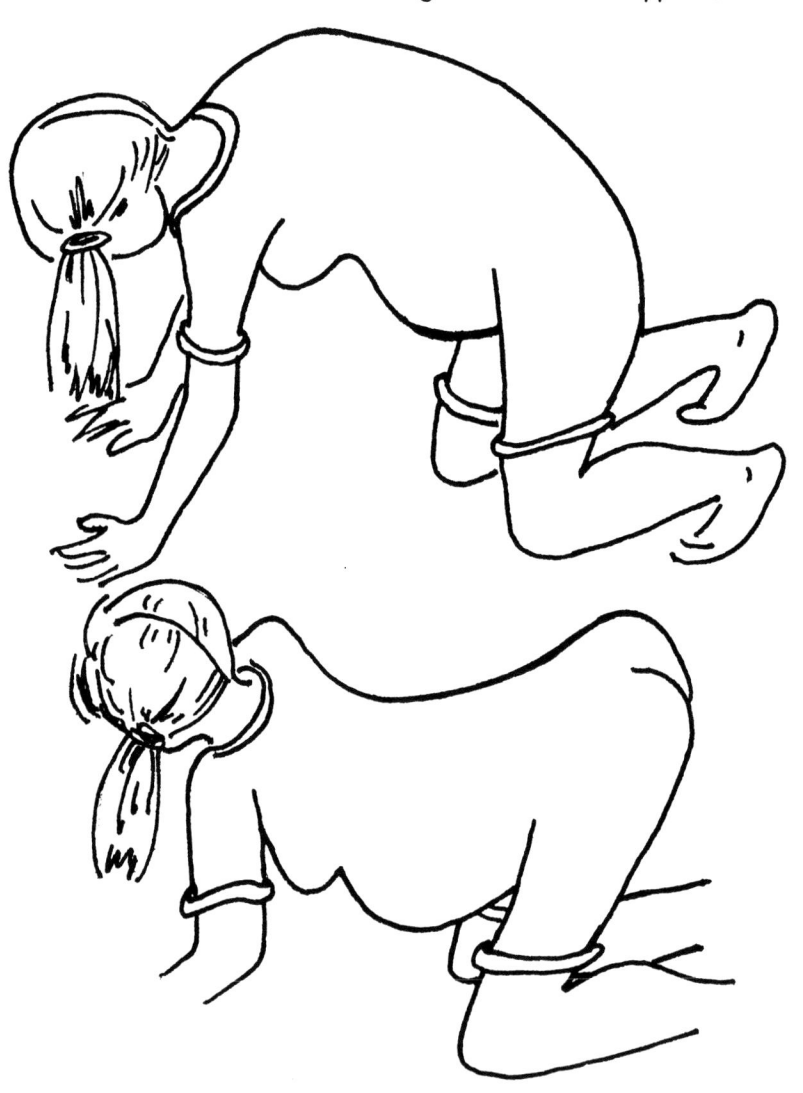

Figure 19. PELVIC ROCKS. Tuck the buttocks under, then swing them back up. Work more at tucking the hips than working the back.

THE SITZ BATH

A sitz bath is taken in a sitz tub that allows only the lower portion of the torso to be immersed in water. "Sitz" is German for "sit," and that's what you do in a sitz bath (see Figure 20).

The sitz is used in Europe to great advantage in pregnancy and childbirth. It is also used for ailments such as hemorrhoids, bad backs, nervousness, and the list goes on. Tubs with high backrests are used to give great comfort. They are usually made of tin, with the skill of an artisan.

A sitz tub will hold about three gallons of water. The user's legs go over the sides, leaving only the buttocks in the warm water. A folded towel put in the bottom of the tub reduces "sit-itis," and if the user's legs are short, a stool is provided or another towel is placed over the edge of the tub to go under the knees. Another container of hot water is close by so the user can dip into it and keep the tub water snugly warm.

Until the Poly-Sitz (my own design) is on the market, a large (#2 or #3 size) galvanized tub can be obtained from a farmer's supply house.

Sitz baths are wonderful for pregnant women. In order for the fetal head to traverse the snug birth canal with minimum discomfort to the mother and baby, the lower uterine segment and the vaginal floor must relax and soften. The business of the day tenses and tones body muscles, but there must also be a time of complete relaxation for this tone-building to be complete.

Sitting with only the buttocks in warm water for one half hour daily during the entire pregnancy puts focus on the birthing area only, not on the

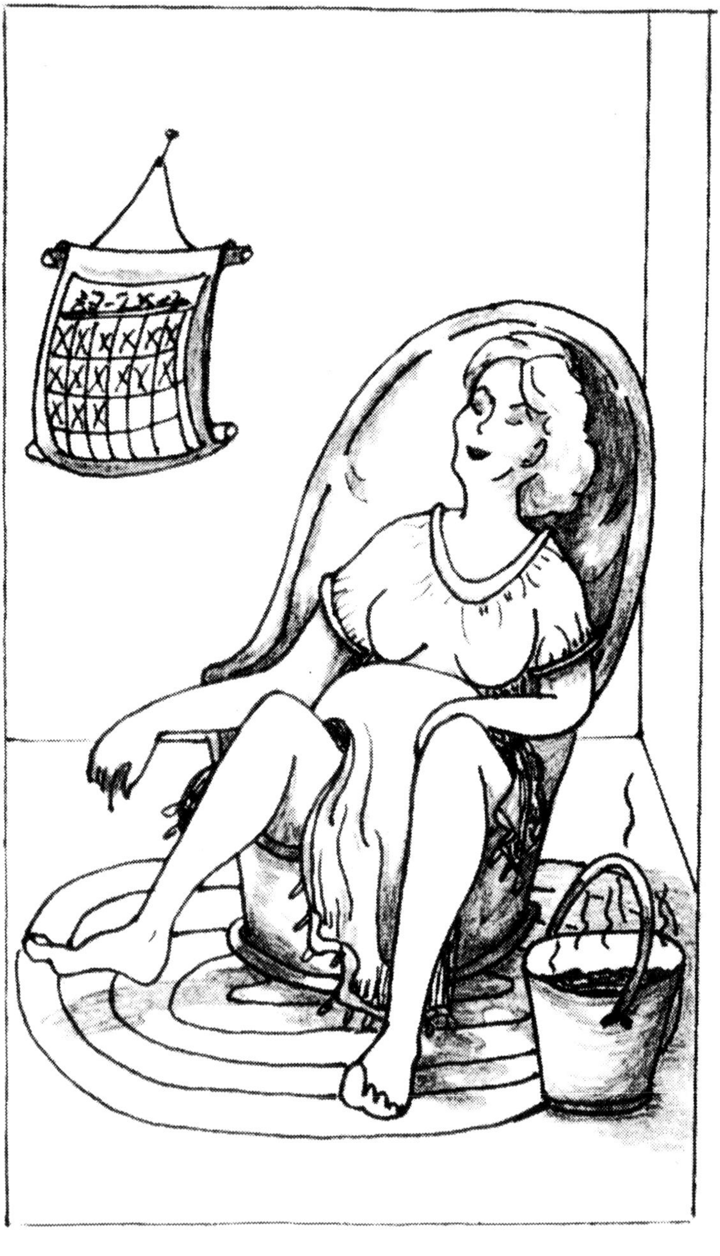

166   POLLY'S BIRTH BOOK

Figure 20.   THE SITZ BATH.

whole body as with a tub bath. The sitz provides the birthing area with at least a half an hour of total relaxation. The warmth of the water and the sitting position also open the bony structure of the pelvic canal, as does the weight of the baby and amniotic fluid. The sitz bath is great preparatory therapy for childbirth. Mother soon becomes addicted to the sitz because it feels so good and because it relaxes her so much.

The last six weeks of gestation, sitz baths are called for twice a day for at least half an hour.

Sitz baths are also comforting and healing after the birth of the baby, especially when there has been suturing or when a tenderness lingers in the birth area. Suturing material is water soluble, but should not dissolve, even with soaking, before about the seventh day. The cleanliness the sitz provides is essential to prevent infection. The relaxation imparted contributes to the joy of the birthing experience and to the prompt issuance of the mammaries. So, enjoy!

NOTES

[1] John A. and Leah Widtsoe, The Word of Wisdom: A Modern Interpretation, rev. ed. (Salt Lake City, Utah: Deseret Book Co., 1950), pp. 134-36. The "Word of Wisdom" refers to Section 89 of the Doctrine and Covenants of the Church of Jesus Christ of Latter-day Saints.

[2] Paul Smith, M.D., and Charles Smith, M.D., lectures.

[3] Ibid.

[4] Richard A. Passwater, Ph.D., "The Advantages of Calcium Ascorbate," short essay [Orangeburg, New York: American Health Products Co., Inc., n.d.].

[5] Where the tonic (restoring) property accompanies the astringent (constricting) quality of herbs, I have found no adverse effects in vasoconstriction (restriction of blood vessels) that are usually found with synthetic astringents.

CHAPTER 10

CHANGES DURING PREGNANCY

PHYSICAL CHANGES

Breast Changes

From the beginning of pregnancy, the breasts become firmer, more tender, and a little enlarged. Breast pigmentation darkens and accumulates, and features white spots. **Colostrum** begins to collect in the mammary glands and is secreted, often during the entire pregnancy. (This substance is especially nourishing to the newborn and sustains the baby beautifully until mother's milk comes in. Colostrum also cleanses meconium from the baby's bowels.) Do not pick the dried specks of secretion from the nipples. This will leave them raw and tender. Vigorous rubbing with a towel following a bath will remove whatever needs to come off.

Stretch Marks

Pink streaks that later turn silver are caused by the extension of the skin over the growing uterus and by skin that grows quickly and is stretched in places such as the buttocks, the upper thighs, and the breasts. Few women get by without them, though I delivered several babies for a lovely mother of fifteen children who gained normally during each pregnancy but NEVER developed stretch marks.

As stretching occurs, the skin tends to itch. Sometimes sitz baths can relax nervous tension and give some relief. Olive oil or marsh mallow tincture (preserved with pure vegetable glycerine) applied to itchy areas may bring great relief. Vitamin E and aloe vera are helpful. BF & C Ointment has good reports. Creams and lotions may also bring relief; however, read labels for harmful ingredients. Elastin creams have been developed to minimize discomfort from stretch marks. Don't be afraid to try your own concoctions. If you find something that works, pass the word along.

Weight Gain

The greater concern should be the quality of food eaten rather than weight gained during pregnancy. Expected and acceptable weight gain is from about ten to thirty pounds.

The average infant weighs 7 to 7 1/2 pounds at birth. Add to that other products of conception: the placenta, 1 pound; amniotic fluid, 1 1/2 to 2 pounds; breast enlargement, 3 pounds; additional blood, 3 to 4 pounds; body fat and increased body fluid, 4 pounds. This gives an estimate of legitimate weight change in pregnancy. (For complications expected when excessive or sudden gains in weight occur, see Chapter 8, Diagnosis of Pre-eclampsia.) A gravida may gain only nine pounds and also have a wholesome outcome.

Excessive weight gain poses problems for the gravida and fetus during pregnancy and labor. Uterine inertia is more likely if a woman is overweight, because of poor muscle tone and the overdistention of the uterus created by a large infant. Overweight women usually have bigger babies. Delivery is also much more difficult. A gravida can lose weight without harm to herself or her baby is she does it with care and good nutrition. With careful observation, the vegetarian diet (with heavier proteins consumed prior to 2:00 p.m.) and a daily exercise program should bring good results.

PHYSICAL COMPLAINTS

Drowsiness

For the first three to six weeks of pregnancy, many women feel very sleepy. They sleep and sleep and sleep. A woman's body is shifting gears when she is first pregnant; her hormones are changing and her body is preparing to carry and deliver a child. Go ahead and sleep. It will be good for you, if it is not overdone. This extreme sleepiness, however, should not last the entire pregnancy, though many tire more easily during pregnancy.

If a woman feels tired and dragged out all the time, she may have one or more of the following problems:

1. She needs more iron or more vitamin B complex.

2. She is having her babies too close together.

3. She needs more iodine or more minerals in general.

4. She needs more rest.

During pregnancy, especially when the mother gets heavier, a short nap every afternoon may be necessary, particularly for mothers who already have small children. You should nap when your children nap instead of telling yourself that you have to get the wash done or dinner made or the rug vacuumed while you have a chance.

Nausea

It is believed that nausea comes in pregnancy for different reasons in different people. Improvement seems to come with increased intake of vitamin B_6 supplements and foods. In fact, injections of vitamin B_6 (1 to 2 cc daily, OR AS NEEDED) are often given prior to the time nausea gets out of hand and begins to dehydrate the mother. It appears that if a woman has made a point of eating and maintaining sufficient B vitamins in her system prior to pregnancy, her likelihood of nausea is lessened, if not eliminated. Again, others say that the "shifting of gears" of hormonal activity also tends to upset the digestive system. (See also Chapter 11, Persistent Vomiting.)

Constipation

Prior to birth or in the postpartum period, flaxseed tea with LB Tonic will gently move the bowels and heal and nourish colonic tissue. You can gather and prepare your own tonic with the following herbs: 1 part each of barberry bark, goldenseal, cayenne, ginger, lobelia (seed), red raspberry leaves, turkey rhubarb root, and 2 parts of cascara sagrada. Powder the mixed herbs and fill "00" capsules, then take as needed. Recommended dosage: two capsules in the morning and two again at night. Flaxseed can be sprinkled on cereal and used in a number of culinary preparations to great advantage.

Also, an enema of 1/2 teaspoon capsicum and 1 teaspoon garlic powder in water will bring good evacuation. Cool water enemas will not cause the nausea that warm water does. Elimination must be kept under control. Roughage, raw foods, walks, and exercise help prevent constipation. Constipation becomes more of a problem in late pregnancy when pressure against the bowels increases. Nervousness is also directly related to constipation in all ages. Here again, walks, B vitamins, sitz baths, quiet times, and rest help immeasurably with constipation due to tension.

Diarrhea

If the bowels are too loose, accompanied by rawness and tenderness at the anus, irrigate with water containing two tablespoons of powdered slippery elm. Prior to meals, drink 1/3 cup warm water with 1/2 teaspoon powdered slippery elm stirred quickly with a fork long enough to mix the herb. Drink immediately before this bland, pleasant-tasting tea jells. It coats and soothes both stomach and gastrointestinal tract as it heals. Garlic with parsley perles should be taken with goldenseal to take care of the cause of the diarrhea. Four to six perles and six capsules of goldenseal a day will usually solve the problem.

Frequent Urination

During the first trimester frequency of urination is increased, due to the placement of the uterus. Midterm micturition (urination) is normal, then the increased frequency returns during late pregnancy. The ureters also increase in size and tend not to empty completely. This increases the chance of urinary tract infection (see Chapter 11, Conditions Mistaken for Threatened Miscarriage).

Fainting

Fainting is rare but does occur. If a mother has no cardiac impairment, fainting can be caused by:

A rapid fall in blood pressure.

Pressure of the uterus on the blood vessels returning blood to the heart (pelvic veins and inferior vena cava), retarding circulation.

Sitting or standing up too quickly.

Standing for long periods of time, especially in hot weather.

Hot baths (warm baths are sufficient; a really hot bath will raise the baby's temperature).

Fatigue.

Stuffy rooms.

Crowded places.

Tight clothing.

Eating too much.

Eating meals that cause flatulence (gas in the intestines).

Fainting probably is not serious unless it results in injury from the fall.

Back Ache

Back ache is usually caused by:

> Vertebrae that are out of alignment, however slightly.
>
> Poor posture adopted in attempt to balance weight changes during pregancy.
>
> Poor muscle tone.

Pelvic rocks (see Chapter 9, Pelvic Rocks, Figure 19) strengthen back muscles. A rest each day, sensible shoes, good posture, and a comfortable bed that is firm will do much to prevent back aches. Some people with "bad" backs do not respond well to waterbeds. Others do. (See also Chapter 9, Stomach and Back Exercises; Chapter 15, Back Adjustments.)

Leg Cramps

It is possible for leg cramps to disrupt needed rest during pregnancy and to distort the peaceful progression of labor, if not enough calcium has been ingested throughout pregnancy. Taking LaVay's Pregnancy Tea and eating properly will prove to be valuable habits. Lying too long on the back (especially during labor) prolongs pressure on circulation to the extremities and may cause distress even though calcium intake has been sufficient. Frequent rests with the feet up are helpful. Lobelia tincture applied to the legs and massage will help. Recently it was reported that deer tallow gives immediate relief. If you have this on hand, rub the tallow into the muscles.

Heartburn

Heartburn usually begins during the third trimester as the fundus rises with fetal growth. The baby crowds the stomach, pushing food or gastric juices up into the esophagus, causing heartburn. When the fetus drops (lightening), there is usually some relief, but little can be done to give total relief until the baby makes its entrance into the world.

Acid neutralizers such as Rolaids or Tums give relief to some women. DO NOT TAKE ACTIVATED CHARCOAL, because it absorbs the NECESSARY acid as well as the EXCESS acid. (Some people will respond to sips of peppermint or red raspberry leaf tea.) If you find a healthy answer to this problem, pass it on.

Excessive Hunger

Most women get hungry more often when they're pregnant or lactating. At times an expectant mother may feel ravenous; other times she may not want a lot of food at all.

If a woman is very, very, hungry frequently, she probably isn't eating the right foods. If she's eating a well-balanced diet, she won't feel hungry all the time. A "hungry mom" may need to increase her intake of minerals and to be aware of her blood sugar level. Hypoglycemics NEED to eat small meals often.

Anemia, Other Deficiencies

A pregnant woman is likely to have three kinds of deficiencies, especially if her diet is poor. These are deficiencies in iron, protein, and folic acid.

Iron deficiency (anemia). Lack of iron in the blood is the most common kind of deficiency. The maternal and fetal bodies demand an increased amount of iron--up to 1,200 milligrams during the months of gestation. The fetus stores iron in its liver the last 10 weeks; it needs iron for the formation of blood cells in the bone marrow and to secure against anemia early in life.

The mother's need for additional iron becomes more acute two to four weeks before confinement. If the mother does not have enough iron and she hemorrhages, loss of additional blood at delivery could be fatal. She also has an increased need for iron during lactation. She should take at least 15 milligrams of iron per day (with vitamin C, to increase absorption). Several natural formulas available bring excellent results, and are much more compatible with one's system. (Avoid ferrous sulphate--it has dangerous side effects.)

Vitamin B_6, magnesium, folic acid, and vitamin E deficiencies can also cause anemia, but extra iron intake will not correct these forms of anemia; the culprit deficiency must be remedied. Nutritional deficiencies are not the only causes of anemia. Chronic blood loss also causes anemia. Symptomatic peptic ulcers, hemorrhoids that occasionally bleed, and heavy menstrual flow can all cause serious blood loss. Corrections should be made and the iron supply built before pregnancy begins since it is more difficult for some people to build and maintain adequate iron during gestation.

A symptom of anemia is paleness. Because anemic people do not have the rich network of capillaries near the surface of the skin, they look pallid. Make-up can hide this pallor in women. Inspection of the mucous membranes of the mouth and gums and of the lower eyelids may reveal pallor.

WHAT TO DO:

FOODS THAT REPLENISH IRON are: okra, asparagus, beets, lettuce (not iceberg), egg yolk, artichokes, kale, spinach, mustard greens, tomatoes, dates, prunes, blackberries, rice, strawberries, cabbage, whole wheat, carrots, grapes and grape juice, molasses.

HERBS THAT REPLENISH IRON are: stinging nettles, mullein leaves, strawberry leaves, Irish moss, sweet acorns, poppy seed, both yellow docks, huckleberry, dandelion, burdock, meadowsweet, comfrey, fenugreek, barberry bark, agrimony, century, raspberry leaves, quassia chips, wheat grass, kochia, parsley.

A caution is in order here. Prolonged ingestion of too much iron, especially from unnatural sources, results in iron deposits in the skin or in organs such as the heart, pancreas, liver, and kidneys. The deposits can cause impairment of function. Extreme overdoses can be fatal.

Protein deficiency. If protein is deficient, there will be abnormal development of the fetus. Protein is essential, but don't overdo this. High intake of protein is recommended by some doctors. Other doctors say the consequence of storing undigested protein is too great. Between 25 and 40 grams per day is very adequate to maintain pregnancy and to develop the teeth, bones, and muscles of the baby.

WHAT TO DO:

Protein can be found in nearly every food we eat. Some sources are richer, of course:

nuts, beans, cottage cheese, yogurt, fish, etc.

Folic acid deficiency. The fetus needs folic acid with B_{12} for good blood development and to lower the chances of abnormal development or mental retardation. Also, with a deficiency of folic acid, urinary infection is twice as common and premature labor is two to three times as common.

WHAT TO DO:

FOR FOLIC ACID DEFICIENCY: raw vegetables, yeast, and supplements of folic acid.

Vitamin C deficiencies. In order for the fetus to utilize iron and folic acid, it needs vitamin C. Vitamin C also aids in stress, so the demands of pregnancy may call for the mother to take a minimum of 1,500 units of calcium ascorbate a day. (She should maintain this dosage during lactation.)

WHAT TO DO:

FOR VITAMIN C DEFICIENCY: tomatoes, green peppers, citrus fruits (especially if you live where they grow), acerola cherries, rose hips, pineapple, pomegranates, plums, grapes, apricots, carrots, rhubarb, turnips, potatoes, cabbage, onions, peas, spinach (raw).

Hemorrhoids, Other Varicosities

Hemorrhoids are varicosities that develop in the rectum. I believe they are caused by numerous contributing factors, but primarily by a "bad" liver (liver dysfunction). They become especially likely if good elimination is not maintained. With the weight and pressure of a growing fetus,

Changes During Pregnancy 179

hemorrhoids may arise for a short period, even if a woman is on a good program. Bearing down during second stage of labor often causes hemorrhoids to protrude from the anus.

Enlarged veins in the legs and/or vulva are also varicosities. Occasionally, a large blood vessel in the groin will gather blood and become hemorrhoidal and very uncomfortable. The pressure in the area during gestation adds to the distress. Any such development, no matter where it occurs, is cause for concern. Though potentially dangerous because such vessels can rupture, they can be treated and corrected to a great degree without sugery, or until surgery can be safely undertaken.

Rupture of any varicosity will produce profuse hemorrhage, but rupture rarely happens. (A midwife should have hemostats on hand to clamp off any rupture during childbirth until it can be sutured. Hemostats have appropriate teeth for this job.)

WHAT TO DO:

> To prevent homorrhoids, as much as possible, the mother should eliminate most breads, noodles, etc., from her diet and stick to raw foods as much as she can. Good nutrition and exercise keep the lymph system, the circulatory system, and the liver functioning well. This is important so that kidneys, bowels, lungs, and skin can rid the system of wastes, and the rest of the system can then receive nutrients it needs. During pregnancy, blood vessels are laboring under overloads, but by receiving the calcium and other minerals that keep them elastic and firm, they can better handle the pressure of restricted circulation that pregnancy may bring on.

If hemorrhoids do develop, the mother should get cayenne into her diet regularly. Even 1/4 teaspoon, in water or juice, two or three times a day will help. Cayenne races through the blood stream and moves the old and collected blood in the swollen tissues. Too much fiber in the diet can cause diarrhea and in turn can cause hemorrhoids. Natural wheat cereals are a good "regulator" if fiber alone has proven to be too strong.

The solution to varicosities is to strengthen the blood vessels, shrink them, tighten them up, and allow other vessels to carry the circulation so that no one vessel takes on more than its share of blood.

Great relief and some toning can be accomplished with sitz baths, and peripacs where the varicosity is located; a change in diet, a liver cleanse, and a mild, ongoing bowel cleanse are helpful. Frequent rests with feet up and knees supported are musts.

White oak bark tincture can do wonders for varicosities of the vulva when applied to a sanitary napkin and used daily or overnight. Saturate the pad and keep it warm on the area affected, one-half hour twice daily, or overnight. (See Appendix D, For Varicosities of the Vulva, for instructions on how to prepare this tincture.) White oak bark, an astringent, may be used as freely as you would sage tincture made the same way.

Another help is 400 IU's of vitamin E in lecithin capsules taken orally with two LB's (liver and bowel herbal formula) at night to keep the bowels soft and gently moving. It is important to take capsicum (cayenne) with blood disorders. Capsicum moves rapidly through the blood stream and will coagulate at a wound, but it will also dissolve clots in the blood very nicely. One capsule twice a day is sufficient for varicosities. More than three capsules a day may cleanse some people too stringently over a long period of time. Other people will need that much and more.

Again, 75 percent of your plate should be raw fruits and vegetables, while you avoid white flour products and white processed sugar. Blood-building foods, herbs, and supplements are a must.

Thumb Therapy for Varicosed Legs. Never rub varicosed legs. There is an excellent therapy that can be safely used following a week's intake of cayenne in the diet. The person affected with the pressures and soreness should lie face down, shoes and stockings off. The therapist begins by placing a thumb only at the center back of the leg, just above the ankle. Very little pressure is applied as one thumb after the other crawls up to the hip. One thumb is placed on the leg, the other thumb is placed right above it, TOUCHING the first. The first thumb leapfrogs the second, then this is repeated in rather rapid succession up the leg. Always start at the ankle with each thumb TOUCHING the other as it travels. As you approach the back of the leg behind the kneecap, skip over the kneecap area (about three inches of the leg) and proceed. Extend the thumb work to the top of the thigh. This can be done three times on each leg, twice a day, for tremendous relief. There is no rubbing done, no significant pressure.

Vaginal Discharge

Good vaginal hygiene practices should be carried out at least on a weekly basis. A quart of warm water with 2 T. vinegar will clean and maintain the slightly acid environment needed in the vagina to ward off infections. This douche, with CLEAN equipment, is refreshing and helps to prevent unclean odors from that area. DURING PREGNANCY, DO NOT USE A BULB SYRINGE OR LIFT THE ENEMA WATER BAG HIGHER THAN YOUR SHOULDERS (to prevent high fluid pressure and air embolism). In addition, do not insert the nozzle farther than three inches into the vagina.

Itching of the vulva or vagina may be caused by a yeast infection or by lack of good hygiene. Daily baths are important. Soap and water, then a good rinse with clear water, will alleviate itching produced by perspiration and leukorrhea. Pat dry and apply petroleum jelly to areas that have become tender or raw.

Acidity does discourage infection, but may cause itching. A very acid discharge can be dispelled with a douche of red raspberry leaf tea or with 2 to 3 T. bicarbonate of soda in one quart of warm water.

Yeast Infection

A white, flaky, vaginal discharge, accompanied by itching and much discomfort, indicates a yeast infection. Yeast infection thrives in dark, warm, moist environments and most women will have this condition in the vaginal cavity at one time or another during their lives, particularly during pregnancy, when the amount of vaginal discharge usually increases. Treatment must be persistent because the infection recurs easily. Efforts to keep the vagina slightly acid will help prevent this condition.

WHAT TO DO:

Take 1,000 mg of niacinamide for a week or until the infection subsides. Also, acidophilus ("super" strengths are available now) is reported to bring good results.

Vinegar douches daily: 2 T. to one quart warm water (DO NOT use a bulb syringe).

Use a douche of black walnut hull and myrrh teas. A small tampon saturated in the black walnut oil or tincture and left in overnight is beneficial (see Appendix D, Black Walnut Tincture). (If tampons are the SLIGHTEST bit uncomfortable, do not use them.)

Garlic powder douches are also effective (see Appendix D, Garlic Powder Douche).

Ginger (1 tsp.) and goldenseal, lobelia, parsley, marsh mallow root, or red raspberry, made into strong teas (each with 1/4 cup glycerine added to each cup of strained tea), will also help if used to saturate a tampon or as a douche.

PSYCHE

A most important psychological phenomenon takes place as an expectant mother ponders over the miraculous changes that are taking place inside her. The wonder evokes anticipation, and anticipation awakens all kinds of expectations, questions, plans for the newcomer, and motivation to do everything possible to have a healthy, happy baby.

Numerous studies continue to support the idea that a person's mind can have amazing degrees of control over the functions of the body. Obviously, the cheerful person repairs and heals a great deal faster than a depressed person. However, psychic influence reaches even further than this. Fear is known to constrict breathing passageways of the body, and complete relaxation can release tensions that obstruct bowel evacuations or obstruct the progress of labor in childbirth. Researchers claim that the emotional make-up of an individual often predicts the kind of birthing experience a woman may have; that is, whether she is high or low risk.

It is important to be optimistic, to learn a great deal about the power, strength, and intelligence of one's body. While being good to your body and by treating it well, EXPECT that it will perform correctly. After all, is not that why one works so hard to cooperate with the mechanisms of pregnancy and birth?

The Chinese, I believe, call the state of pregnancy "Happiness in me." And it is quite true that "A merry heart doeth good like a medicine."

CHAPTER 11

DISORDERS IN PREGNANCY

DANGER SIGNALS

When a woman is pregnant, her body changes dramatically. Many of these changes are normal and to be expected, but certain changes can signal danger. Your client should be instructed to call you if any of these signs appear:

1. Vaginal bleeding, no matter how slight.

2. Swelling of face or fingers.

3. Severe, continuous headache.

4. Dimness or blurring of vision.

5. Pain in the abdomen.

6. Persistent vomiting.

7. Sudden escape of fluid from the vagina.

8. Chills and fever.

The most serious consequences of these signs are discussed in this chapter.

VAGINAL BLEEDING, ABDOMINAL PAIN

Any amount of vaginal bleeding at any time during pregnancy could be dangerous. Bleeding may or may not be accompanied by abdominal pain. In early gestation (first and second trimesters), problem bleeding might include spotting-to-hemorrhage proportions from several causes: abruptio placenta, a malformed fetus aborting, placenta previa, ectopic pregnancy, intercourse--all of which can initiate spontaneous abortion. In late (third trimester) prenatal periods, bleeding can come from abruptio placenta and placenta previa, particularly. Also, antenatally, a light-to-heavy spotting can come from a rigid cervix that is beginning to dilate prior to, or in connection with, early labor.

Abruptio Placenta

As the name suggests, with **abruptio placenta** an abrupt separation of the placenta from the uterine wall occurs before the baby is born. This can take place anytime during pregnancy, even in parturition. Essentially, there is usually intense pain associated with the abruptio placenta. This particular separation begins near the CENTER of the placenta as opposed to the edge, as it sometimes does in parturition. EXCRUCIAT- INGLY SHARP PAIN is the first signal. It is caused by pressure from the hemorrhage as it forces further separation. Maternal heart rate rises rapidly and the gravida goes into shock. Rarely is she able to get to the hospital in time to save herself, much less the baby.

The main difference between life and death in this type abruptio placenta and the one that occurs during labor is that help is on hand in childbirth and can begin rendering first aid. The second difference is that many times the abrupt or premature separation during labor begins along the edge and can be somewhat confined or discouraged by the contractions against the fetus, causing compression which somewhat disallows a continuation; therefore, the time and the circumstances add to the potential safety of the baby and mother. Also, the mother rarely feels pain associated with the edge or marginal abruptio separation because of some discomfort with the normal contractions going on in her labor. In the first instance, if time allows, C-section is the only answer, with indications in some cases for a complete hysterectomy to save the mother. Occasionally C-section is called for in the parturition situation, and at that time usually both infant and mother are saved. Sometimes the infant is compromised (life preserved, but the baby is damaged in some way).

WHAT TO DO:

>Give the mother 1 teaspoon cayenne in 1/2 cup COLD water and TRANSPORT AS QUICKLY AS POSSIBLE. Notify hospital to be prepared for abruptio placenta. This is life-threatening.

Placenta Previa

Marginal Placenta Previa. **Placenta previa** has reference to where the placenta has embedded in the uterus at the beginning of pregnancy. With **marginal placenta previa,** the conceptus implants in the lower half of the uterus (**low-lying placenta**), and as the placenta grows, it develops NEAR OR INTO THE MARGIN (border area) of the internal os. When the baby's head dilates the cervix, there may or may not be bleeding; however, there is the tendency for the placenta to present with or ahead of the fetal head. If the placenta

188 POLLY'S BIRTH BOOK

is presenting first, the oxygen supply to the baby will be cut off, so the midwife prevents this from happening. This type of placenta previa can usually be handled adequately at home.

WHAT TO DO:

>If there is a small amount of bleeding and birth is imminent, give shepherd's-purse tea and simply watch the perineum to detect if the placenta is trying to present with the head. It will differ in appearance from other tissue in that there is a dark bluish red color beneath a shiny membrane. You may not detect this dystocia until the head starts to bulge open the vagina and vulva, at which time you continue to push the placenta back behind the head (with one finger) until the head precedes the placenta.

>**Placenta Previa Proper.** This occurs when the placenta grows ACROSS OR OVER the internal os of the cervix, in any degree. BETWEEN THE SEVENTH AND NINTH MONTHS, the weight of the baby and the stretching of the uterine wall in antenatal days will cause the placenta to break or detach in several places, bringing various amounts of bleeding. Spotting at this time should be reported to a physician, who will usually hospitalize the mother—perhaps even for several weeks. NO ONE SHOULD PALPATE INTERNALLY, EITHER VAGINALLY OR RECTALLY. A mere touch can disrupt the site and cause profuse (even fatal) bleeding. The baby must eventually be delivered cesarean, but it is important for the mother to carry the baby as close to term as possible, to give the fetus additional days of maturity. When it is no longer safe to retain the baby, C-section is performed.

WHAT TO DO:

IN THE EVENT OF SPOTTING, NO ONE SHOULD PALPATE INTERNALLY, PARTICULARLY DURING THE THIRD TRIMESTER OF PREGNANCY. Bleeding at this time (as opposed to the slight bleeding which sometimes occurs at the onset of labor) is indicative of placenta previa proper and can be life-threatening to both mother and fetus. NOTIFY A PHYSICIAN. Cold HVC (honey, vinegar, and cayenne, in water) should be taken for bleeding. Vitamin E (600 to 800 IU), vitamin C (calcium ascorbate, 2,000 mg), and shepherd's-purse tea (three cups) should be taken DAILY to help sustain mother and baby and to prolong the time before delivery. (Prematurity is a major cause of infant death in this situation.) DELIVERY MUST BE IN A HOSPITAL, BY CESAREAN SECTION.

The parturient is ALWAYS transported when undue bleeding occurs early in labor. Labor in the hospital can be monitored to determine whether the fetus is being compromised with any amount of bleeding. The advantage is that at any moment the bleeding reaches unacceptable proportions, and the fetal heart rate indicates too much stress, an immediate cesarean section can save both mother and baby. Otherwise, if labor progresses without undue stress, vaginal delivery is possible and is preferred.

Ectopic Pregnancy

A conceptus that implants anywhere outside the uterus is called an **ectopic pregnancy**. This abnormality usually results in the loss of the embryo by the second month, though there are exceptions.

In a tubal pregnancy (the common ectopic pregnancy), signs of a normal pregnancy will have occurred; however, ABDOMINAL TENDERNESS sets in between the third and fifth weeks. Discovering this condition early may make it possible to salvage the uterine (fallopian) tube and ovary. A vaginal exam to the side of the cervix will reveal a displaced uterus and a lump or bulge where implantation has occurred.

Excruciating tenderness is experienced at the cervix during intercourse, internal palpation, or when defecation (bowel movement) is attempted. Fever up to 101° F is usually present. There may be spotting, heavy bleeding, or no bleeding. Abdominal pain usually spreads to the shoulders.

Another way to determine this condition is to look into the sclera. If there is a tubal pregnancy, the small blood vessels that originate at the outer edge of the sclera (at about four-thirty or five o'clock) and travel in toward the iris will demonstrate midway a strangulation effect. The constriction in the vessel will resemble a knotted ball of string with the end pointing up.

As the conceptus grows, the tubal lining gradually ruptures. (There may be in the sclera short, red, blood vessels shooting out from the strangulation, much like a child's drawing of the rays going out from the sun.) A sharply rising pulse rate will indicate either internal or excessive bleeding. IMMEDIATE HOSPITALIZATION IS IMPERATIVE: the mother's life is in danger.

WHAT TO DO:

    Treat for shock and bleeding with HVC, transport. If rupture has taken place, removal of the ovary is probably necessary.

Unexplained Spontaneous Abortion

Hemorrhage that occurs without any pain or warning--usually during an early period of pregnancy--is considered "accidental" and most often is caused by low implantation of the placenta. It may occur when the gravida is sleeping and she awakens to find herself lying in a pool of blood. Sometimes it ceases only to recur again at another time when she least expects it. Then again, the initial bleeding may be so profuse as to prove fatal to her or the embryo. Or, she may have a rather continuous, small discharge of bleeding. This is usually caused by placenta previa and is the cause of many early miscarriages. First aid herbal preparations for bleeding are certainly in order. Because of the bleeding and the compromise made to the infant in many cases, nature will cause the abortion.

In rare instances bleeding ceases, never to return. In this case the placenta, embedded at a more normal site, (though partially separated) somehow retains, undisturbed further, and pregnancy is carried out to term.

It is believed that bleeding and premature labors are many times brought on by overstressed and overworked mothers, accidents, or lack of hesperidin complex, vitamin C, and progesterone (especially indicated if bleeding recurs and if the mother has aborted repeatedly[1]). The latter may often be the answer to many unexplained spontaneous abortions which have been caused by premature separation of the placenta. Lack of hesperidin complex accounts for the tiny blood vessels at the placenta site breaking under stress of greater capacity loads demanded in growth. At other times nature will naturally expel a nonviable fetus.

Being at a disadvantage to know for sure which of these causes may be at the root of bleeding or cramps, immediate action is called for in an effort to prevent the miscarriage if possible.

Threatened Spontaneous Abortion

If miscarriage precipitously occurs during the FIRST trimester, it probably can be handled adequately at home. The major concern with this spontaneous abortion is hemorrhage. If during the SECOND or THIRD TRIMESTERS miscarriage threatens, and is not prevented, hospitalization is advisable due to the fact that trauma equipment may save a viable baby's life. If life-saving is not possible, legal entanglements may stem from supposed neglect on the part of attendants and parents.

The following suggestions will usually prevent miscarriage if applied at the ONSET of symptoms and if a fetal malformation or defect is not promoting the loss. Such a loss is usually merciful.

WHAT TO DO:

With contractions (cramping) alone:

1. Immediate and complete bed rest (use bedpan) until at least two days past any cramping. The mother may then ease into normal activity; she should not lift anything heavier than a broom.

2. One cup strong catnip, shepherd's-purse, and false unicorn tea; then 1/2 cup every 20 minutes until cramps have completely ceased. (Catnip tea for a week afterward; continue Pregnancy Tea.)

3. Lobelia tincture on bottoms of feet, under arms, over abdomen (for contractions).

With bleeding:

1. Immediate and complete bed rest (use bedpan).

2. Elevate the end of the bed or the mother's hips. The mother should put her feet on a heating pad or heated brick. Place an ice pack[2] on her abdomen until the bleeding stops. It is important to keep her warm.

3. One cup strong catnip and shepherd's-purse tea; then 1/2 cup every 20 minutes until 8 to 12 hours after bleeding stops.

4. Vitamin E (200 IU) hourly for eight hours.

5. One cup false unicorn tea (room temperature) with 1/4 teaspoon cayenne, 3 to 4 times a day.

6. Lobelia tincture on bottoms of feet, under arms, over abdomen (for contractions).

7. Continue daily intake of Pregnancy Tea.

8. Inspect clots that pass to determine whether the conceptus may have aborted. If loss of blood exceeds two cups or continues longer than an hour, transport. (Midwives can usually control hemorrhage in less than 10 minutes in normal childbirth. Sometimes spontaneous abortion can be more complicated.)

9. When things are under control, the mother should remain in bed and continue taking

her teas for at least a week past the last show of blood. Goldenseal (three times a day) will help guard against infection. The mother may then ease into light activity, but should lift nothing heavier than a spatula for three weeks.

Conditions Mistaken for Threatened Miscarriage

Abdominal distress, unrelated to pregnancy, is often confused with threatened abortion. If cramps do not shortly assume some regularity and increased frequency, as in normal labor, the discomfort may be due to: (1) an inflamed appendix, (2) infection in the urinary tract or bowels, or (3) some type of bowel obstruction.

Appendicitis. Appendicitis pain is fairly localized, about two inches to the right of the navel. An inflamed appendix may have to be removed, even during pregnancy, so it is important to determine whether this is the cause of the discomfort. A woman who suspects she has appendicitis should not aggravate this condition with an enema. A slow, deep push on the site of the appendix that is ABRUPTLY RELEASED will cause intense pain and help confirm appendicitis. This can be accompanied by a white blood count.

Infection. Infection in the bladder or urinary tract is often obscure until it becomes advanced. It then produces pain which spreads throughout the abdomen, and is associated with fever as the infection spreads.

Herbs with their own penicillinlike properties, such as comfrey, goldenseal (in capsules), and garlic powder (in enemas), are excellent infection fighters for most people. Astringent herbs, such as juniper berry, yellow dock, and sanicle can be taken (in teas) for the kidneys.

Check with your physician if you are unable to bring an infection under control, particularly when you are pregnant.

Bowel obstruction. For bowel obstruction, use gentle massage therapy along the ascending, transverse, and descending colon. Take cool water enemas with garlic (to kill bacteria) and cayenne (to stimulate peristaltic nerves to evacuate feces) and LB Formula to soften and move stools. Be sure to replace friendly bacteria with 1/3 cup acidophilus following meals for a few days.

EDEMA

It is normal for a pregnant woman occasionally to have some edema of the legs and feet because of the extra weight on these extremities and the resulting pressure on circulation. Nature compensates by collecting water to protect these areas. However, swelling can be a sign of toxemia if it appears in the face and hands or above the abdomen (see Chapter 8, Diagnosis of Pre-eclampsia).

Drinking water does not cause water retention; however, lessening sodium in the diet helps solve part of the problem. Herbal diuretics are safer and are said to strip less potassium from the system than do synthetic products. Kidney herbs and the right foods are the real answer in most instances.

SEVERE, CONTINUOUS HEADACHE

The severe, continuous headache occurring anytime during pregnancy can be caused by one or more of several things: tension, constipation, spinal misalignment, swelling of the pituitary gland (swelling is common in pregnancy), or visual problems that may be corrected by seeing an eye doctor. Any discomfort is disparaging, and causes can usually be discovered by the process of elimination. This malady may also be caused by advanced stages of high blood pressure which most certainly can bring about the consequent loss of mother and child if not treated immediately. If each possible cause has been treated and the headaches persist, it may be due simply to pituitary swelling. The worse thing about this is probably the discomfort, and headaches many times can be relieved by putting the feet in hot water for 20 minutes.

VISUAL DISTURBANCES

Visual disturbances may be brought about from the swelling of the pituitary gland or from ocular problems; however, the more serious problem occurs if blood pressure associated with hypertension or toxemia is causing the retina of the eye to separate. Again, any danger signal is nature's way of saying that all possibilities of problems need to be checked and dealt with properly. Hypertension cannot be neglected without serious consequences resulting.

PERSISTENT VOMITING

Persistent vomiting is usually caused by vitamin B deficiencies, particularly vitamin B_6. It may last four to eight to twelve weeks or even, in rare cases, for the entire pregnancy. The key to dealing with this problem, as always, is to work on it before it gets out of hand.

Some of the consequences of persistent vomiting can be dehydration, loss of weight--or even

starvation of both the mother and the baby--
toxemia, and coma. Toxemia may occur because
toxins in the body are not eliminated through the
kidneys. The kidneys need fluids in order to
function properly, so if a pregnant mother cannot
keep down liquids, toxins accumulate. Sometimes
slight jaundice sets in. The amount of urine
excreted may lessen and show signs of albumin (a
protein), casts, and even fresh blood. All these
consequences indicate retention of toxins and
serious problems.

Vomitus that looks like coffee grounds means the
stomach has bled from the wretching. This is
serious.

WHAT TO DO:

> Treatment of vomiting should begin as soon as
> possible. If the problem is already serious
> or is beginning to be, and vitamin B_6 in a 10
> cc vial is obtainable, the mother should have
> intramuscular injections of 1 cc (or more) per
> day as needed for two to three days, then
> usually every third day after that or whenever
> the nausea returns. It is almost impossible
> to overdose on the B vitamins. They are water
> soluble and easily assimilated or discarded.
> Persons whose diets have not met minimum B
> vitamin requirements suffer from numerous
> maladies, such as tiredness, nervousness, and
> anemia, just to mention a few. A thick, dry
> tongue is one advanced symptom of vitamin B
> deficiency. If the gravida has symptoms of an
> extreme nature, 2 cc B complex daily, indefi-
> nitely, would not harm her. However, it seems
> reasonable that when her condition improves
> remarkably, the dosages can be reduced dras-
> tically or eliminated altogether if a balanced
> diet is taken for maintenance. (At this

printing, both the 10 cc and 30 cc vials of B_6 cost about $5.) Usually the doctor will write a prescription for a 30 cc vial. (SYNTHETIC B vitamins or single doses that are too large CAN cause a "flush" or rash.)

Also:

1. Lobelia tincture rubbed on the feet, under the arms, and on the abdomen lessens the tension and spasmodic triggering of vomiting.

2. An enema, with squawvine tea or clear water, will help replace liquids.

3. Separate ice trays from squawvine, red raspberry leaf, catnip, and alfalfa (a good digestive aid) teas can be frozen, then made into slushes and eaten slowly.

4. The mother should eat several small meals a day; toast between the small meals.

5. Greasy foods, meats, or food disagreeable to her taste should be discouraged.

6. She should increase her intake of B complex, vitamin C, and zinc, if she can keep it down.

7. Olive oil can be rubbed on her entire body two to three times a day for nourishment if starvation is evident and intravenous fluids are not available.

8. Foods and drinks should be either very hot or icy cold--lukewarm foods are nauseating.

If jaundice, delirium, steadily rising blood pressure to levels of 130 mm Hg or above, fever of 101° F or more, or if hemorrhaging of the retina occurs, the gravida may have to have a therapeutic abortion in order to save her life. (A retina hemorrhage is indicated by dark red spots or brushlike strokes in the retina. These signs mean her blood pressure is so high that it is destroying capillaries in the eyes and will soon destroy sight.)

To PREVENT the problem of persistent vomiting in future pregnancies, have the mother increase her intake of B complex (at least thiamine [B_1]), vitamin C, and zinc.

PREMATURE MEMBRANE RUPTURE

Occasionally in the third trimester the amnion will rupture, seemingly for no reason at all. A watery dribble or flush will appear. A dribble usually means the rupture has occurred high in the uterus; a flush indicates the rupture occurred near the external os. Sometimes this occurs during or following intercourse.

If the membrane ruptures prematurely with a slow dribble (as opposed to a rush of water) two to six weeks before due date, and the mother does not go into labor within 48 hours, most doctors induce contractions with Pitocin. This they do because they fear that if the baby is not born soon, infection (previously prevented by the protective bag of waters) will set in and endanger the life of both mother and baby.

In home birth, we try to assist nature in dealing with the problem. It may prevent the mother from going into premature labor and help to heal the rupture if you have her do the following:

200 POLLY'S BIRTH BOOK

WHAT TO DO:

1. Go to bed immediately and stay in bed. Use a bedpan. Turn, but don't toss in bed. Do not raise to elbows.

2. Drink catnip tea in a strong concoction every half-hour.

3. Alternate the catnip tea with red raspberry leaf, alfalfa, and comfrey tea, every other half-hour.

In 8 to 24 hours, the rupture will heal and the water will replace itself so that the mother's pregnancy can continue until term. However, the mother should remain in bed AT LEAST 24 hours after the time the healing takes place.

IF THE RUPTURE OCCURS WITH A RUSH OF WATER instead of just a dribble, the same treatment is used, unless the umbilical cord has prolapsed. A prolapsed cord demands immediate attention: the life of the fetus is endangered. Specific instructions are in Chapter 16, Prolapsed Cord.

CHILLS AND FEVER

Chills and fevers are usually associated with infections or contracted diseases. If you respond nicely to certain home remedies you have been successful with in the past, you may be able to handle some of these situations very well. Otherwise, consult your physician, especially during pregnancy—he deals with diseases.

WHAT TO DO:

At the FIRST SIGN of soreness, nausea, or whatever, attempt THEN to terminate its effect and its development so the baby will remain unaffected.

The very best of first aids is to make sure the eliminative systems are open and working well. Also, first aid begins with something that will kill bacteria, etc., and something that will get into the blood stream and lymph system right away. You may already have any number of home remedies that work for you; if not, here are a few. Find one that works for you and your family; add it to your home nursing file to be passed on to others:

1. Particularly effective in combatting illness is a garlic enema: 1 teaspoon powdered garlic to each quart of tepid water. Warm water enemas usually make you nauseous. One-half teaspoon to one tablespoon cayenne can be added to great advantage. It does not sting inside your body. The anus only may sting following evacuation for about 19 seconds. Time it yourself!

2. For my family, goldenseal with echinacea taken three to four times a day kills infection fast and settles the stomach—if you take it at the first signs of nausea.

3. Pick (if during the growing season) nine big leaves of fresh comfrey, cut and juice in blender. Add this to 1 1/2 pints of boiling water, 1/2 teaspoon myrrh powder, and 2 tablespoons Celestial Seasonings Sleepytime Herb Tea (or chamomile,

spearmint, lemongrass, passion flowers, blackberry leaves, orange blossoms, hawthorn berries, skullcap, rosebuds, and tilia flowers—or as many as you may have of them). Steep for 20 minutes, strain, and add 1/3 cup pure vegetable glycerine. Cool until it can be sipped with comfort while you curl up in bed with a good book.

4. REST is important. Give your energies back to your body to heal itself.

Fever

5. A low-grade fever is sometimes helpful to your system. A prolonged or high fever is less safe. One way to bring down a fever is to soak 1 tablespoon chia seed in pineapple or grape juice, then drink it. Or, rub lobelia tincture over the liver area and at the base of the skull. Cool water packs applied to the backs of legs, foot therapy, and cold sheet treatments may be resorted to for a persistent fever.[3]

Sore throat, cough

6. Swab a sore throat with pure apple cider vinegar. Alternate with drinks of hot catnip and comfrey tea mixed with the juice of half a lemon, 1/2 teaspoon butter, 1 tablespoon honey (to taste), and 1/4 teaspoon ginger. Something else that is very soothing to a sore throat is to wash and eat all the greenest celery leaves you can find. A couple of handfuls at the onset of a sore throat will usually solve the problem of an irritated, "nonstrep" throat. It takes a culture of

throat mucus to determine a "strep" throat. Strep throat needs immediate attention.

7. Drink hot teas of comfrey, purslane (rich in vitamin A), and amaranth. Plant amaranth in your potted plant boxes for the winter. Chew the buttons; swallow the juice only for great relief of the throat. Wild amaranth (redroot) will do wonders in a cough syrup. Hound's-tongue syrup is also excellent for coughs. Cough syrups are made for the family in various ways. My favorite one does not capitalize on sweetness, but on the soothing of vegetable glycerine.

Colds

8. A highly recommended remedy for colds is to soak barley and wheat for 24 hours using twice as much water as grain, then drink the water. Use a humidifier to increase the humidity in winter, get plenty of rest, take megadoses of vitamins C and A.

NOTES

[1] The mother should increase her intake of calcium ascorbate with minimum dosages of 350 mcg hesperidin complex and 600 IU vitamin E daily during and between pregnancies. Use in conjunction with the Good Program.

[2] An ice pack can easily be made to have on hand by saturating a hand towel with water and storing it in a sealed plastic bag in the freezer. One isolated, but ingenious, mother in this situation sent her daughter to a nearby cold stream for a few small, flat rocks.

[3] See also Robert S. Mendelsohn, M.D., How to Raise a Healthy Child . . . In Spite of Your Doctor (Chicago: Contemporary Books, Inc., 1984), Chapter 7, "Fever: Your Body's Defense Against Disease," pp. 66-79.

CHAPTER 12

CONDITIONS AFFECTING PREGNANCY

RH FACTOR AND HEMOLYTIC DISEASE

Science has expanded our insight into blood group factors, particularly the Rh system, changing what was once considered a fairly simple subject into quite a complex one. We still have some gaps in our understanding that we hope further research will fill in. Following is a very limited explanation. More detailed information can be obtained from another source.

A mother's immune system is a marvelous thing. However, on occasion the very thing which helps protect her against disease, infection, and foreign substances can pose a hazard to the child within her. Theoretically, if the baby has an **Rh** or another **blood group factor** present in its blood (inherited from its father) which is lacking in the mother, and a significant amount of these genetically incompatible red blood cells enter the mother's circulation, the mother may create antibodies to eliminate this "foreign" substance. If this happens, she has become **sensitized** to that particular factor.

In practice, in almost all cases (95+%) of Rh incompatibility, the mother lacks the dominant D Rhesus gene: she is termed R**h negative;** that is, her blood does not react to the antirhesus immune serum. Her baby (and the father) is **Rh-positive:** its blood contains this gene and reacts positively with the serum.

If enough Rh-positive fetal red blood cells enter the mother's circulation, the D Rhesus gene stimulates antibody formation in the mother. (An Rh-negative mother who is sensitized already has these antibodies in her blood as a result of a previous birth, miscarriage, blood transfusion, etc.) When these maternal antibodies in turn gain access to the fetal circulation, they accelerate the destruction of the fetus's own red blood cells and the baby may be born with a **hemolytic disease** (hyperbilirubinemia, erythroblastosis fetalis, etc.).

Today, Rh-negative mothers who deliver Rh-positive babies are given human anti-D gamma globulin (e.g., **RhoGAM**) to protect them from forming antibodies which might adversely affect future pregnancies. This is given intramuscularly (usually 1 cc) within 72 hours postpartum.

With the advent and availability of RhoGAM, the chance of a baby suffering from a hemolytic disease due to Rh incompatibility is greatly decreased. According to **Williams Obstetrics,** "Hemolytic disease of the newborn should now be a problem almost totally limited to Rh-negative women who were sensitized before anti-[D] globulin was available and to the 2 or 3 per cent of Rh-negative women who become sensitized without apparent cause."[1]

Rh-hemolytic disease usually occurs in the third or later pregnancy. The mother's antibody build-up can be tested so that the best course of action may be determined. In most cases the birth of an affected infant can be anticipated. An exchange transfusion at birth or even an intrauterine transfusion may be necessary for a severely affected baby.

Home births can be planned for Rh-negative women who have not been sensitized. In a home birth setting, a sample of the baby's blood is obtained (from the cord) so the baby's blood type and Rh status can be determined.

(1) After the birth, and before the cord stops pulsating, DRAW 3 TO 5 CC OF CORD BLOOD by inserting a hypodermic syringe needle into one of the cord vessels (all the blood in the cord belongs to the baby). (2) Immediately after the cord stops pulsating, CLAMP THE FETAL SIDE OF THE CORD so the baby will not lose blood. (3) CUT THE CORD.[2] If you do not have a hypodermic syringe, at this time simply strip the residual blood in the cord into a sterile container, such as a boiled baby food bottle. (4) CLAMP THE MATERNAL SIDE OF THE CORD, CAP THE CONTAINER IMMEDIATELY, AND DELIVER THE FETAL BLOOD SAMPLE TO THE NEAREST BLOOD BANK, HOSPITAL, OR LABORATORY. It should be labeled with the names and phone numbers of the mother and back-up doctor so RhoGAM can be obtained for the mother if the baby is Rh-positive.

RhoGAM is expensive--at this writing 1 cc is over $100. IT MUST BE GIVEN WITHIN 72 HOURS TO BE EFFECTIVE.

Even the baby born in good condition must be watched for signs of jaundice. The jaundice which is a sign of hemolytic disease usually occurs within the first 12 to 36 hours following birth, unlike the "normal" jaundice seen about the third or fourth day after birth. (In home births even this third or fourth day jaundice is unusual.)

An interesting phenomenon has been called to my attention. On three different occasions in my midwifery classes as we discussed the Rh factor someone told the class her Rh status had changed. These women had each begun their childbearing years Rh-negative. When they had continual problems with pregnancies, they began seriously to build their blood and their general health.

In each case physicians, not the mothers, discovered a change in the Rh status. The doctors were astounded and called for additional tests and reports. Family doctors who had been treating these women for years shook their heads and admitted that they could not understand why a mother who had been Rh-negative for years was now Rh-positive.

At first I smiled at these stories. Surely mistakes had been made. But I continued to become aware of others (six to date) to whom this had happened. In another class, a woman raised her hand and said, "That is not impossible. I am like those women. I used to have Rh-negative blood, but for the last six years my status has been positive."

These women all shared something in common. In each instance, these women had concentrated on purifying and building their blood by changing their diets so they had exceptional nutritional intake. They did the following kinds of things:

1. They ate fruit (or vegetables, if hypoglycemic) for one week, then followed with what is essentially the Good Program (see Chapter 9). They ate fresh, raw (as often as possible), home-grown foods and foods uncontaminated by additives or sprays. They also eliminated sugar, tea, coffee, alcohol, and

soft drinks, as well as white flour, prepared boxed foods, and other refined products from their diets.

2. They used the herbal lower bowel tonic (LB) and had occasional enemas to keep their bowels evacuated thoroughly during body cleanses.

3. They used herbs to cleanse and build the blood. Several of these mothers gave periwinkle special credit: they drank one cup of periwinkle tea per day. Other herbs also used were capsicum, angelica, blue cohosh, goldenseal, peppermint, borage, coriander, sorrel, mistletoe (between pregnancies), holy thistle, tansy, valerian, vervain, hawthorn berry, bloodroot, and wheat and other grasses. Sometimes they added supplements (see pages 82-84 in **A Superior Alternative**).

4. They ate foods that built blood: grape juice, molasses, beets, etc.

No one knew how long it took to bring about the change in Rh status, since she did not know such a thing could be done and did not keep a record. More research needs to be done in this matter; in the meantime, it certainly will never hurt anyone to clean and build up her blood.

DIABETES MELLITUS

Pregnancy is affected by diabetes in the following ways:

1. Chance of spontaneous abortion or premature delivery is slightly increased.

2. Toxemia during pregnancy is augmented (increased frequency and severity).

3. Fetal death in utero before onset of labor is much more common than in normal, nondiabetic gravidas.

4. Incidence of excessive-sized infants (ten pounds or more) is many times that of normal gravidas. The excess weight is not just from fat, but from endocrine imbalances. The result can be a number of mechanical dystocias during labor, and thus an increased rate of C-sections.

5. Hydramnios (excessive amniotic fluid—more than two liters) is common. Premature birth is more likely with hydramnios; a 50 percent fetal death rate follows. Prolapsed cord is much more frequent.

6. Congenital malformations are more frequent.

7. Lactation may be inhibited in some cases.

8. Neonatal period is associated with special hazards, such as hypoglycemia and anoxia.

Pregnancy also makes the treatment and control of diabetes difficult for the following reasons, among others:

1. Unpredictable changes in sugar tolerance alter levels of insulin required.

2. Vomiting confuses the dietary program and may provoke acidosis.

3. During labor, muscular exertion alone may so deplete the glycogen (sugar) reserve that the diabetic may need quick and sharp alterations in carbohydrates and insulin, resulting in unpredictable delivery outcomes.

4. A gain in sugar tolerance after birth and sudden hypoglycemia are common.

5. Lactation upsets blood sugar, hormonal, and other balances in the body. This and also infection (even mild) may bring on acidosis and coma quickly in the mother.

Because of increased pituitary activity and intense endocrine changes, the four periods of time when women are likely to have low carbohydrate tolerance are: puberty, menstruation, pregnancy, and menopause.

If the mother is not diabetic and she wants to avoid having these borderline periods develop into more serious or permanent problems, it is wise for her to adopt a good health program—one she can follow faithfully--in spite of hereditary factors.

If you are not sure whether the expectant mother has diabetic tendencies, ask her the following:

1. Is there a history of diabetes in your family?

2. Have you ever had any unexplained stillbirths or neonatal deaths?

3. Have you had one or more unexplained premature labors?

4. Have your babies weighed more than ten pounds? Has each baby weighed more than the last?

5. How old are you? (The incidence of diabetes increases sharply with age; 35- to 45-year-olds are more vulnerable to low sugar tolerance.)

6. Do you frequently have excessive thirst or a metallic taste in your mouth?

7. Do you gain more than 30 pounds during pregnancy? (Is she overweight?)

8. Have you ever had hydramnios? (Does she now?)

9. (Does she have signs of pre-eclampsia?)

If her answers suggest the possibility of diabetes, have her check with her doctor. Blood sugar levels, not just urinary sugar levels, are important in diagnosing this condition.

Gestational diabetes comes about in women who have no prepregnancy evidence of the disease. During pregnancy, abnormalities in glucose tolerance—and sometimes even clinical diabetes—appear. Most often these changes are reversible with a strict dietary program, and after delivery the evidence of diabetes rapidly disappears. Recurrence of sugar in the urine indicates that blood sugar tests should be made, unless there is a simple explanation for the excess sugar (such as a recent "sugar binge"). If certain blood sugar levels are present or persist, the gravida should be under the observation of her physician.

You, as a midwife, must NEVER ACCEPT THE RESPONSIBILITY FOR A KNOWN, PREGNANT DIABETIC IN A HOME BIRTH. Silent acidosis is the cause of many unexplained fetal deaths, and acidotic coma is responsible for almost all maternal deaths in this complication of pregnancy. Acidosis may accrue, but show few or no symptoms.

If the disease is well controlled, vaginal delivery (in the hospital) is better than a

C-section, because diabetics are poor patients for operations.

If you must deliver a diabetic mother, under extreme, unavoidable circumstances, expect hypoglycemia and anoxia in the newborn. If possible, you must feed the infant immediately. Twitching, convulsive movements or cyanosis in the newborn all indicate hypoglycemia.

RUBELLA

Rubella is rare, but it does occur. If it is contracted in the first trimester of pregnancy, there is a likelihood of damage to the fetus about one-sixth to one-fifth of the time. The risk of malformation from rubella after this period is relatively slight. If a NONPREGNANT woman is not immune to rubella, the decision is hers to make whether to ask for the innoculation. When vaccination is given, the woman MUST NOT become pregnant then, nor for three months after being vaccinated, because she may develop the disease and her fetus would be vulnerable.

VENEREAL DISEASE

America is in an epidemic state of venereal disease. A recent study indicated that syphilis and gonorrhea are on the decline since herpes has become epidemic and is so easily passed from one individual to another. Since venereal diseases are highly contagious, they pose serious hazards for the mother, baby, birth attendants, and all those caring for mother or baby. Venereal diseases are not always easily detected. Dormant or not, all venereal diseases can affect the fetus before, during, or following birth. Fetal mortality is high. While a midwife would not accept such a case knowingly, in an emergency she may be required to give aid to anyone. Always keep sterile, disposable gloves in your kit for such circumstances. Be wary of any unfamiliar sores, foul-smelling discharge, lesions, or rashes, and be aware also that there may be no outward signs of these diseases apparent. Take EVERY aseptic precaution and expect fetal complications. Care is essential to prevent blindness. Dilute silver nitrate or an equivalent should be put into the infant's eyes immediately following birth. Bathe the baby with warm mineral water or an herbal astringent prior to dressing it. As soon as possible, bathe yourself with disinfectant diluted in water. Use calendula tincture to wash up to your elbows until you can get a bath and clean clothes. (Use a germicidal solution to wash your clothes in afterward.)

It might be helpful to add here that seldom will a woman ask for home birth who realizes she has a disorder or condition that would term her high risk. When a midwife finds a potential candidate with unfamiliar symptoms, she will refer her to the back-up doctor. The medical community will respect and accept the midwife who not only performs a valuable service, but who knows her own limitations as well.

NOTES

[1] Louis M. Hellman and Jack A. Pritchard, **Williams Obstetrics**, 14th ed. (New York: Appleton-Century-Crofts, 1971), p. 1039.

[2] Opinions differ about how to handle the cord of the Rh-negative mother. Some cut the cord immediately; others allow it to cease pulsating. It is easier to obtain an adequate blood sample from the cord while it is still pulsating. After the cord has been cut, DO NOT STRIP THE RESIDUAL BLOOD TOWARD THE BABY.

CHAPTER 13

BIRTHING SUPPLIES

PORTABLE MATERNITY KIT FOR THE CAR

It is wise for families to keep in the car at all times a portable first aid kit that contains maternity supplies. These can be purchased or made up at home. A list of things in the kit should be made and put on a label that can be seen from the outside. Everything, including the bottles of liquid, should be packaged securely in a box.

An ideal kit would contain the following:

- 1 small woolen blanket; to fold beneath the mother.

- 2 half-sheets; for drapes and emergency use.

- 2 towels, 1 washcloth; for amniotic fluid absorption, cleaning of the mother, etc.

- 2 pair sterile gloves (unbroken packages); for attendant's use.

- 1 dozen packages disposable (moist) handwipes; for washing hands, cleaning the perineum, and general use.

Birthing Supplies

1/2 gallon water with germicidal solution in it; to disinfect anything that becomes accidentally contaminated.

2 sterile umbilical clamps (or sterile 10-inch shoestrings, strings, or cloth tapes); for tying the umbilical cord.

1 2-ounce bulb syringe; for suctioning the baby, if needed.

1 pair scissors (sterile) or adequately packaged razor blade or disposable scalpel; for cutting the umbilical cord.

1 heavy-duty plastic bag (one-gallon size, zip-lock or with a tie); for the placenta.

4 sanitary napkins; for the mother's use.

1 or 2 receiving blankets; for wrapping the newborn.

1 quart sterile water; for drinking and other needs.

1 8-ounce, leakproof container with 1/2 tsp. capsicum, 1 T. vinegar, and 1 T. honey inside. Pour the sterile (boiled or distilled) water into the container, mix, and give to the mother as soon as the head is out; for shock, bleeding, and to replace body fluid. (Can be used whenever needed during labor or postpartum.)

All linens should be sterilized. Small items (in their sterile wrappings) can be placed in the center of the linens, then rolled up and tied. These will be free from travel dust when put in a plastic bag and snuggled in one end of your box.

Plastic bottles of liquid will also be protected in the other end of the box. Seal and label the box.

HOME BIRTH SUPPLIES

Here are materials the couple planning home birth should have on hand. They should be prepared well in advance. Since they may be used again and again, either by you or your daughters or neighbors, you should have extras of many items in your home storage. Many disposable things are available now, but they may not always be; therefore, practical suggestions are given for making your own reusable items. These are much less expensive in the long run.

Disinfectant cleansing agent.

Plastic sheet. Should be big enough to cover the entire birthing bed (see Figure 21). Painters' plastic covers are inexpensive. Large, clean, garbage bags that have been cut open, shower curtains, or plastic tablecloths are also fine. Use a disinfectant to sterilize used items.

Newspaper pad. Twenty-two open sheets, taped at the corners, make a fine pad for supporting Mother's buttocks during delivery so that the baby isn't born into the bed. Newspapers also absorb moisture very well.

Protective pads, 2-feet-by-2-feet. These are used on the birthing bed and to protect the bedding for the next few days after birth. You can make several washable pads by sewing a towel to oilcloth or plastic. Toddler disposable diapers, opened flat, can be used. Commercial disposable underpads are also available.

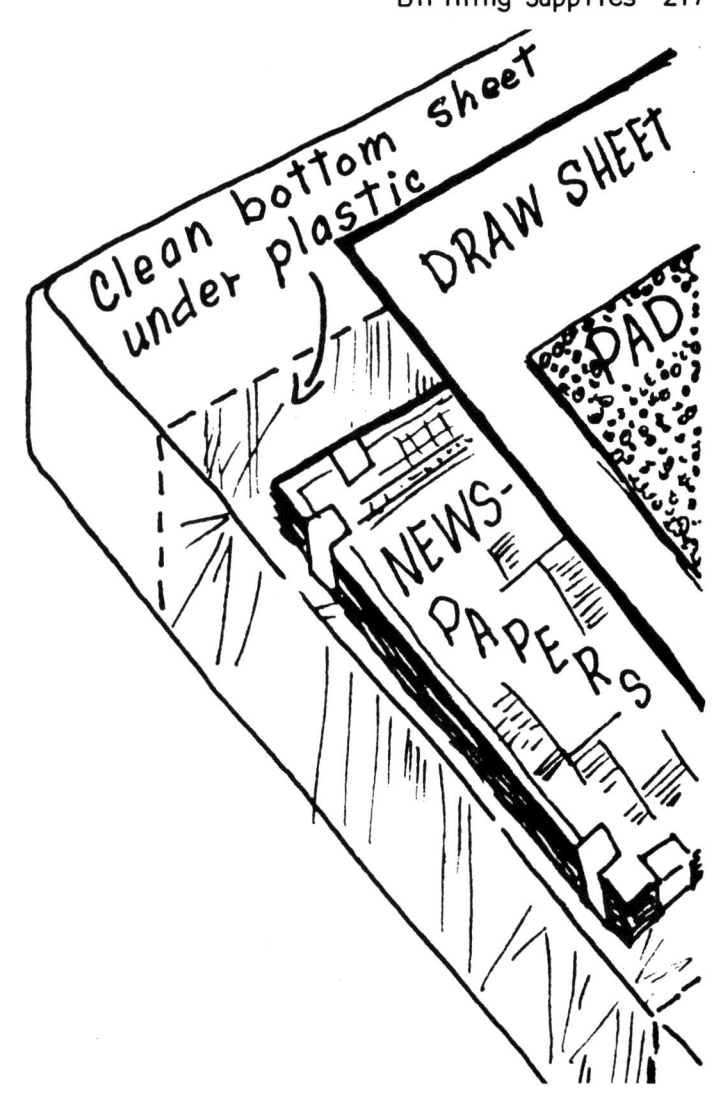

Figure 21. THE BIRTHING BED. The draw sheet is a full sheet, folded and tucked tightly over the plastic sheet and newspapers. A changeable pad is then placed under the hips. Following birth the draw sheet, newspapers, and pad are removed. Fresh draw sheets and pads should be used for two to three days, as needed.

Large towels, 6 to 8, including at least 2 white ones. These are used to keep the birthing area clean during parity. The white towels are important in detecting any meconium staining when the water breaks.

Flannel cloths, 16-inches-by-16-inches, 8, or **sterile cotton** (1-pound box); for bleeding emergencies.

Sterile gauze, 1 box. This is available in individually wrapped packets or in a 4-inch-wide roll. It is used to support the perineum while the baby's head is crowning, and to apply the olive oil with when cleaning the baby. Pieces of old flannel or bird's-eye diapers (sterile) work well.

Hand towels and washcloths, several; for peri-pacs and general use.

Sanitary napkins, hospital size, 1 box. Sanitary napkins can also be made from soft cotton fabrics. Fabric napkins should be soaked in tepid water, washed (or boiled) in soap and water and a little bleach, and rinsed very thoroughly, dried, and folded for reuse. Unlike the convenient but often expensive commercial napkins, these are reusable.

Sanitary belt(s). These can be homemade from folded, 2- to 3-inch widths of any sturdy material, or by using nonrolling elastic and safety pins.

Nightgown(s).

Nursing bra(s).

Enema equipment.

Large pans, 5 quart or larger, 2 or 3; for emergencies (ice packs for bleeding or a warm tub bath for a traumatized baby).

Stainless steel pan, 4 quart or larger; for boiling water for teas and for sterilizing purposes.

Olive oil, 1 full quart; for rimming and for cleaning the baby. The bottle should be unopened and unused. Storage in the refrigerator will prevent the oil from turning rancid.

Herbal supply. The mother should not rely on the midwife for herbs she might need in parturition. She should have on hand all the herbs listed under the midwife's kit, plus:

- Red raspberry
- Comfrey
- Alfalfa
- Marsh mallow root
- Blessed thistle
- Catnip
- Fennel seeds
- Polly-Jean Five-Week Antenatal Formula (leftovers)
- Calcium

Plastic bags, several boxes; for immediate use and long-range storage. You will need large (20- to 30-gallon), medium (5-gallon), and small (sandwich size) bags. You can use the larger bags to store your supplies in after they have been readied. You can use the sandwich bags (preferably zip-lock) to store small amounts of herbs and capsules, so large containers won't have to be opened. A plastic bag inside a large paper shopping bag can be used to catch the placenta following birth, for easy disposal.

Alcohol, 1 small bottle.

Umbilical ties, 2. Each tie should be 10-inches long and sterile. Soak them in alcohol for one hour, then dry them on a sterile towel and store them in plastic. Cord, string, twill tape (sewing), umbilical tape, umbilical clamps, or even small, thin shoelaces can be used.

Scissors, sterile; for cutting the cord or other materials.

Ear (bulb) syringe, 2-ounce size, new, sterile; for suctioning the baby, if necessary.

Layette; for baby.

Diapers. Store your favorite kind of diapers. If you make your own, 100% cotton flannel offers the best absorption. A bolt or two of this is an excellent storage item. Bird's-eye material absorbs well and provides more air circulation for summer use. They also dry quickly after washings. Some mothers like the prefolded diaper that eliminates a lot of folding after washes.

Diaper pins, 1 dozen. The extra pins are handy if abdominal bands are used for mother and/or baby. Pins are an excellent storage item.

Baby bottles, 4-ounce, 1 or 2; for teas and for emergencies.

The birthing supplies should be cleaned, disinfected, and carefully stored in an easily accessible place, perhaps with other emergency kits. Placing them in plastic and then in labeled cardboard boxes helps keep them dust-free and ready to use should they be necessary at a moment's notice. DO NOT GET OUT YOUR SUPPLIES UNTIL YOU ARE SURE TRUE LABOR HAS BEGUN.

To clean the sheets, pillowcases, towels, cloths, etc., whether they are new or used, wash them in hot water (after bloodstains have been removed in tepid water) with any good soap or detergent and about one cup of Clorox (or equivalent). Rinse everything two or three times and dry them on a clothesline in the sun--wash the line off, first-- or in a hot dryer. Then fold the linens, without letting them touch the ground, furniture, or floor, and put them into an unused storage bag. Tie the bag securely and store it until needed. This procedure should be repeated after every birth. ALWAYS BE AS CLEAN AS IS HUMANLY POSSIBLE.

THE MIDWIFE'S KIT

ESSENTIAL ITEMS

> **Scrub supplies:** nail clippers, hand soap (Safeguard, Dial), disinfectant (pHisoHex or similar), fingernail brush, and something to clean under the nails with.
>
> **Sterile, disposable gloves.** These must be stored in quantity—they may become hard to obtain. As many as 3 to 7 pairs of gloves (or more) may be used at each birth.
>
> **Lubricating jelly or olive oil.**
>
> **Fetalscope/fetascope.** There are several styles available, including a wooden model made in Europe. As with other instruments, preferences as to style and size usually vary.

Stethoscope. A stethoscope and blood pressure cuff are essential first aid items for any home.

Blood pressure cuff (sphygmomanometer). I prefer the model which combines the bulb, valve, and gauge (manometer) into a single unit which is held and operated in one hand.

Speculum, stainless steel, medium size, adjustable; essential when visual observation of the vaginal and cervical area is necessary.

Catheters, 3 to 5; for manually emptying the bladder. Also, include a plastic or rubber catheter which has been altered to accommodate reinsertion of a prolapsed umbilical cord (see Chapter 16, Prolapsed Cord, illustration).

Thermometers, 1 oral and 1 rectal. Take into account the need for extra batteries whenever battery-operated equipment is used.

Tape measure, inch/centimeter, retractable; for measuring fundal heights, newborn heads and lengths, etc.

Instrument kit. Some midwives prefer to carry their instruments in a covered, stainless steel instrument tray. Others have made compartmented kits. I separate and carry my instruments in flap-pocket purses, made of heavy material, which have ties that go around the outside. These ties keep the instruments from moving, and thus from becoming scratched, entangled, and possibly damaged. The entire kit can be placed in the oven for sterilization. The type of kit used is not important, but that your instruments are: (1) accessible, (2) well-taken-care-of, (3) ALWAYS STERILE BEFORE USE, and (4) used only in a proper manner. Be sure to protect your instruments from children, and children from your instruments.

Sterilizing tray.

Germicidal sterilizing agent. This is particularly useful in the event a midwife is called from one birth to another in close succession or when any of the equipment becomes contaminated at the scene of the birth. Other disinfectant uses, in addition to instrument sterilization, make this an important item to carry and store. Sterilize your instruments in a germicidal solution, an autoclave (if available), a large pressure cooker (10 minutes at 10 pounds pressure), or an oven (225° F for 2 hours).

Rochester-Pean hemostats, 10- to 12-inches, curved, 2. These hemostats have plenty of serrated clamping area and locking handles. They are used when the cord is wrapped tightly around the neck when the baby's head is born. (6- to 8-inch Kelly forceps may be sprung when used on very fat cords.)

Kelly hemostatic forceps, 6- to 8-inch, curved, 2; for possible ruptured varicosities. These ruptures are unlikely, but a midwife must be prepared for any eventuality. (**Hemostats** are a type of forceps designed to check hemorrhage; they have finer-grained teeth that will not damage blood vessels.) (See Figure 22.)

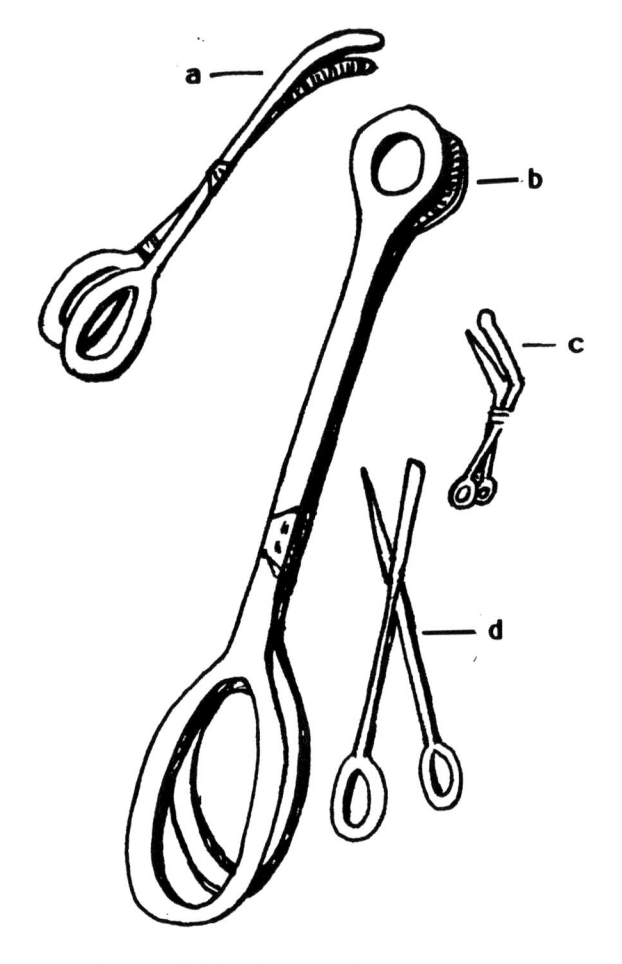

Figure 22. INSTRUMENTS FROM THE MIDWIFE'S KIT. (a) Kelly hemostatic forceps have a relatively long, curved clamping area. (b) Keyhole (ring) forceps hold cotton, gauze, or tissue without puncturing. (Each forceps has a locking device so tissue can be secured while your attention is drawn elsewhere.) (c) Bandage scissors are used to cut gauze, cotton, etc. (d) Sharp/blunt scissors can be used for episiotomies and for cutting the cord.

Keyhole (ring) forceps, 9 1/2- to 12-inch, 1. The serrated rings do not perforate tissue and can be used for removing fragments of membrane or for retrieving and clamping possible broken cords pulled back into the birth canal.

Allis forceps, 7 1/4-inch, 1; used for rupturing (safely) membranes late in labor.

Bandage scissors, 5 1/4-inch, 1; especially good for cutting materials.

Sharp/blunt surgical scissors, 5 1/4-inch, 1; for episiotomies. These have a straight blade; the blunt tip protects the baby when they are in use. Properly guided, they can be used to rupture tough membranes.

Suturing equipment. Every family's first aid supply should have suturing equipment available, whether any member of the family knows how to use it or not. In an emergency, someone--without supplies in hand--may be skillful in their use and can come to the rescue.

Suturing forceps (needle holder), 1; has a small head for working in tight places.

Needles, half-circle, regular or thread-bonded. Check supply catalogs for various sizes and styles of needles and needle points. For most perineal needs, I prefer the precision point or taper point needles, bonded with size 3-0 (000) surgical thread. (These needles do not have cutting edges.)

Surgical threads. See Chapter 18, Suturing Materials.

Thumb (tissue) forceps, 1; to hold tissue while suturing. These cause pain if the area being sutured has not been deadened. They are excellent for pulling splinters (even glass) from fingers and toes!

Herbs and supplements:

> Shepherd's-purse
> Lobelia (herb and tincture)
> Blue cohosh
> Mistletoe (European or American)
> St. Johnswort
> Capsicum (cayenne)
> Ginger
> Calendula tincture
> False unicorn
> Valerian tincture
> Vitamin E with lecithin (capsules, in oil)
> HVC (honey, vinegar, and cayenne mixture)
> Magnesium phosphate

Umbilical tape, clamps, or 10-inch ties. Store a supply of whatever you like best: umbilical clamps, umbilical tape, cord, string, twill tape (sewing), shoelaces. All umbilical ligatures should be sterile.

Bulb syringes, 2-ounce, sterile-packaged, 2 to 3; for suctioning the newborn. Store a supply. NEVER REUSE ON ANOTHER BABY.

Suction tube, or similar aspiration apparatus (such as the DeLee suction catheter).

Argyrol, silver nitrate compound, or equivalent; used in the infant's eyes at birth to prevent V.D.-caused blindness.

Penlight, with extra batteries.

Flashlight, with extra batteries.

Wristwatch, with a second hand (or simultaneous hour, minute, and second display); A MUST.

OPTIONAL ITEMS

Infant bag resuscitation mask ("Ambu bag"); has a self-inflating squeeze bag that allows only safe amounts of air into the baby's lungs.

Portable oxygen unit.

Umbilical scissors, for cutting the cord without slippage. The scissors have a circular blade area.

Utility tongs, 8-inch, straight; for picking up instruments without contaminating them.

Scale, for weighing the baby. The Chatillon IN-15 hanging scale is compact and accurate.

Otoscope, for examining the ear canal and eardrum.

Ophthalmoscope, for examining the inner eye. These useful home nursing instruments (otoscope and ophthalmoscope) come in a set, if desired.

CHAPTER 14

ANTENATAL PREPARATION FOR BIRTH

PREPARING FOR CONTROLLED CROWNING

Four weeks before due date, a husband can help his wife prepare for the fetal head to pass through the vaginal opening by stretching the area a little each day. He should first scrub thoroughly with warm, soapy water and a brush, rinse, then dry his hands with a clean, unused towel. (Anytime anything passes through the vaginal opening, the possibility of introducing harmful bacteria is high. Germs abide in the area surrounding the vaginal opening because urine and fecal matter pass from that area. Baths and the scrubbing of hands are important to prevent infection.)

At the same time each day, the husband should take fresh, warm olive oil, lubricate his hand, and insert the palpating index and middle fingers gently about 2 to 3 inches, stretch the perineum just slightly, and hold it for a moment. Done every day, this stretching dilates the opening little by little until the whole fist can comfortably fit in it by due date. If a day or two is skipped, the opening may regress.

If the gravida is tense and a bit rigid, the husband should lay a folded, clean, very warm, wet hand towel over the entire perineal area. A ginger bath will also help her to relax. If she is too tense, these procedures may be easier if they follow her daily sitz baths or a nap. Her promptings and guidance must be adhered to strictly. If the stretching causes more tension and distress than is profitable, it should be discontinued.

Also important at this time are the sitz baths on a two-a-day schedule and the prenatal exercises (see Chapter 9, The Sitz Bath, Exercise). These will help facilitate the preparations being made by nature for Baby to come.

DETERMINING FETAL POSITION

Three to four weeks before due date, begin to determine the position of the fetus within the uterus. **Presentation** refers to the part of the fetus which "presents" (or will present) itself to be born first. In a **cephalic presentation,** the head is the **presenting part.** Usually the head is flexed downward so that the **vertex,** or crown of the head (see Figure 23), presents first; thus, the **vertex presentation** represents the common, normal presentation. (As such, the term "vertex" is often used to signify the head-down position.)

When the buttocks or feet are down, a type of **breech** or **footling presentation** follows. Ninety-five percent of the time the breech, or buttocks, will be in the fundus, though, and the head will be down. (Remember that one in six primigravidas will carry her baby breech until the 32nd week, when it will usually turn to a head-down position.)

A **transverse** (as opposed to a **longitudinal**) **lie** is one in which the fetus is primarily in a horizontal position, as sometimes occurs in multiple births, lending itself to an **arm** or **shoulder presentation.**

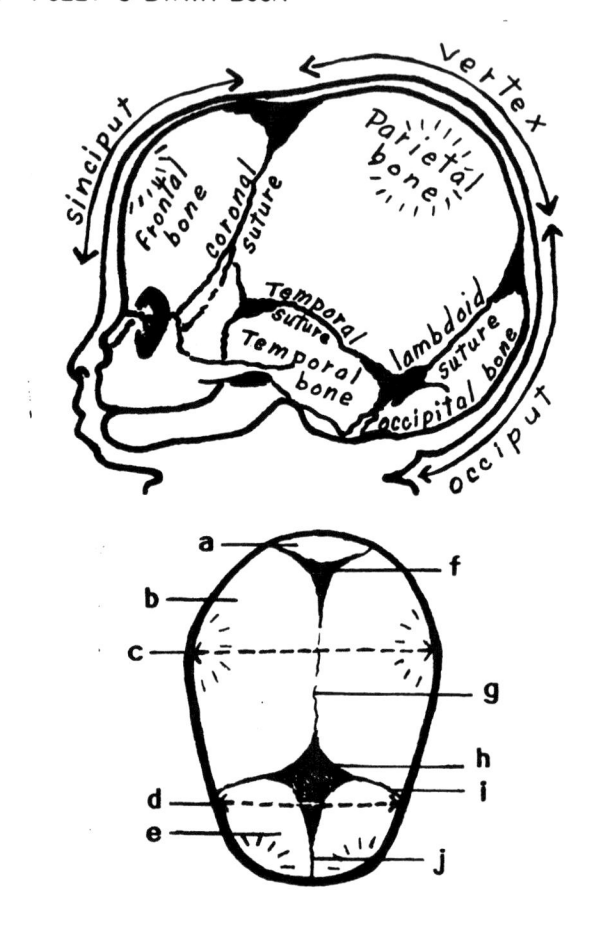

Figure 23. THE FETAL HEAD, SIDE AND TOP VIEWS. (a) occipital bone, (b) parietal bone, (c) the biparietal diameter (between the parietal eminences, or "bumps" on the sides of the head) is about 3 3/4 inches; (d) the bitemporal measurement is about 3 1/4 inches across; (e) frontal bone, (f) posterior (lesser) fontanel (back, smaller soft spot), (g) sagittal suture, (h) anterior (bregmatic or greater) fontanel (front, larger, diamond-shaped soft spot), (i) coronal suture, (j) frontal suture. The flexibility of the membranous spaces between the bones (fontanels, sutures) contributes to how easily the head molds in the birth canal.

Discovering which way the fetus is situated within the uterus at term will give the midwife an idea of what the presenting part, and consequently, the mechanics of birth, will be for that particular baby. Positions from left to right may change often prior to and during early labor.

To determine fetal position, first palpate on the abdomen. Face your client's head--she will be lying down, of course—and lay your hands on the sides of the uterus. With your client's knees slightly bent, you can feel more deeply into the abdomen. Apply a bit of pressure with your palms and fingers to find the baby's hips or the head. The buttocks will be round, but not as round and firm as the head. The thighs are also detectable. The head will be movable, but not the breech.

Sometimes the uterus is a little rigid, making palpating more difficult. If your client is relaxed, you can press firmly and make slow, deep movements and not hurt her. Avoid quick or sudden, jablike movements. Obesity or an excessive amount of amniotic fluid will also make palpating more difficult. If you can find the contour of the fetal back and follow its curvature to the head, it is possible to hold the unengaged head between the fingers and the thumb. Walk the fingers over the abdomen from one side to the other to find the fetal extremities: knees, elbows, and sometimes heels or toes.

Use the fetalscope to assist you with your findings. Loudest, clearest fetal heart tones are found between the baby's shoulders. If the loudest heartbeat (and therefore, the baby's shoulders) is between the mother's navel and thigh, the baby is in good position for labor and delivery.

The baby's back and **occiput,** or the back of its skull, are in line with each other. The position of the occiput IN RELATION TO THE MOTHER is used to identify the **position** of the vertex baby, particularly at the onset of labor. Always remember that where the occiput is found tells the tale.

For example, if the baby's occiput is on the MOTHER'S left side, it is in a "left occipital position." Depending upon whether the occiput is rotated toward the mother's front (anterior), side, or back (posterior), the baby is in an anterior, transverse, or posterior position. Thus, a baby whose occiput is on its mother's left side, toward her front, is in **Left Occiput Anterior (LOA) position** (see Figure 24). His back will also be in the left, anterior portion of the mother's abdomen, and his small parts (knees, elbows, feet, hands) will be opposite (on the mother's right, posterior side). Perhaps only a hip or thigh will be detectable. The buttocks will be up, in the fundus. Clearest fetal heart tones should be on the mother's left, about halfway between the bend of the thigh and the navel.

If the occiput is on the mother's right side, toward her back, the baby is in **Right Occiput Posterior (ROP) position.** His back will be in the right, posterior portion of the mother's abdomen, and his small parts will be left and anterior. (The small parts are very easy to find, with peaks and valleys as opposed to the solid rim of the back.) Buttocks will be up, in the fundus, and clearest heart tones should be heard on the mother's right, more toward her side.

With breech and face presentations, the sacrum and chin (mentum) are used to designate the baby's position (for example, Left Sacrum Anterior, or Right Mentum Posterior).

LOA	LOT	LOP
ROA	ROT	ROP

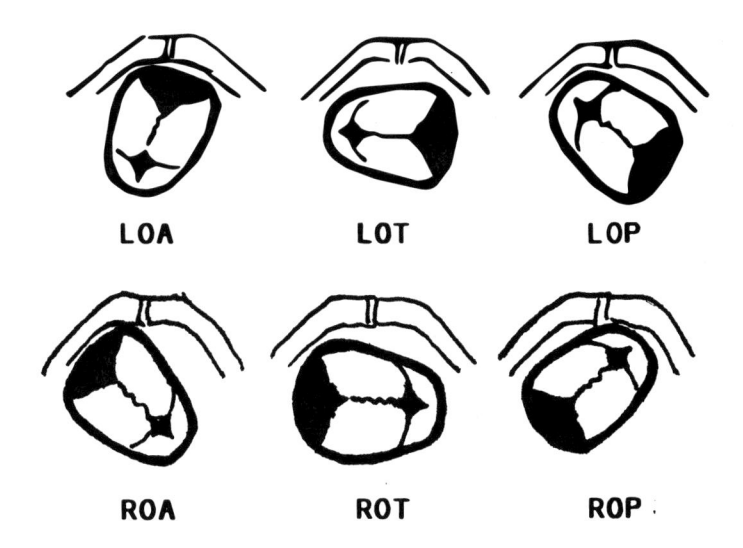

Figure 24. OCCIPITAL POSITIONS (as seen from below). The position of the vertex baby at the onset of labor is designated by the location of the fetal occiput in relation to the mother's pelvis—left positions are to the MOTHER'S left, not the attendant's. **Shown above are:** Left Occiput Anterior, Left Occiput Transverse (the most common position), Left Occiput Posterior, Right Occiput Anterior, Right Occiput Transverse (the second most common position), and Right Occiput Posterior. Positions in which the occiput is directly anterior (Occiput Anterior) or directly posterior (Occiput Posterior) are rare.

DETERMINING ENGAGEMENT

With the primigravida, the fetal head usually has become engaged two or three weeks before term. This pressure helps the pelvis to relax open a little more in preparation for birth. Strangely enough, seldom does the multipara experience engagement of the fetus until labor sets in.

When the fetal head settles down into the pelvis, it is considered to be **engaged**. When the attendant, or doctor, says, "The head is down," she MAY MEAN that the head, as opposed to the breech (buttocks) is down, OR that engagement has occurred or is occurring.

At the last two weeks, the head almost always is in a vertex position. With the mother lying down, step beside her and face her feet. Place your hands on her abdomen, your fingers pointing over the pelvic arch. Have your client breathe out while you feel deeply into the pelvis. Palpate with both hands for the baby's head. If the head is not engaged, it may be fairly high and it will be very moveable. In fact, while you are palpating, the baby may decide to change positions and you may have to "round him up" again. If your finger tips can cup the head, it is above the pelvic arch and not engaged. If the head is engaged in the bony canal, it will not be mobile and will be most difficult to feel. Before engagement, you can grasp most of the roundness of the head. If your finger tips fan out because you cannot find the roundness of the head, the head is at least partially engaged. You will feel only the occipital portion of the head, and the rest will be obscured because it is partially down and under the pelvic arch. Sometimes the head is so deeply engaged that you will feel the shoulder just above the pelvic arch and you may think it is a foot, so reaching deeply under the brim of the arch is necessary to make sure of the diagnosis.

If there is any doubt, an internal exam will determine whether the head is engaged. There is no round hardness--not just firmness--quite like a baby's head. Even though you will be feeling the head through cervical tissue, the hardness is easily discerned. If you touch the head with the tips of your fingers and it bounces, it is "floating," or not deeply engaged.

If the head does not engage when it should, it may be that the lower uterine segment, cervix, and vaginal floor have failed to soften sufficiently to allow the head to sink into the pelvis. Often the primigravida is tense and not sure what to expect. The excitement of it all keeps her from truly relaxing. This is why sitz baths on a double-time program are so very important the last few weeks of pregnancy, or even during labor.

An incidence of multiple fetuses can also prevent engagement, as may **hydramnios** (an excessive amount of amniotic fluid) or a **cephalopelvic disproportionment**. The latter means that the pelvis is too small to accommodate passage of the head, or is contracted somewhat. There may be a combination of any of these, and all may indicate the need for special skill in delivery or even possible cesarean delivery. Engagement may be delayed if the head is tilted at the neck too far to one side--perhaps because of a low placenta--placing the sagittal suture too close to the symphysis pubis or the sacral promontory (**posterior** or **anterior asynclitism**).

Cephalopelvic Disproportionment. Rarely will one encounter the problem of the fetal head being too large to fit into the pelvic inlet. It does sometimes appear in interracial marriages and especially in the case of **hydrocephalus** (the abnormally large, water-filled skull). A trial labor is usually allowed (except in instances of hydrocephalus), and if it proves futile, C-section will be needed.

To determine if there is a disproportionment between the size of the fetal head and the pelvic inlet through which it must pass, palpate abdominally a few days before term (one to two days, or before hard labor sets in). Face your client's feet (again, she is lying down), put your fingers and thumb around the baby's head, then push down and slightly backwards (in a direction to simulate a flexing of the head). The posterior portion of the head will come into close contact with the sacral promontory. See if you can slide the baby's head under the brim of the pelvic arch. At the same time, feel with the first two fingers of the free hand to see if the head is above the brim. If the head seems to give and NO PART OF IT OVERLAPS at the pubic symphysis, then it should be able to engage on its own. If you feel any of the fetal head when it is supposed to be underneath the arch, then home birth is inadvisable.

UNDERSTANDING THE PROCESS OF LABOR

When the first stage of labor sets in, it means your body has received the right hormonal changes and signals to begin the expulsion of your baby. Muscles in the abdomen begin a beautiful, rhythmic pattern that will push and guide your baby through the birth canal in a slow enough way to minimize discomfort and fast enough to promote safety for you and your baby. This will usually take from six to eighteen hours, depending on your individuality. (It can take much longer without too much risk.)

You will learn to relax and enjoy the most interesting and divinely programmed activity in which you will ever be involved. Quietly observe each step as you learn to cooperate with your body in giving birth. Such interesting things happen to cause a safe journey through the birth canal. Our marvelous bodies work in a most natural way to bring this about. See if you can identify some of these orchestrations. You may even find yourself turning or twisting or wiggling in motions that seem to help the baby on its journey.

Those around you will remind you when to just relax, when to bear down, and when to pant, and they'll help you understand what is taking place in the moment. Your attendants will know how to assist you when you need help and what to do that you may not be able to do for yourself, such as applying some marvelous therapies.

Although you may have read much about birth, you will learn firsthand how it all comes to pass. There will be compassionate, skillful, and intuitive people giving you every care needed to bring the birth to a safe conclusion.

Should the need arise for additional or outside help, they, with you, will know at what point this should be done. Transporting plans are fixed in mind, and care will be taken to do it as carefully and as expeditiously as possible. A driver will have been chosen, the gas tank filled, the route to the hospital planned, babysitters arranged for, and the doctor notified with phone numbers already posted. No panic or hurry should upset a change in plans; the new plan will be simply executed by all concerned. You have taken precautions throughout pregnancy to give birth safely to a healthy baby and the Lord will bless those efforts.

The attendants will check the baby's position and all vital signs that will give clues to the condition and progress of labor. They know how to determine dilation and engagement of fetal parts and they know how to tell if any abnormality has begun to set in, along with what to do about it. They will know whether your body is just being poky and taking its time or whether there is an obstruction or uterine inertia taking place.

Rest assured that this baby you are wanting also wants you, and will indeed assist in its own birth in many ways.

MECHANISM OF LABOR: VERTEX PRESENTATIONS

An overview of the process of birth follows. Since the fetal **vertex** is the presenting part in almost all births, the vertex presentation is used to illustrate the mechanics of labor. (It is helpful if the mother can realize and appreciate what is happening within her body during labor.)

The **mechanism of labor** is usually divided into a series of steps, movements, or changes in position the fetus must undergo in order to be born (see Figure 25). Though each step describes a different action, the first four actions are not necessarily separate from each other; they may be occurring at the same time. They are:

1. DESCENT.

2. FLEXION.

3. ENGAGEMENT.

4. INTERNAL ROTATION.

5. EXTENSION AND CROWNING AT THE VULVA.

6. EXTERNAL ROTATION (RESTITUTION).

7. EXPULSION.

Descent. None of the meaningful mechanisms of labor can take place until lightening—the first actual step in descent—has occurred one or two weeks before labor. After labor sets in, all contractions contribute to the descent of the fetal head, even those performing the necessary dilation of the cervix. During first stage, contractions cause the uterine muscles to exert pressure on the amniotic fluid, which in turn exerts pressure on the whole baby in a gentle but firm way to cause dilation and descent (see Figure 26).

Flexion. As descent occurs, the baby's head finds resistance here and there (from the cervix, the walls of the pelvis, the pelvic floor), and it is a good thing it does, because this resistance acts as a pair or hands, if you will, that curl the body and flex the head, causing the fetus's chin to go down onto its chest. This flexion thrusts the occiput forward and leaves the smallest possible diameter of the head to lead the way through the birth canal. The circumference of the engaging part of the head in a well-flexed, vertex presentation is about 11 inches. If the head comes through poorly flexed or at a wrong angle, it will need about 13 to 14 inches! (Brow and face presentations are a consequence of poor flexion.)

Engagement. Technically speaking, when the widest portion of the normally flexed head (**biparietal diameter**) has passed through the pelvic inlet, **engagement** has occurred. Unless there has been an unusual elongation of the head, if the foremost portion of the head is at or below the level of the ischial spines (**zero station**), the head is **engaged**. (Stations are used to indicate position within the birth canal; see Figure 27.)

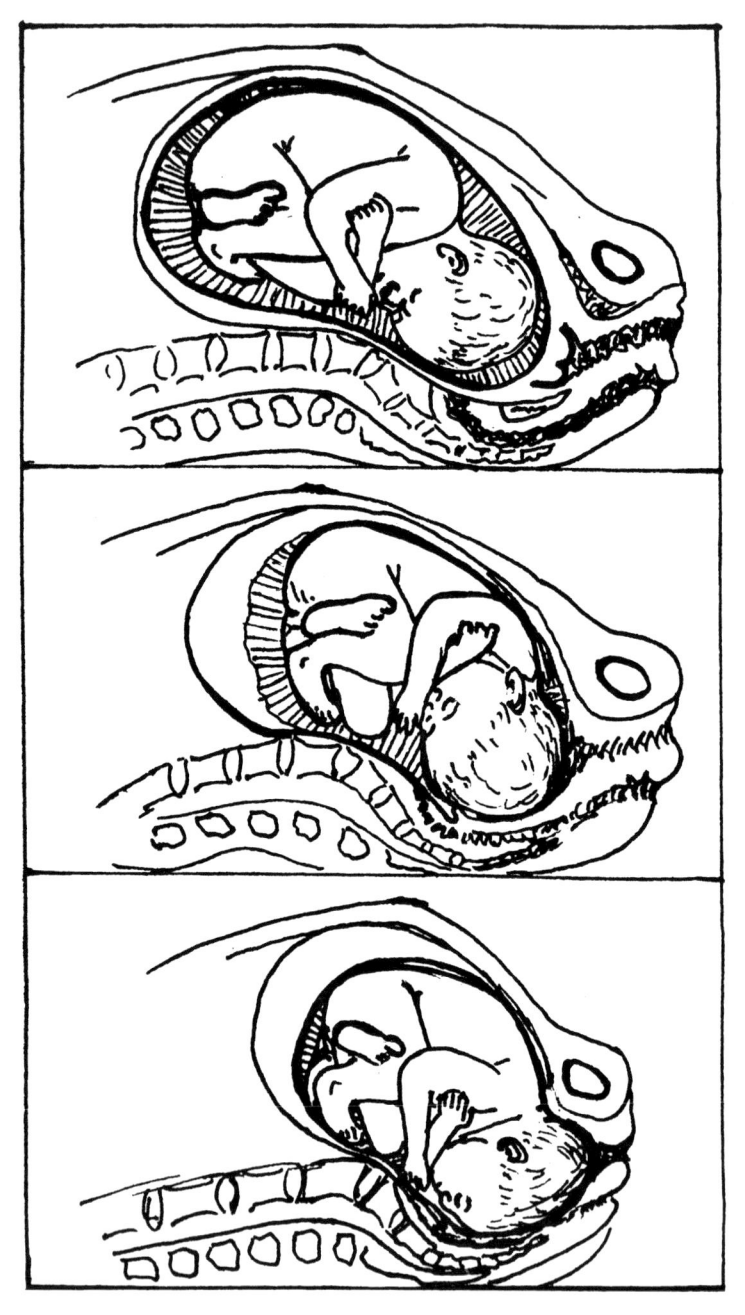

Figure 25. MECHANISM OF LABOR: LOA POSITION.

Antenatal Preparation for Birth 241

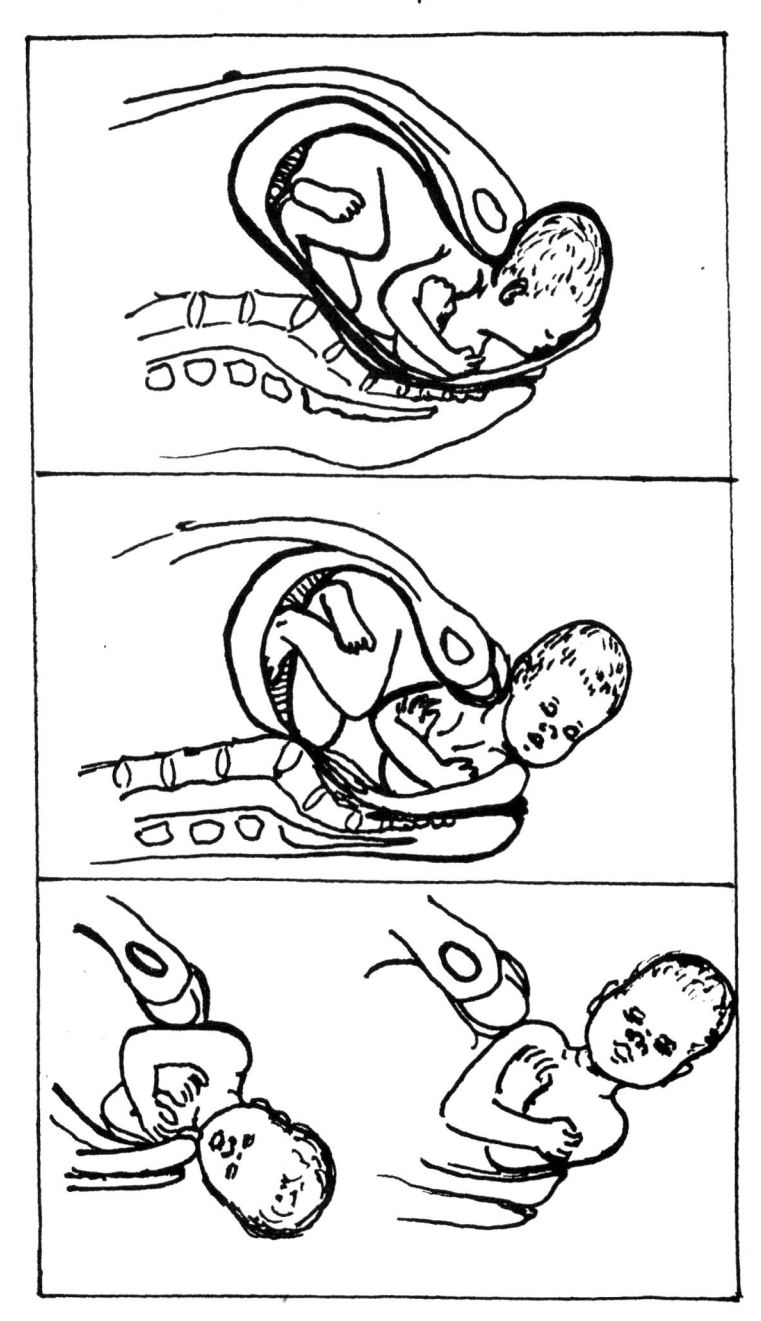

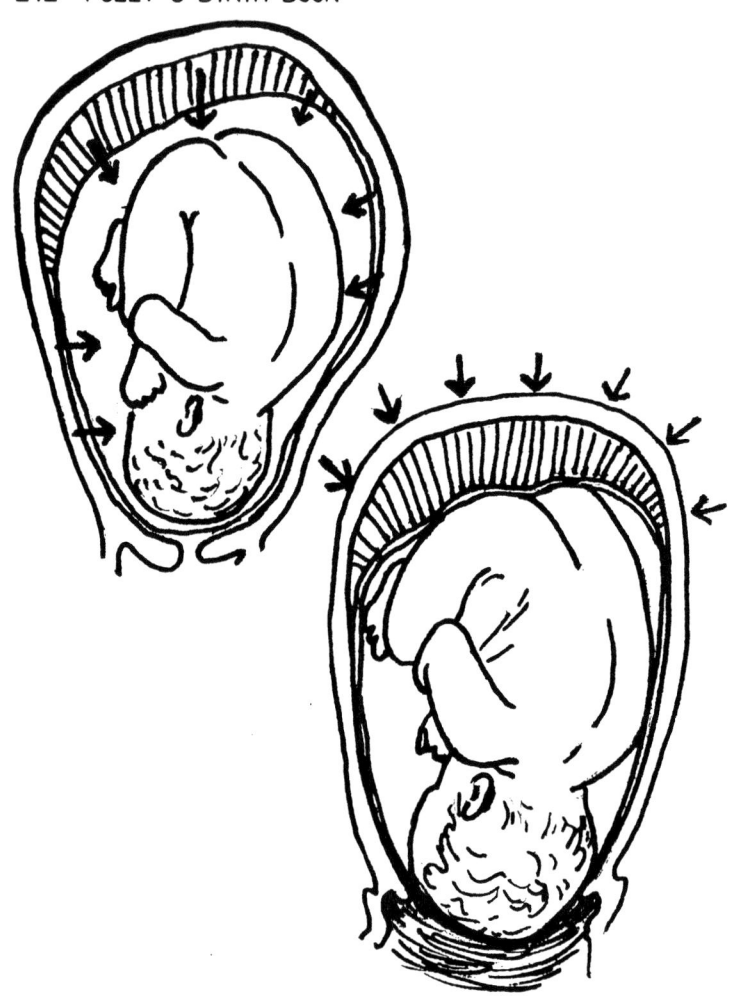

Figure 26. DIRECTIONAL FORCE OF CONTRACTIONS. (**top**) In early labor, the pressure of contractions focuses on the amniotic fluid, equalizing pressure on the baby and assisting with dilation; however, contractions also cause a slight interference in placental circulation. (**bottom**) Expulsion of the fetus is aided by pressure of abdominal muscles and the diaphragm on the baby's buttocks. When the membrane is ruptured, placental circulation interference is increased during contractions.

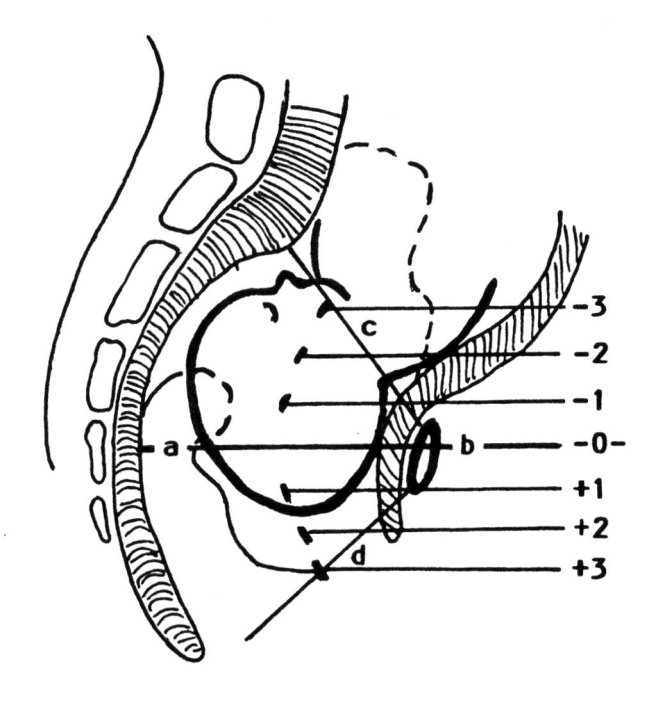

Figure 27. STATIONS OF PROGRESS IN THE BIRTH CANAL. (a) ischial spine, (b) symphysis pubis, (c) pelvic inlet, (d) pelvic outlet. The ischial spines (-0- station) are about halfway between the pelvic inlet and outlet. The birth canal above and below the spines is divided into thirds (or fourths) to facilitate more accurate assessment of the progress of the presenting part. When the lowest portion of the presenting part reaches the ischial spines, it is said to be at zero station and engaged. When the presenting part reaches the pelvic outlet and the perineum, it is said to be at +3 station. As the head distends the perineum and is ready to crown, it is at +4 station.

When the wide part of the head reaches "0" station—the narrowest and tightest fit within the pelvis—an **internal** or **initial crowning** occurs. (A second, **external crowning** occurs when the head emerges through the perineal tissue, outside the vaginal cavity.)

Internal Rotation. The musculature of the pelvic floor and the placement of the ischial spines encourage a rotation of the fetal head to an **occiput anterior position** (see Figure 28). No matter what occipital position the baby starts out in, almost always the head rotates to the anterior until the occiput is up and the face is down. This is the position of the head both when it exits the pelvic outlet and when it is born.

The heads of babies that start in either a **left** or **right occiput anterior** position rotate 1/8 of a turn (45 degrees). Those in **occiput transverse** positions rotate 1/4 of a turn (90 degrees), and those in **occiput posterior** positions rotate 3/8 of a turn (135 degrees).

Exceptions to this normal rotation occur only about 5 percent of the time, when the occiput slips down into, or rotates into, the hollow of the sacrum posteriorly. The baby goes on to be born face up. Bear in mind, though, that the great majority of occiput posterior babies spontaneously rotate anteriorly, especially with good contractions, good flexion, and good muscle tone.

Extension. As the head reaches the part of the birth canal that extends upward (see Figure 29), the head must "deflex" and extend upward, too. This places the base of the occiput in contact with the inferior edge of the symphysis pubis. The uterus exerts pressure posteriorly, and the resistance of the pelvic floor acts anteriorly to

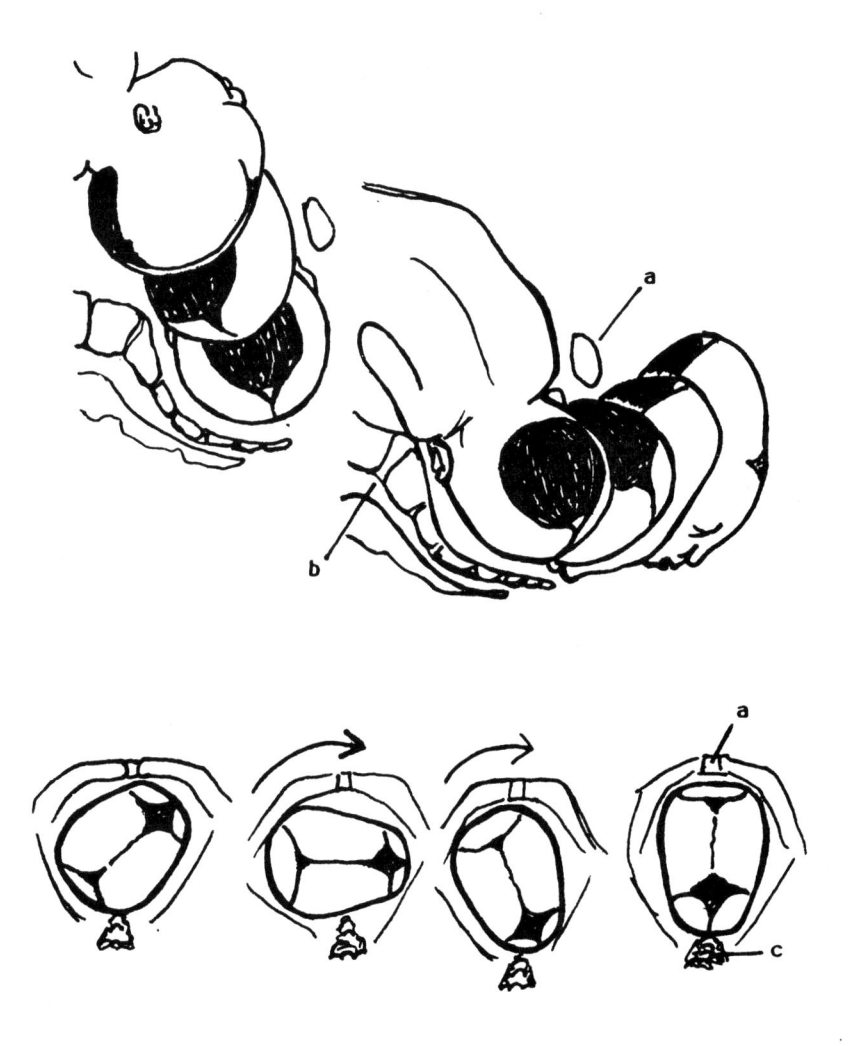

Figure 28. ANTERIOR ROTATION: ROP POSITION. (**top**) Descent, engagement, and extension of the fetal head as it presents. (**bottom**) Rotation of the fetal occiput, as seen from below, is made in 45° angles. (a) symphysis pubis, (b) sacral promontory, (c) coccyx (tailbone).

cause extension of the head. The baby is now on its way up and out at the vulva. (If the face begins to extend too soon, the attendant's hand will exert just enough pressure to encourage the occiput forward, helping to prevent laceration.)

Crowning at the Vulva. After the occiput crowns externally, the forehead, nose, mouth, and chin, in that order, sweep over the inside tissue of the perineum proper (below the vulvar opening), then emerge. The head drops down after it is born, and the little chin lies over the anal region of the mother, waiting, we hope, for the attendant to check for the cord to see whether it is around the baby's neck. (If the contractions do not wait, the attendant asks the mother to pant until this is done.)

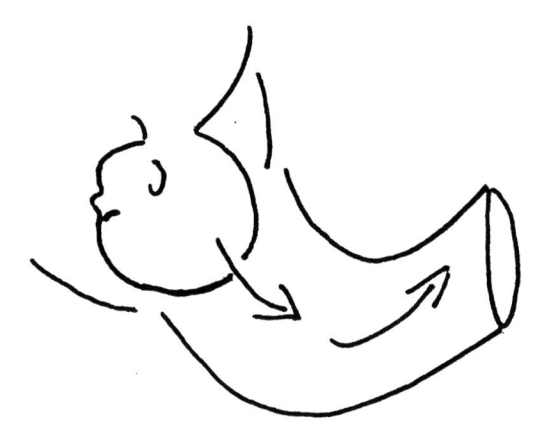

Figure 29. THE CURVE OF CARUS. The fetus travels DOWN, then back UP to be born.

External Rotation (Restitution). The baby's body is on its side, in the canal. Once the head is out, it "makes **restitution**," or turns so it is again facing forward according to the direction of ITS body. (If the occiput was directed originally toward the left, it (the occiput) rotates toward the left ischial tuberosity, and if it was originally directed toward the right, it rotates toward the right ischial tuberosity).

Expulsion. The shoulders (the anterior one is usually first) deliver, and the rest of the body slips right out.

UNIT III

Parturition

Before I begin the discussion of labor, I want to emphasize the importance of letting nature take its course. I am very proud of the first midwife I trained, because she learned this important lesson well: **WHENEVER POSSIBLE, wait for nature to take care of problems that arise.** Do not hurry birth!

Too many birth attendants try to hurry a poky birth. Pokiness is okay as long as some progress is being made, as long as vital signs are good, and as long as complications are not developing. My friend who found this to be true said to me once: "I didn't know you could wait 'that' long for the baby to be born and it would still be all right. My inclination would have been to hurry the mother to get the baby out once you could see the head. Now when I know when all is well, I can wait without fear because I trust nature."

Contractions, whether mild or more vigorous, were geared to expel the fetus, and normally will fulfill their measure with finesse.

CHAPTER 15

FIRST STAGE OF LABOR: BEGINS WITH THE ONSET OF LABOR AND ENDS WITH FULL DILATION

WHEN TO CALL THE MIDWIFE

A pregnant woman, especially a first-time mother, may not know when she is in labor. As a midwife, you need to teach her to call when one or more of the following signs appear:

1. **"Show" of blood-tinged mucus.**

    This indicates that the mucous plug has passed from its protective station at the external os of the cervix. This may precede noticeable contractions or it may come later in labor. The mucous plug is mucus that has adhered to the external os to protect the membrane. When it is disturbed by changes in the cervix (dilation), it breaks loose and slips out (see Figure 30).

2. **Her "water breaks."**

    The membrane containing the amniotic fluid (the **amniotic sac** or **"bag of waters"**) may

252 POLLY'S BIRTH BOOK

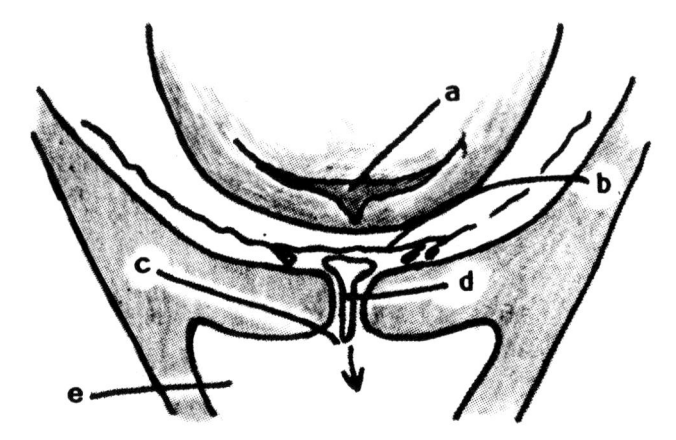

Figure 30. THE MUCOUS PLUG. (a) small (posterior) fontanel, (b) amniotic membrane, (c) external os, (d) mucous plug, (e) vagina. When dilation begins, the mucous plug separates and slips out. Changes in the cervix may cause slight bleeding, and the plug itself may be blood-tinged.

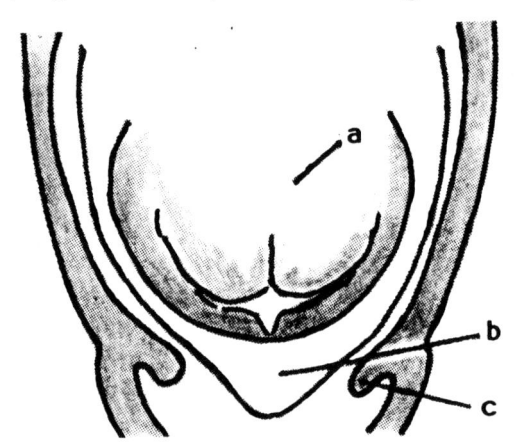

Figure 31. FOREWATERS ASSIST DILATION. (a) fetal head, (b) forewaters (amniotic fluid in front of the fetal head), (c) cervix. The force of contractions causes the forewaters within the membrane to bulge into the external os. This assists dilation of the cervix and is much easier on the fetus and mother.

rupture near the onset of labor. It is hoped that the membrane will remain intact until second stage labor, because it acts as a cushion to absorb the brunt of contractions that otherwise can be hard on the baby's head and the mother (see Figure 31). If the membrane breaks and a rush of water issues, sometimes the water carries with it the umbilical cord. This can be very serious and must be dealt with immediately (knee-chest position, etc.; see Chapter 16, Prolapsed Cord).

Rupture of the membrane does not necessarily mean that labor will begin immediately. However, it can, and it usually does begin within a few hours. Concern is felt when labor has not begun AT TERM within 24 to 48 hours following rupture of the membrane. The primary concern is that infection will arise. The amniotic fluid is protective, and when much of it has gone--and especially when examinations are made--bacteria are easily introduced. Extreme caution is the key and the fewer the exams by ANYONE, the better, until labor sets in. Showers are preferred over tub baths until true labor begins.

3. **Fairly regular and persisting contractions.**

These are unlike the abdominal tightenings, called **Braxton Hicks contractions,** which cause little, if any, discomfort, and which a mother may experience any time, particularly after the seventh or eighth month.

It is not always easy to recognize mild, true contractions, especially for primigravidas, who have never felt them before. Contractions that are dilating the cervix (true labor) may at first feel just like Braxton Hicks contractions (sporadic contractions throughout pregnancy that increase in frequency and may become partially rhythmic near term). Be understanding when your client calls and is confused about whether what she is experiencing is real labor. Reassure her that everyone experiences this uncertainty.

True labor contractions have a pattern in which the contracting action draws in the abdominal muscles. A thickening fundus creates pressure, and together they push the baby toward the cervix to dilate it large enough to accomodate the passing of the fetal head (or the presenting part). This action gives the feeling of tightening, drawing, and pressure of abdominal muscles. Some women describe contractions as incredible pressure and tightness, but not pain (however, most parturients experience increasing discomfort as labor progresses). True labor contractions will become somewhat regular, with shorter intervals and greater length and intensity as labor progresses.

4. **Persistent back ache.**

If the mother has done her pelvic rocks every day, back aches will not likely accompany pregnancy. Yet, as her due date approaches, a persistent back ache can be a sign of labor. Back aches occur at different times during some labors, or perhaps not at all. They almost always occur, however, in posterior labors.

If a back ache persists--even though the mother's back is properly aligned (see this Chapter, Back Adjustments) and she is rested-- she may be in labor. A warm tub bath will not make true labor go away, although at times there may be a temporary lull before labor steps up. Then again, the warm tub bath may hasten labor.

Any one of the above signs, or these signs in combination, are enough to indicate that a birth attendant should be notified. When the gravida calls, expecting that labor is in progress, ask two or three pertinent questions. "Has your water broken? Did it dribble or did it flush out? How close are your contractions? What is the duration (length) of each contraction?" (The DURATION of contractions is more important than the FREQUENCY of them.) An in-person assessment will reveal a clearer picture of the gravida's labor.

THE MIDWIFE ARRIVES

After you have arrived at your client's home, you can usually determine whether or not she is in true labor within an hour or two. This decision is critical, for if true labor has commenced, the all-important duty of "being there" has also begun, not because there is danger of the baby arriving right away necessarily, but because you play an important role in successful labor. You are able to detect any potential problems arising, within safe time limits, and you offer much security and reassurance to the anxious couple.

Upon arriving at the home, the midwife seldom routinely goes about her work. An overall assessment of the mother's physical and psychological state will determine whether the midwife takes the mother's blood pressure first or times her contractions, whether she calms her down first or checks possible dilation, whether she must act quickly to discover a possible cord prolapse or even whether she should prepare the mother for immediate transport to a hospital.

When you determine that the mother is in true labor, assess her emotional and physical state and reassure her. Orient her about what steps you and your assistant(s) will be taking to get ready for the birth. You should explain to all those present at the birth what you expect of them and what they can expect from you. You should warn them that as the second stage of labor approaches, you must take full control of all that is happening, including coaching.

Ready your equipment and supplies, including teas, and make up the delivery bed. (Midwives soon learn to wait until true labor is determined before they make the bed. Then linens will not have to be washed again if labor has proven to be simply preparatory or "false" labor.)

Keeping a Labor Log

A good midwife keeps a progress report of labor. It can be done in longhand on forms or in a notebook. The date, time, place, mother's name and age, and which birth this is go at the top of the report. This is later filed with all her pregnancy records, since it may be helpful with succeeding pregnancies. (A copy may become valuable as a sentimental contribution to the child's journal or history, to go along with a cassette recording of his first cries and the excited comments of everyone during the first half-hour of his life, the first pictures, etc.). The time during labor serves as an excellent opportunity to teach an assistant or trainee the ramifications of a well-attended birth. She may make the entries under your supervision. Each time anything of significance occurs, or if something is done for the mother, note the time and make a very specific, but concise, entry. Vital signs are always recorded. Comments about the mother's condition are noted when appropriate.

When, on occasion, the midwife is tempted not to bother with records, she must also remember the legal benefits they serve. In the case of complications or death, a record of appropriate steps that were taken will be available.

Timing Contractions

The duration of a contraction in the home setting is still measured from the onset to the strongest point or peak only. Stop timing as the contraction begins to fade away. Early contractions usually last about 30 seconds and may be irregular. They will begin to last a full minute as transition from first to second stage approaches. Sooner or later contractions usually assume some regularity of frequency: 10, 5, 3 minutes apart. Seldom are their intervals completely regular or precisely on time. Don't be surprised if the duration, regularity, or intensity of contractions diminishes considerably upon your arrival at the home. Your presence helps the mother to calm down.

Noting Vital Signs

Part of labor assessment comes with taking the mother's vital signs. Excessive changes in her blood pressure, temperature, or pulse rate and respiration will indicate that an adverse health condition is developing which would affect delivery. Slight increases in pulse rate, respiration, and blood pressure will mean only that the woman is affected by the anticipation of the birth and the performance of labor. Listening to the baby's heartbeat will tell you if the baby is alive and well or if labor is posing a stress. An occasional check of fetal heart tones throughout labor is wise. As second stage approaches, and thereafter, more frequent auscultations should be made, especially if any indications of stress have been noted.

Position and Engagement

Early in labor you need to palpate externally to determine the baby's position so you can anticipate the sequence of events that will follow. When you check internally for dilation and effacement, you can verify your findings and note whether engagement has taken place. The direction of the fetal sagittal suture (between the two fontanels) is a useful positional landmark. (See also Chapter 14, Determining Fetal Position, Mechanism of Labor.)

Dilation and Effacement

The cervix is a canal about 2 centimeters long, between the uterus and the vagina. This channel is "taken up" (retracted) into the lower uterine segment; it is shortened and thinned out until the former canal is a mere opening, only paper-thin—a process called **effacement** (see Figure 32). (The cervix is 50% effaced when it is 1 cm long, and 100% effaced when it is thin.) The cervix also **dilates**; that is, the opening widens.

Following hand scrubs, check for dilation and effacement occasionally during labor. (Be sure fingernails on your examining hand have been clipped short!) The cervix has begun to soften or already is very soft. It may or may not be thinned out. The palpating fingers seemingly must reach "to China" to find the external os in

First Stage of Labor 259

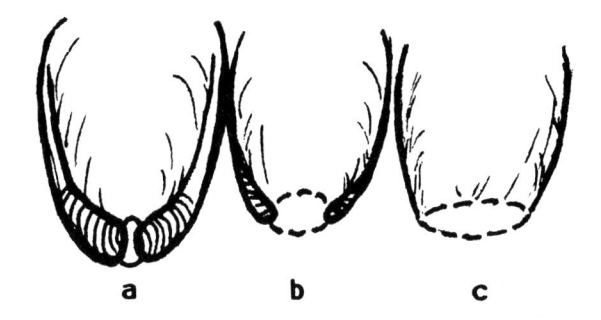

Figure 32. EFFACEMENT OF THE CERVIX. The cervix shortens and thins in preparation for passage of the baby. (a) pregnant uterus at term, (b) normal effacement and dilation at mid first stage, (c) complete effacement and full dilation at the conclusion of first stage.

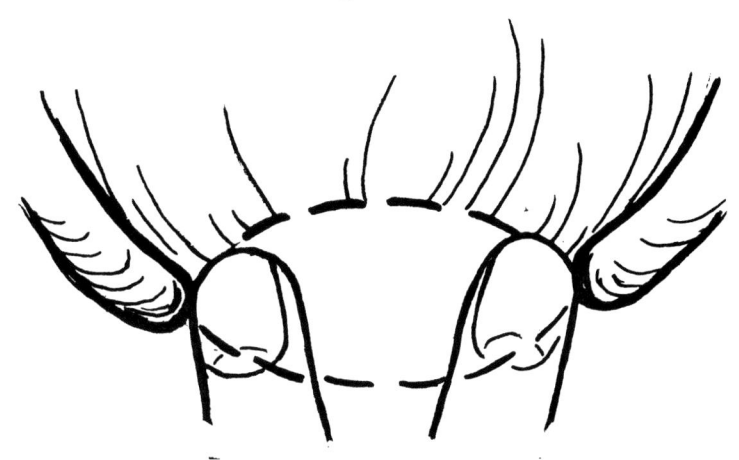

Figure 33. MEASURING DILATION OF THE CERVIX. The cervix (external os) is 5 centimeters (halfway) dilated. Dilation is measured by estimating the diameter of the cervical opening in centimeters. Finger widths can be used to estimate the number of centimeters. (Three finger widths are about 5 cm, more or less according to individual finger sizes.) Dilation is considered complete at about 10 centimeters.

EARLY LABOR sometimes, as it may not be in the center at the far end of the vaginal canal. It may be up and under and slightly on the right side of the uterus (attendant's right). It feels much like the anal opening if it has not thinned out. With complete effacement the edges (rim) are flat and as thin as paper, so patience must be exercised to find the rim of the cervix. Note not only how far dilation and effacement have progressed, but also whether the cervix is thinning out evenly.

To determine amount of dilation, place your finger tips in the opening and make a mental note of how many finger widths could fit there comfortably (see Figure 33). Do not go inside the cervix (it is elastic), just measure from rim to rim, from one side to the other. You should be familiar with how far apart your fingers are at each centimeter measurement. Practice and experience help. If you palpate through one or two or three contractions, you can observe whether the contractions are dilating the cervix (you should feel the cervix stretching open wider with the contraction).

CAUTION: On occasion the fibrous material of the cervix has broken down somewhat; it has stretched in pregnancy and this has caused superficial "rings" or breaks in the tissue on the surface of the uterus. These rings feel much like the paper-thin rims of the external os at various dilations. DO NOT MISTAKE THESE FOR THE CERVIX (EXTERNAL OS) AND MISJUDGE A DILATION THAT IS NOT THERE. Experience will help you distinguish from superficial rings.

Dilation is complete when at 9 to 10 centimeters (perhaps it will need more) the cervix can accommodate passage of the fetal head.

(Engagement of the fetal head can begin prior to full dilation, but deep engagement usually happens following full dilation as prolonged contractions force the head past -0- station.) A primigravida may take four to 24 hours or longer to dilate completely.

It is not unusual for a multipara to be dilated two or three centimeters as much as six to eight weeks before labor ensues. Some women may dilate almost completely without even knowing it over a period of one to two days. (This is typical of women who have taken the five-week antenatal formula.)

I have delivered a few women whose tone was so good after a third to eighth child that the cervix was like that of a primipara right up to softening and retraction of the cervix. Home birth mothers who have prepared well for the birth will make comments such as, "Are you sure I'm doing anything? I'm not hurting at all!" When you assure her she IS dilating, she will add, "Boy, THIS is the way to go! I never dreamed it could be like this!"

Enemas and "Prepping"

If true labor has been established and the gravida has not had an enema, now is the time for her to take one. (Fecal matter can obstruct labor as well as contaminate the birthing area when she bears down later in labor.)

Very long pubic hair is clipped shorter, but there is no need to "prep" (shave) home birth mothers. (In fact, shaving may increase the rate of maternal infection. There certainly is no reason for shaving in terms of the health of the mother or baby.) It is imperative that the perineum and pubic area be bathed, unless a precipitous birth is in progress. In that instance, pour clean, warm water over the pubic area if there is time.

Setting the (First) Stage

Engage in light and pleasant conversation with the mother and those present at the birth while you wait for first stage to pass. Take advantage of teaching moments if the couple is curious. They should be interested and are usually full of questions. Be truthful, but reassuring. Do not go into gory details about complications, which probably will not appear and will only program the gravida with fear. Do not use the word "pain" in describing contractions. "Discomfort" or "pressure" are more accurate adjectives and will not teach her to think in terms of pain.

During the first stage of labor, the mother may engage in light activity such as walking around the home or yard, or working at nonstrenuous tasks. She may do this until contractions become more intense and she is dilated 5 to 8 centimeters. She may want to rest while sitting occasionally, but her dilation will be accomplished in one-third less time if she is in a vertical position during first stage. The **drive angle** works to an advantage (see Figure 34).

If the membrane does not rupture and the cervix is not too far back, you will be able to feel the membrane tense and bulge at the external os with each contraction. If the membrane breaks, check for possible prolapse of the umbilical cord. This can be very serious and must be dealt with immediately. Cords do not prolapse very often.

The mother may feel like bearing down at certain times during the first stage of labor, but you

First Stage of Labor 263

must not allow her to do so until she is fully dilated. Bearing down prematurely CAN lacerate the cervix.

Be patient. Experience will tell you how often to check dilation and how often to take a fetal heart tone (FHT). Usually once every hour or two is sufficient in early labor.

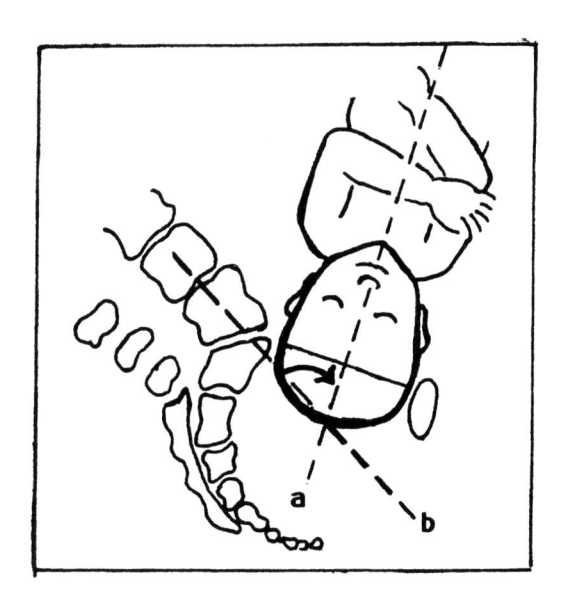

Figure 34. THE DRIVE ANGLE IN LABOR. (a) longitudinal axis of the fetus, (b) axis of the maternal spine. An advantageous drive angle (**arrow**) may be achieved by permitting the mother to remain standing on her feet (or walking around often) during first stage of labor. Progression of labor is better when the drive angle is between 60 and 80 degrees (standing or sitting upright) than when it is 45 degrees or less (lying down).

Dilation should continue to progress to more likely assure a safe outcome. If dilation or progress of labor at term or postterm halts for more than two to six hours, you need to find the reason why. If you have checked everything you know to check (urinary output, position of the baby, the abdomen and cervix during contractions for the proper performance of muscles, progress of the fetal head, etc.), I would suggest that you call another midwife and check to see if you have missed something. (We have spoken often of calling a back-up physician, but sometimes another midwife is equally as helpful. I have received phone calls from midwives all over the country during their labor vigils for just such reasons. As a rule, midwives are happy to consult with each other.)

Just do not allow a LABORING mother to go on indefinitely WITHOUT PROGRESS because sooner or later you are going to encounter problems. The exception is the person for whom all is going well--no distress, but no labor, after having reached five to six centimeters of dilation. The fetus is under no apparent stress, but labor ceases and the mother feels good after some rest and wants to get up and pursue light activity, or just wants to go to sleep and have a good rest. Let her. In this case labor will begin again in perhaps six to ten hours. The important thing is to keep abreast of her condition to ensure that what is taking place is a variation for her labor, but not necessarily abnormal or adverse. DISTRESS IN LABOR WITH LACK OF PROGRESS is the usual clue to an adverse condition that needs help.

AIDS FOR THE LABORING MOTHER

There are several natural things a midwife can do to help the mother relax and to help her labor progress. If it seems that the attendants are to be "on the move" doing things continually during parturition, this is not so. Therapies and such are taught for use when the need for them arises, and they can be extremely helpful in making the laboring mother comfortable.

Femoral Pressure Points

One set of **femoral points** is found at and under the forward angle of the crest of each ilium (see Figure 35). Place your hands with fingers foward over your own hips as if you were going to "read someone the riot act!" Swing them about three inches toward the toes and press down with the middle fingers, and they will very likely land right on the femoral points on each side of the

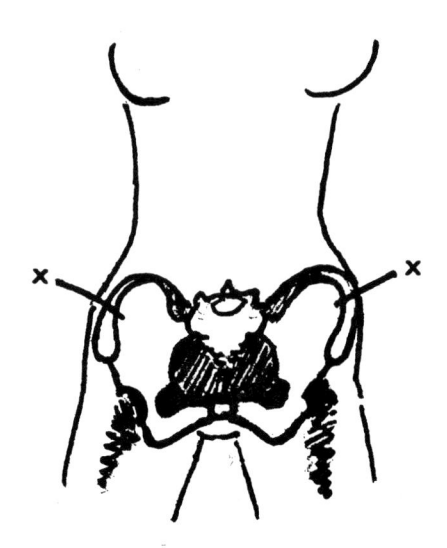

Figure 35. FEMORAL PRESSURE POINTS. One set of femoral pressure points (x) is found where the crests of the ilia turn inward.

body. Find these points on the mother where the bone of the crest of the ilium turns down toward the toes. To relax the mother during or between contractions, dig gently into the underside of each point and press with about four pounds of pressure until all tension releases (about 2 to 3 minutes). The nerves at this spot, when pressed, relax the muscles across the abdomen. (This therapy is useful when a gravida is tired or experiencing too many Braxton Hicks contractions during pregnancy. Add sitz baths and gentle foot rubs for excellent results.)

Sacral Pressure Points

If there is a long, narrow birth canal, a posterior presentation, and/or back labor, pressure to two **sacral points** will give much needed relief from discomfort (see Figure 36). The midwife, her assistant, or the father can apply 2 to 4 pounds of pressure to each side of EITHER the first or second sacral dimples. This is done as follows:

> The sacral vertebrae of the spinal column are found below the lumbar vertebrae, in the flat area across and above the buttocks. Between the vertebrae are dimplelike areas into which will fit the tips of your thumbs or fingers. Pressure here on each side of the spine gives great relief. Hold pressure in the dimples during contractions. Do this until each contraction subsides.
>
> With any back labor, someone's hand, palm up, may be slipped under the parturient's back when she is lying down, just below the small of the back. During contractions, simply cup the hand. Finger tips will give pressure to one side of the spine; the heel of the palm

First Stage of Labor 267

will give pressure to the other side of the spine. If the mother is standing during contractions, apply pressure to these dimples with the thumbs. The parturient may want to lean against the doorpost, a chair, or a dresser during such times.

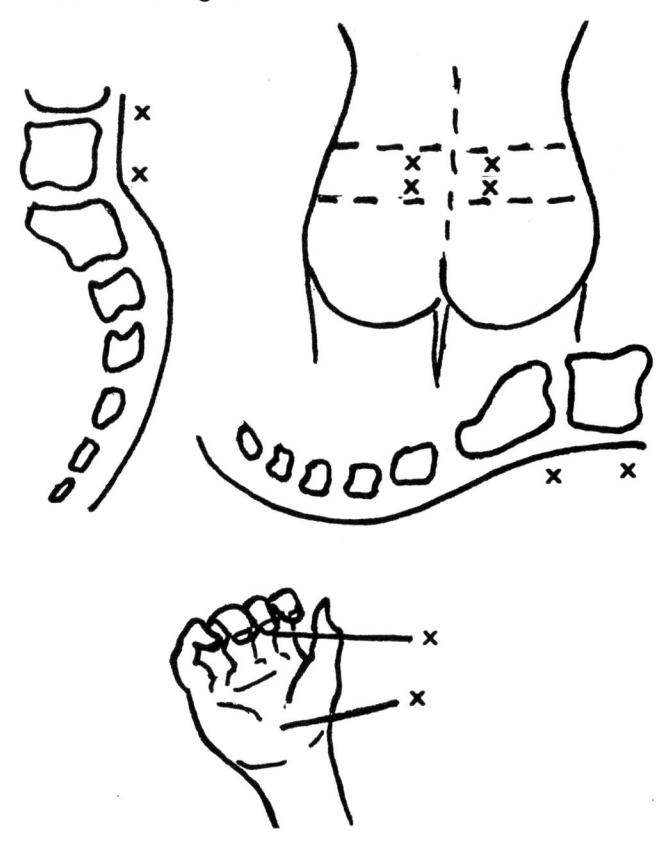

Figure 36. SACRAL PRESSURE POINTS. Shown here are three views of the sacral pressure points (x) in standing and supine positions, and the places on the hand (x) that hold the points when slipped under the parturient in supine position. Apply pressure to either the upper or lower set of points, whichever is more effective.

The parturient will guide your hand to the correct position, for she knows where relief is utmost.

This therapy may be needed during the last two-thirds of labor.

Back Adjustments

Second and third trimesters often bring on tired and sore backs due to postures assumed under the heavy loads of pregnancy, and nothing is more distressing than to go into labor with pain already in the hip, leg, back, or neck. Muscle tension in these areas should be released and the spine should be properly aligned and comfortable. Such problems can distort progress in labor and greatly magnify any discomfort associated with delivery.

Two or three simple maneuvers will often remedy this problem. (Never apply these techniques following accidents or injuries which may have broken bones or seriously misplaced parts. This calls for treatment from experts.)

Soreness between the shoulders can be drastically reduced by having the gravida kneel on the floor and lean over a flat chair seat. Place your hands to the sides of the spine (never ON the spine) at midthorax or at the highest peak (usually right where the bra fasteners meet). Your RIGHT HAND will be closer to you, an inch away from but alongside the spine, with fingers pointing to your left. Your LEFT HAND will be placed alongside the far side of the spine, an inch away, with the fingers pointed in the opposite direction (see Figure 37). Keep your elbows rather straight. Pressure is applied rather deeply, but with a quick, springlike motion with the flat palms of the hand. A GENTLE TWIST OF THE PALMS INWARD (toward the assistant's body), given as the spring action is applied, will relieve the tension-drawn muscles that have maladjusted the spine.

This adjustment may be applied to spots 2 to 3 inches closer to the neck (NEVER ABOVE THE SEVENTH CERVICAL VERTEBRA, the last vertebra to move when the head is bent forward) and to spots 2 to 3 inches toward the waist. The "popping" noises that are heard help you to know the adjustment was made.

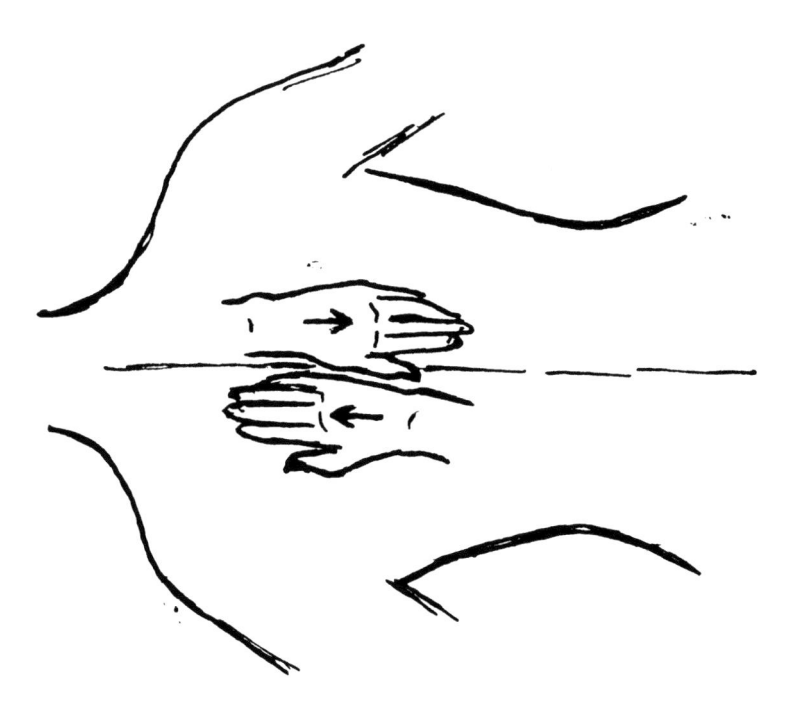

Figure 37. UPPER BACK ADJUSTMENT. Pressure of the thrust comes from the shoulders and is directed through the heels of the hands. The elbows do not bend. Very slight movement is made in the directions of the arrows.

If the gravida will take a deep breath, exhale slowy, and relax, your adjustment is made BEFORE she inhales again. If she is really relaxed, there is absolutely no pain associated with this maneuver. You cannot injure her with 4 to 10 pounds pressure applied thusly if you do not put your palms directly over the spine and if you release the pressure immediately.

A lumbar roll can be done by the gravida herself. She stands erect, swings both arms (near shoulder level) to her LEFT as far as she can. Then while vigorously swinging them back to her RIGHT, she lifts her RIGHT knee as high as possible with a vigorous swing up and toward her LEFT shoulder. IN OTHER WORDS, HER KNEE SWINGS INTO THE DIRECTION HER ARMS ARE COMING FROM. THEY CROSS DIRECTIONS SIMULTANEOUSLY. The arms are then placed to her RIGHT and the LEFT knee is lifted and swung in one smooth, lift-swing action.

This adjustment can also be done another way. The gravida lies on the floor and turns on her side. The bottom leg remains straight, the top leg is drawn up to a point where the foot hangs over the knee of the bottom leg. It helps if someone will hold her top knee ON THE FLOOR to keep it from moving as she makes her upper torso swing backward. She clasps both hands together, shoulder-level, then pulls the upper elbow back to the floor with a quick thrust. Afterward, she gets on her opposite side and positions herself as before to repeat the maneuver in the opposite direction.

Still another way to accomplish the spinal roll is to seek someone's help. The gravida lies on her side as before, with the upper (or both) knees drawn halfway to the abdomen. IF SHE WANTS THE UPPER BACK ADJUSTED, SHE HOLDS EACH OF HER

SHOULDERS WITH OPPOSITE HANDS. The assistant, who is kneeling at the gravida's front, places one hand, midforearm, on her top arm and pushes backward to balance her directly on her side. (If the assistant were to let go of her hold, the gravida would be so balanced she would just as likely roll one way as the other. That is where she should be to get a good adjustment from the following action.) The assistant now places a hand, or inside of elbow, behind the top hip and in one motion vigorously pulls the hips forward and rolls the shoulders back toward the floor.

Do not force the shoulders TO the floor, although some very limber people will indeed easily obtain this position. The whole idea is to roll the spine. You may have unintentionally done this as you have sat behind the wheel of your car and turned to look to the rear to safely back the car out of the driveway. That is all that is happening in this maneuver.

IF THE GRAVIDA WANTS A LOWER BACK (LUMBAR/SACRAL) ADJUSTMENT, while on her RIGHT side, she will place her LEFT hand on her LEFT side at her WAIST. Her RIGHT hand will clasp her LEFT arm on top of the wrist. The assistant holds the gravida's top hand firmly and rolls it only slightly backward, while forcing the HIPS forward. In this position the "twist" occurs from the waist down and adjusts the lower back. A deep "clunking" sound comes from this maneuver if the back is "out" in this area.

Cervical Rimming

You may gently rim the cervix now and then to assist stubborn areas or scar tissue on the cervix to thin out evenly. This can reduce labor time up to 1 1/2 hours.

Rimming is done, during contractions, after dilation to 3 1/2 centimeters, and is simply a gentle "smoothing" of the cervix with lubricated tips of one or two fingers. Your finger tips should not enter the cervix; rather, they rub the exterior edge, or rim, of the cervix, beginning in the center of the thicker rim and smoothing toward the thinner sides until the contraction subsides. If the parturient feels you rimming, you are working too hard. You may be a source of tension or even damage to the area. Rim gently, as needed, until full dilation.

Hydrotherapy

One of the most comfort-giving therapies is that done with warm water. Hydrotherapy is extremely helpful to ease discomfort, soreness, and tension. When hydrotherapy is used, immediate relaxation occurs, soreness abates, and labor progresses with much less distress. Sometimes herbs are used in the water for additional benefits (see Appendix D, Herbs for Hydrotherapy).

Sitz Baths. Sitz baths are discussed in detail in Chapter 9.

Tub baths. Tub baths can be used profitably during early labor. When the parturient is dilated to 3 1/2 or 4 centimeters, give her a warm tub bath (in a thoroughly clean tub) and a cup of blue cohosh tea to drink. She may rest in the warm tub for 20 to 30 minutes. Some parturients do most of their labor in a tub, if labor is not too long (though some women tire if they are in the water too long). There may be a lull in labor for an hour or so after this relaxation, then often good, strong labor will set in. Some practitioners deliver breeches in tubs of deep, warm water to obtain fluid warmth and support to the body and extremities (this doesn't leave room to safely maneuver the baby, though). Others deliver vertex births in tub baths.

Peripacs. Peripacs are a "girls best friend" when she begins to build tension as labor assumes greater proportions. Nothing seems to relax a parturient as much as warm peripacs, used occasionally in late first stage and especially in second stage prior to birth. To make a peripac, dip a hand towel, folded twice, into very warm, sterile water (or water treated with herbalseptic, calendula tincture, etc.). Wring it out loosely and hold it against the parturient's thigh to test the warmth. If it is comfortable to her, apply it to the whole birthing outlet until it begins to cool. Repeat this perhaps once or twice, then cease until needed perhaps once or twice more. You'll find she will relax from head to foot. This kind of relaxation lessens discomfort and expedites birth.

Foot Therapy: The Uterine Reflex

The midwife may use foot therapy to aid in dilation and to take the "edge" off the mother's discomfort.

Years ago, when I first began attending births, a therapy instructor told me that while she was giving birth to her last baby she became aware that there was probably an area on the bottom of the foot that, if found and worked carefully, would assist in childbirth. She insisted that the next time I, or any of those I worked with, delivered a baby, we should check out this possibility. I was the lucky one to discover not only the place on the foot but the advantages to using this spot in affording the parturient much comfort.

This spot on the foot, which I called the **uterine reflex**, is worked with the thumb in a circular motion during contractions, using olive oil to reduce friction. Olive oil does not dry up as quickly as hand lotions do, so your thumb and her foot last longer before tenderness develops. The use of some kind of lubricant enables one to rub more deeply into the muscles and tissues.

Over a 12-hour labor, I discovered the following thing as I worked the uterine reflex:

1. The spot we are concerned with is found at the top center of the pad of the heel (see Figure 38). As the uterus contracts, there is a corresponding, mild, sphincterlike action in this spot on the heel. When the uterus contracts and puts pressure on the cervix to make it dilate, the uterine reflex opens, leaving a rather deep, fluidlike feeling within the spot on the heel. As the contraction reaches its peak and subsides, the muscle structure in the uterine reflex closes up and becomes firm again.[1]

2. When the reflex is worked in conjuction with rimming the cervix (past 3 1/2 centimeters dilation), uniform thinning of the cervical rim--and therefore, labor--is facilitated considerably.

3. Through monitoring of the uterine reflex, a contraction can be detected 3 to 5 seconds before the parturient becomes aware of it, just as a person who is palpating internally can feel the beginning of a contraction when the cervix tenses.

4. Working on the uterine reflex will give considerable relief, lessening the discomfort of

First Stage of Labor 275

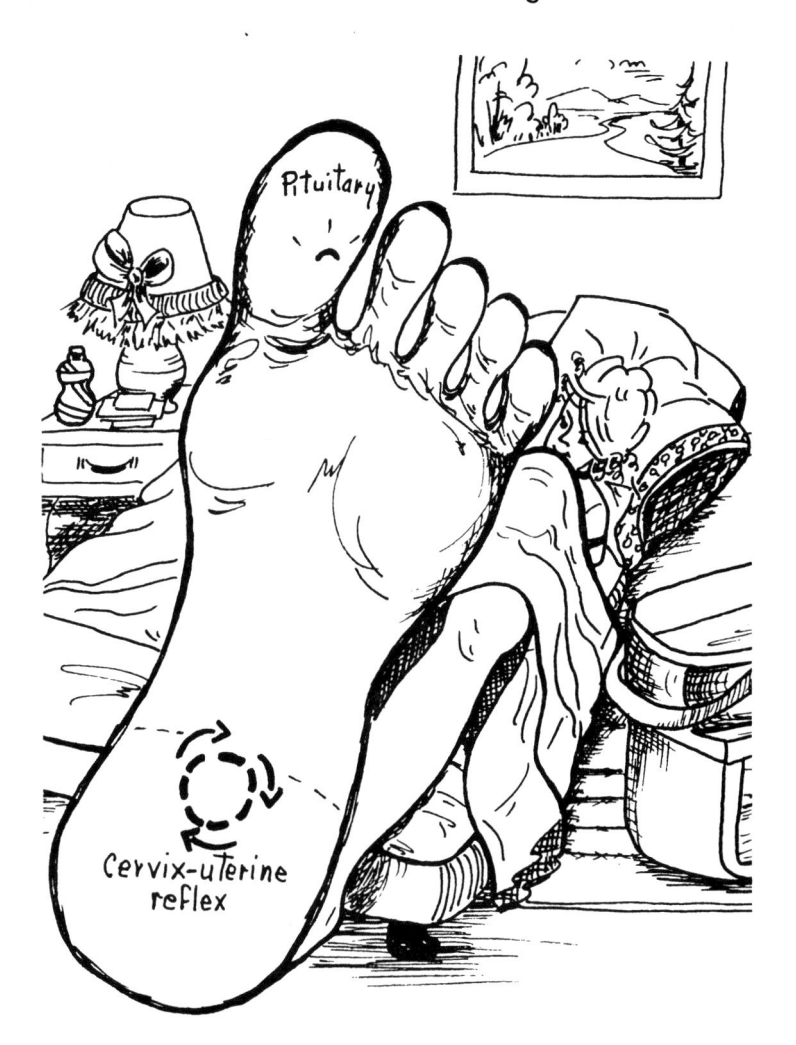

Figure 38. FOOT THERAPY. Working the uterine reflex, particularly during first stage labor and, if needed, during placental separation, is a blessing to laboring mothers. The pituitary pressure point should be held in cases of breech birth until the birth is completely accomplished to prevent uterine inertia from setting in following the birth of the fetal torso.

contractions. The parturient may become so dependent on the relief given that she will call you to your station immediately if she finds you not there when the next contraction begins. When the reflex is worked properly, with depth and firmness of pressure throughout contractions, the parturient is able to relax much more and to cope VERY WELL with the stronger contractions.

5. Working the reflex assists in a cephalic (head) presentation when labor is prolonged, and in frank and complete breech presentations (after 3 to 5 centimeters dilation).

6. There seems to be a cervix-perineum correlation, because if a woman has had two or more episiotomies, or has had many cervical tears during past deliveries, effort to work the uterine reflex is usually wasted. Apparently the scar tissue that results from an episiotomy and from tears inhibits the nerve interaction necessary for the reflex to work as it should. Only one parturient in ten who has scar tissue build-up may still receive help, if her skin is very thin.

7. At 5 centimeters the uterine reflex no longer closes back down between contractions, but remains open and soft. It is possible to determine with great accuracy that dilation has reached this point by using the reflex.[2]

8. Husbands and family members can pick up foot therapy very quickly. Usually in just a short time their fingers become deft at working the foot.

9. While working the heel, you will soon discover that the reflex on one foot feels different

from the reflex on the other foot. Upon close examination, you will find that one side of the uterine reflex on one foot is thick. The cylindrical opening that is round and full on the other foot is not round at all on this foot. This irregularity denotes the SIDE of the body where the placenta is. The approximate PLACENTAL SITE (**placenta reflex**) is indicated by the placement of the irregularity on the circle.

10. When a placenta is slow to separate, work the foot where the placenta reflex is found to encourage separation.

11. Once you have taught others to use the uterine reflex, one of the questions you will be asked is, "What is that little, round knot in the center of the reflex?" Look and you will find them working the opposite foot from the placenta reflex. You will smile. You already know that after the baby is born the little round knot will no longer be there!

12. We have found that when we use rimming and uterine reflex therapy, we rarely encounter anterior lips, unless one is already established upon arrival at the scene. Working this reflex may indeed assist in dispersing the lip.

So, do not discount the integrity or the immense value of this therapy in childbirth. Find someone who is an expert at working the uterine reflex and learn from him or her, then make good use of your skill for the parturient's sake. We have only begun to find the many natural things to be learned about our bodies and their capacity to teach us if we will only pay attention.

Lobelia Tincture

Lobelia applied externally is an excellent aid in childbirth because of its painkilling and relaxant properties. Taken internally, more than one cup of lobelia TEA at the earliest part of labor may cause nausea. Use the TINCTURE, then, in the following ways:

1. Apply tincture to the lower back.

2. Apply tincture across the lower abdomen.

3. Apply tincture to the bottoms of the feet and to the underarms.

4. Give an enema at mid first stage: use 2 to 3 tablespoons lobelia TINCTURE to a quart of lukewarm water after fecal matter has been evacuated.

NEVER take lobelia tea or tincture orally without a stimulant, such as a pinch of capsicum (cayenne). People respond differently to all substances, and the heart muscles of some individuals could relax too much without a natural stimulant added.

Resting Between Contractions

DURING ANY STAGE OF LABOR IT IS IMPORTANT FOR THE MOTHER TO REST BETWEEN CONTRACTIONS TO CONSERVE HER STRENGTH AND ENERGY. Total rest between contractions is crucial during second stage. Labor was correctly named. It takes hard work to push the fetus through the birth canal, and since the parturient may have begun to tire by second stage, she needs strength and control of both labor and her emotions at this point. She vitally needs rest, so remind her to take 1 to 3 deep breaths and to rest in between each contraction. This replenishes the oxygen supply that is somewhat depleted during sustained bearing down.

Any time during first or second stage labor, the parturient should avoid "craning" her neck (lifting or extending the chin). This affects and applies tension to certain back muscles, which in turn decreases sacral mobility, lessens space for the uterus, increases pressure on the main blood supply to the uterus, and aggravates maternal discomfort.

I've seen some midwives encourage mothers to cry if they feel like it during transition and second stage. I do not. There are times when venting emotions is healing, but when a parturient gives way to her emotions with more than a tear or two or more than a groan during a difficult push, she loses momentum. She loses her "oomph" in the strength of her push. She may also have a letdown in her confidence.

Giving way to emotions at this time may lessen a woman's ability to continue as creatively as at first and may cause her to feel disappointment in her efforts. When you assist her to "keep her chin up," she will feel proud that she did not cry.

One girl who had told me several times about her low tolerance for pain explained we'd have to "scrape her off the ceiling." But with help, she didn't even shed a tear and was very brave indeed. The greatest of all was her pride when, with a little support, she surprised herself and was able to handle birth most successfully. Your supportive role here is imperative so that you can help her to cope.

Coaching: The Relax-Rhythm Method

Coaching parturients to relax will erase 70 to 100 percent of their discomfort in labor. I have helped numbers of women who had some discomfort but absolutely no pain.

Coach the mother's breathing as contractions come on. She should be encouraged and praised when she does well. The husband often makes a tremendous coach. He can learn this method quickly with your help, and he loves being useful to his sweetheart. (However, the midwife in charge coaches during second stage.)

During first stage, when the contractions become strong and the mother feels the need, begin to coach her breathing. Tell her to expect two "fizzles," or ineffective contractions, before one good one, then two more ineffective ones and another hard one. To be forewarned is to be forearmed, and this information helps the mother know she is progressing normally.

As the contractions grab and work toward the peak of intensity, wait until a contraction is over before beginning to instruct her. Tell her to completely relax while you help her understand what she must do in order to work WITH and NOT AGAINST the contractions. The following tips will assist her in learning the art of relaxation. Have her do the following "sample breathing" only once or twice, so she doesn't expend energy. Place your hand on her abdomen. Have her pretend her lungs are under your hand. Tell her that is where she must breathe from. Tell her to push your hand up as she inhales and to let your hand fall with her abdomen when she exhales.

First Stage of Labor   281

This teaches her to breathe with her abdomen, not with her chest. Her chest should barely move. It takes only a few contractions for her to get the feel of what is taking place and what must continue to happen throughout the rest of first stage. Once she is pushing the hand up with each breath, then she no longer needs to concentrate so much on pushing the abdomen up—she should be used to it. We don't want her to have to "do" anything but breathe. She will not rub her abdomen or do anything of any kind. By breathing this way, she will be able to assist the contractions, she will feel much less distress, and she will gain confidence in her labor. There may be slight variations used if they entail using your energy, not hers.

In Japan, a woman labors alone in a darkened, quiet room where she can concentrate on her relaxation. When a difficult contraction comes along, she picks a musical tone out of the air, as it were, and hums that single note until discomfort passes. When attendants are with her, they also pick up on that tone and HUM ALONG WITH HER until the contraction subsides.

Though the mother now knows how to work with contractions, you still must coach her with EACH CONTRACTION from that point on throughout labor, just as if she did not know how to breathe! You "talk her" into birthing, much as the ground crew in an airport's control tower talks down an airplane during a storm.

The laboring mother may labor in a chair, leaning on the dresser, lying on her left side—whatever is most comfortable and relaxing.

As you coach, you should speak softly in rhythm with her breathing, possibly a bit slower, since the excitement of having a baby tends to make most parturients breathe a little faster than normal. Say something like, "Breathe in . . . and out. Relax your shoulders . . . and out. And in . . . and out. Unknit your brows . . . and out."

If you notice that she holds her fists closed or her shoulders are a little rigid, say, "Open your hands. That's good. Great! And in . . . and out. Drop your shoulders . . . and out. Lift your tummy . . . and breathe out."

When a contraction reaches its peak, stop coaching and praise her efforts.

If she does not quite have the idea, tell her, "You almost had it that time." When she has done it correctly, tell her, "Great! You see how that helps?" Be honest with her. "The contractions will get harder, but you will be able to handle them if you stay this relaxed." Then help her to maintain relaxation. It is important that she not compare the current contraction with past ones. She must STAY IN THE MOMENT, deal only with present happenings.

It is essential that she relax. Dr. Grantly Dick Read says even bending your finger is tensing. We do not want ANY tension during first stage contractions.

If the mother has practiced and feels confident with another method of coaching, perhaps with her husband's assistance, that is her option; encourage her. However, if she seeks your help, the Relax-Rhythm Method is preferred by most.

PROGRESSION OF LABOR

I want to emphasize here again that there really is no such thing as a normal, routinized, now-this-happens, now-that-happens birth. No two births are alike. Every woman's body is different, every unborn child is different, every birth situation has its unique environment. So no textbook or midwife or obstetrician can tell anyone exactly what to expect in every birth. There may be some sensations that almost every laboring mother experiences, but there will always be exceptions. That's why a midwife's skill in observing carefully is so important. She must be able to pick up what is a complication and what is simply a variation with a particular mother.

There are several things that many mothers experience during the first stage of labor, and if you observe them, they can clue you as to how labor is progressing.

For instance, at the end of first stage, for 8 to 12 contractions, most mothers experience more discomfort than any to this point or afterward (as they finish the last stretch, literally, of cervical dilation). The contractions seem harder, but they are not. They are requiring a final stretch of the cervix and are simply lasting longer. Tell a mother this, so she will know that THESE "HARDER" CONTRACTIONS WILL NOT CONTINUE THROUGHOUT LABOR, nor will they remain so intense after full dilation. Tell her that they are a sign that labor is progressing to the next stage. If she knows this, she will be encouraged. This reminder is vital to her psychological support.

Since the intensity of contractions at this point can be hard to take, the mother may be closer to being discouraged than she will be during the entire birth, and she may fear she won't be able to deal with labor any further. Do not be offended if she abruptly rejects a suggestion, her husband's help, etc., at this point. Allow her a few moments to recoup. Assure her that after these few hard contractions, labor will be much different, and she may even enjoy watching her baby be born. Tell her she will feel great pressure, but NOT INTENSE PAIN after this part of labor (dilation) has ended.

A mother may turn her head once or twice from side to side and wiggle or turn her whole torso as if to help the baby's torso engage and traverse its descent through the bony canal. This occurs mainly in multiparas. She will perspire and need a cold, wet cloth on her face or forehead.

Sometimes, after full dilation, expect another lull as labor makes its transition from first stage to second stage. At other times contractions will come, one on top of the other, in sustained succession.

Uterine Inertia

As a midwife, you may begin to suspect uterine inertia if the parturient has labored for three or four or five hours without any progress in dilation. This is called **primary inertia.** (Slow progress may indicate an obstruction; this will be discussed later.)

Uterine inertia occurs when uterine muscles are so bereft of tone and elasticity that they accomplish little or nothing when they contract. The parturient feels the contractions, but they are strong enough only to make her uncomfortable, not strong enough to dilate the cervix or to push the baby out.

First Stage of Labor

Uterine inertia may become a problem any time, especially with fifth and succeeding pregnancies when elasiticity of the uterus may be reduced. Chances of this problem increase if the first three or four pregnancies occur close together. The uterine muscles may be so tired that they are not able to do their job--that is, to produce birth, to crowd out the placenta, and to contract after birth sufficiently to keep the fundus hard enough to prevent hemorrhage.

If the parturient appears to have mild uterine inertia, your experience may tell you not to interfere at all. She may just be a slow beginner. This slowness to dilate, however, does indicate that her labor may be longer than usual, and you might begin to prepare her for that.

The cup of blue cohosh tea and the warm bath will usually step up labor after she has reached about 4 1/2 centimeters dilation. This timing is important.

Let her go wash her hair or prop her feet up and talk to you for a while. Don't hurry things. Slow labors aren't horrible, they're "nature." So just be patient as long as some progress is being made and both maternal and fetal vital signs indicate that all is well. These conditions--PROGRESS and VITAL SIGNS--are the criteria, in spite of the fact that once in a while the mother may labor a couple of days before giving birth. Rest and nourishment are essential to prevent fatigue.

Secondary inertia occurs when contractions stop altogether. At times this happens when contractions are needed most--during second or third stage. If this happens in the hospital, mothers are usually given Pitocin to speed up labor and make contractions harder. If Pitocin does not accomplish progress in labor, physicians will resort either to an extraction birth, or they will resort to C-section. Both the choice of procedure and the procedure itself depend upon: (1) the current trend, (2) the hospital, and (3) the attending physician. Either of these alternatives carries with it substantial risks.

WHAT TO DO:

Secondary inertia is very rare in carefully planned home births. If you encounter it, do the following:

1. Give the parturient sips of HVC[3] with a medium portion of cayenne (about 1/2 teaspoon if she can tolerate that much, 1/4 teaspoon, if not). Composition powder is especially helpful at this time (see Appendix D, Herbal Composition Powder).

2. Or, add spikenard to 1/2 cup of blue cohosh tea and have her sip it.

As long as the fetal heart rate remains strong, you have plenty of time to work to stimulate the uterus in these ways. If a woman has shown a few signs of inertia toward the end of a fairly long labor and then secondary inertia comes on during second stage when birth is imminent, simply let her turn to her left side and go to sleep (for up to one hour) until contractions resume.[4] If they do not resume within the hour, transport, particularly if the mother shows signs of exhaustion.

The mother must rest completely and have complete quiet while her body recharges so she can finish her labor. When she begins to recognize the return of effective contractions (mild contractions may continue while she rests), it is important that attendants not allow her to turn her body or to expend energy in any way. They must do all this for her. She must conserve all her energy for expelling the baby, and she will have contractions and strength enough to accomplish birth.

Special circumstances may add to the possible occurrence of secondary inertia, such as the rigid muscle tone of the ballet dancer or the worn-out and tired muscles of the grand multipara.

The ballet dancer may be unable to truly relax her muscles. Her relaxation is disciplined, forced-- not real relaxation. She may find it difficult to truly calm her whole system. The grand multipara, whose muscle elasticity is poor, may have muscles that are willing, but seem to get their signals crossed and nothing is really accomplished during contractions.

The preventive measure in both cases is to adhere to a well-balanced program during pregnancy. The dancer should restrict her vigorous muscle concert and allow her whole system to learn to relax fully. The grand multipara should build tension by exercising, especially the abdominal muscles, and walking. She might also take Pituitrophin and Utrophin, simple-structured, natural compounds (**protomorphagens**), prepared from beef extracts, that build muscle tone. Also important for her is motherwort tea (or capsules) and a generous intake of the red raspberry, alfalfa, and comfrey teas. They, along with appropriate foods, will help to supply the calcium and protein, etc., that she needs. The five-week formula will greatly assist with prevention of uterine inertia (see Chapter 9, Polly-Jean Five-Week Antenatal Formula).

Obstructed Labor

Anything that prevents labor from progressing is an obstruction. Exceptionally hard labor, prolonged and without progress, is a key to **dystocia** (dysfunction or difficulty of delivery or birth). Different types of obstructions and how to deal with them follow:

1. Two or more ounces of URINE in the bladder.

WHAT TO DO:

> To PREVENT this problem, be sure the parturient voids frequently during labor.
>
> If edema has set in and the parturient cannot empty her bladder, catheterize by gently inserting a sterile catheter, using aseptic technique, into the urethral opening (the small opening above the vaginal opening; see Chapter 6, The Bladder). Even with the utmost sterile precautions, infection can occur, but you can deal with that later.

2. FECAL MATTER in the lower bowel.

WHAT TO DO:

> To PREVENT this problem, give a tepid water enema early in labor.
>
> Give a tepid water enema in conjunction with foot therapy at those points on the feet and legs that encourage bowel evacuations. (If a woman knows she tends to retain enemas involuntarily, be sure to add 1 teaspoon of salt to the water so she will evacuate easily.)

First Stage of Labor   289

3. A MALPOSITION of the fetus, such as transverse (horizontal) lie.

WHAT TO DO:

A sign of this problem is the protrusion of a sausage-shaped, water-filled membrane from the cervix. This may indicate an irregular pressure on the cervix such as with a multiple birth or a horizontal lie, or it may indicate prolapse of the cord inside the membrane. Touch it to see if the latter is the case. You will feel pulsating in the protrusion if it is the cord (see Chapter 16, Prolapsed Cord, for what to do in this situation).

To correct a horizontal lie, find the head and buttocks. Then, through the abdomen, roll the fetus into a ball if possible. Cup the fetal head with one hand to slowly work the head down toward the pelvic inlet while working the buttocks up toward the mother's heart with the other hand. Keeping the fetus in a rolled-up ball is helpful. A back-and-forth, gentle rocking movement may begin the correction.

In a multiple birth, if the second baby is in a horizontal lie, cup your left hand abdominally over the fetal head, reach with your right hand into the vaginal canal, through the cervix (it will be dilated), and get both feet between your thumb, index and middle fingers. Be sure the cord is not through the crotch. Gently pull the feet down in a pull-rest, pull-rest motion so the birth can proceed normally in a footling position. You have much control this way: the anterior (face down) presentation can be chosen easily, and the infant is slippery and can be turned for best results. Proceed as for breech birth (see Chapter 20, Breech Births).

4. TIPPED UTERUS.

A tipped uterus does not allow the force of labor's contractions to push against the cervix, but pushes instead against some part of the uterine wall, delaying dilation and descent. This labor can go on for a day or more, particularly in the primipara.

WHAT TO DO:

> Have the parturient stand for contractions and elevate her right foot on the seat of a chair and lean onto her thigh. This will lift the weight and position of the fetus to tip the cervix down and forward where it should be so that the contractions can accomplish dilation.
>
> If you have not been able to reach the cervical rim while she was lying down on her back, you may have to go through the vaginal canal (with the whole gloved hand) as she stands and leans against her thigh. This is difficult in some cases, but it can be done. When she becomes tired, hold the cervix as someone helps her to lie down. CONTINUE TO HOLD THE CERVIX DOWN. Be gentle, never forceful in this action. (DO NOT tear the cervix with force!) Doing this will aid dilation, since the force of contractions now will be directed correctly and dilation begins. When you release the cervix it will probably rise again, therefore, continue to hold the cervix in place. This may be tiring. Attendants may have to spell each other off to accomplish normal dilation. This will reduce

labor time by several hours, giving relief and encouragement to the parturient.

If a mother giving birth in a hospital has a fetus high in the womb that "will not come down" or a tipped or tilted uterus, she is usually given Pitocin to speed up labor and make contractions harder. If this is done without bringing the cervix around so that it aligns with the birth canal, then the contractions will push the baby's head against the uterine wall instead of against the cervix. Forcing hard contractions by using Pitocin can result in lacerations of the uterus or can build an anterior lip, causing problems in future pregnancies (see Chapter 16, Anterior Lip).

The hospital may even resort to cesarean section following a long, hard labor. A midwife can manually correct this problem in almost all cases. Assist nature instead of giving up on her and resorting to interventions that pose safety risks to both mother and infant.

NOTES

[1] Working the uterine reflex will not induce labor if cervical effacement has not begun. Sometimes the reflex cannot even be found until true labor sets in.

[2] For over a year and a half, before I began palpating internally, I summoned the doctor to test the accuracy of my determination of cervical dilation, using the uterine reflex. Not once was I mistaken. When our back-up doctors discovered that we were accomplishing so much with therapy and other natural remedies, they began to intensify our training. They realized we were able to understand and manage much more and were ready to accept more responsibility in the births than they had thought.

[3] HVC = 1 T. honey, 1 T. apple cider vinegar, and cayenne (in the amount needed for the occasion) in a full glass of tap water. This is, without doubt, the best oral remedy for tiredness or shock. Rice bran syrup is also excellent for quick energy (and for curbing nausea).

[4] When the body saves its resources for what is most vital to life and gives only its overflow to what is not necessary to survival, it is utilizing Humphrey's Law of Conservation. For example, when a person drinks too much alcohol, he passes out. Why? Because if he remained conscious, he would continue to drink and would kill himself by saturating his blood with alcohol. Nature's way of saving his life is to cause unconsciousness. When his body has had a chance to restore itself, he will regain consciousness. Similarly, a mother who experiences secondary inertia has a body that simply cannot go on without recharging by calling upon its own resources. (See Walter B. Cannon, **Wisdom of the Body**, New York: W. W. Norton, 1939.)

CHAPTER 16

SECOND STAGE OF LABOR: BEGINS WITH FULL DILATION OF THE CERVIX AND ENDS WITH THE BIRTH OF THE BABY

EARLY SECOND STAGE

As the midwife in charge, the first thing to do when the parturient begins second stage is to remind everyone present that you must be in full control. Everyone must yield to your judgment in these crucial moments. You know what is going on, and you are the ONLY one who must coach at this time. No one encourages the mother to push or to do anything else except as they are instructed by you.[1]

When you determine that the cervix is fully dilated and the mother begins to have the urge to push, the first stage of labor is over and second stage is beginning. Full dilation of the cervix allows the head to slip through it. The attendant can no longer feel the cervix that has slipped over the fetal head. The parturient may or may not have experienced a normal 10 to 20 minute lull in her labor, called **transition,** between first and second stages.

The first two to three bearing-down contractions assist good flexion of the head and contractions begin to last 1 1/2 to 2 minutes, frequently following one another without ceasing. Primigravidas may be fully engaged and the fetal head is now feeling the resistance of the vaginal floor; thus, tilting and rotation has begun. Multiparas may be ahead of this process--their infants are usually already rotating.

Palpation at this point will determine any change in position of the vertex. Expect the fetal head to rotate 1/8 of a turn successively with contractions as it travels down the vaginal canal, until the occiput is anterior. (The fetal BODY rotates very little at this point, usually. Its shoulders remain vertical as the head turns; then, the head turns back after it is born to align itself again with the shoulders prior to their presenting.) Palpating for the anterior and posterior fontanels (soft spots) will help you to determine progress. You hope to palpate the SMALLER (posterior) soft spot, which indicates that the head is flexed properly and the occiput is presenting. If the head is not flexed, apply pressure to the forehead with palpating fingers during the next contraction. Usually nature does all this for you.

THERAPIES FOR BIRTH CANAL EXPANSION

During second stage, the mother's bearing-down efforts can be eased and assisted through the use of therapies which help the birth canal to expand. Mothers, particularly those with narrow builds, will greatly appreciate the extra centimeters of room.

Pelvic (-0- Station) Expansion

Inferior Symphysis Pubis Touch. When the fetal head seems to have difficulty transcending the bony canal through stations -2 to +2 (see Chapter 14, Figure 27), insert your index and middle fingers, palm up, about 1 1/2 to 2 inches into the vagina until you feel the bony bridge under the pubic hair. Just hold the fingers there. There is cartilage between where the bones meet, and with this quiet, simple touch, relaxation will occur that assists in giving about an extra centimeter of room. No pressure is needed, just a holding touch until the fetal head moves down (see Figure 39).

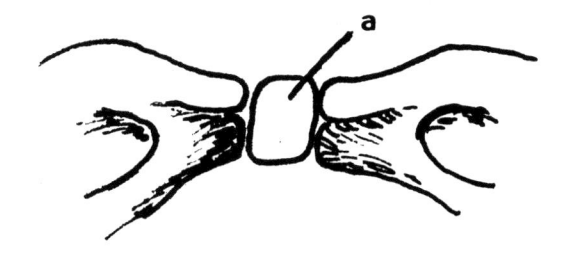

Figure 39. INFERIOR SYMPHYSIS PUBIS TOUCH. During second stage, slip palpating fingers through the vagina to the bony arch found under the pubic hair. Fingers are turned up, and the tips hold the cartilage at the center of the arch, the symphysis pubis (a), with the GENTLEST pressure. Relaxation occurs that allows about an extra centimeter of space for the fetus.

Inferior Sacral Acupressure. For additional room within the canal, palpate externally to the inferior (bottom) edge of the last sacral vertebra while the parturient is on her left side and has her legs slightly drawn up to a comfortable position (see Figure 40). These points are found two inches (right and left) from the middle of the spine, on the underneath side of the last wide vertebra above the coccyx (tailbone). You may have to reach deeply into the flesh. Exert 4 to 6 pounds of pressure to the underneath sides of the vertebra. (Applying pressure with the thumbs to a bathroom scale and practice can help you distinguish the intensity of the force needed.) Direct the force of the pressure toward the middle of the back. This assists in lifting and creating sometimes a full centimeter of room at -0- station and at the sacral promontory. Sustain the pressure until the fetal head feels deeply engaged and is moving on. Relax your pressure between contractions. This therapy relieves back pain occurring at the two upper sacral dimples and gives extra room at the sacral prominence in the birth canal.

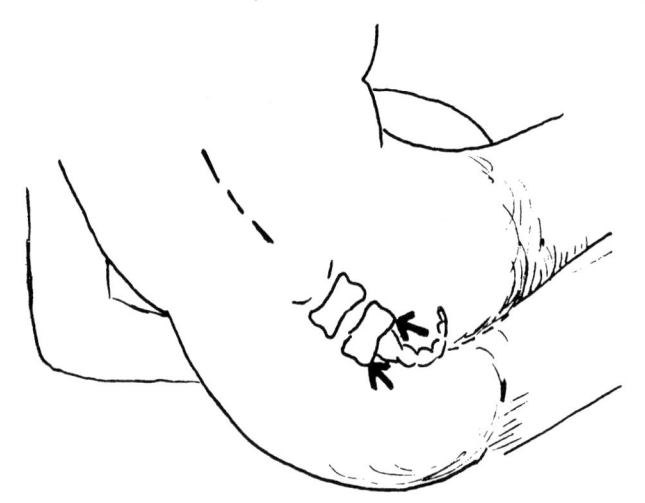

Figure 40. INFERIOR SACRAL PRESSURE POINTS. Four to six pounds of pressure is applied with the thumbs (in the direction of the arrows) to the lower edge of the last sacral vertebra (just above the tailbone) to give an extra centimeter of space at the sacral promontory.

Cervical & Perineal Expansion

Rimming. Rimming, done firmly but gently, is especially helpful as the fetal head passes certain points. It can be done: (1) on the cervix (see Chapter 15, Cervical Rimming, and this chapter, Anterior Lip), (2) inside the vaginal opening as the head appears, and (3) on the perineum as the face sweeps internally over the perineum proper (see this chapter, Controlled Crowning). More uniform expansion of tissue is accomplished when rimming is correctly done.

Peripacs. Warm water peripacs are of great immediate help when used periodically during second stage if this stage is taking longer than about 45 minutes (see Chapter 15, Hydrotherapy). Expansion of tissue and of the bony structure of the birth canal results when total relaxation is accomplished. Hydrotherapy here is unquestionably profitable.

ANTICIPATING, PREVENTING, AND CORRECTING PROBLEMS

At this stage in labor, it is possible for complications to show up. Just in case they do, be prepared to manage them properly.

Fetal heartbeat is taken frequently if any doubt about it arises. Excessive fetal activity can be a sign of fetal stress, so any time the mother notices the baby moving more than usual, auscultate (listen to its heart). Any change in FHR--20 or more beats above or below normal for that fetus--is significant. A drop of 10 to 20 beats during contractions is significant if in 10 seconds there is not a normal recovery between contractions. If this happens, have the parturient turn to her left side to labor for a while.

This will relieve some of the pressure on the fetus and provide more oxygen. If this correction helps, and it usually does, she may even deliver on that side.

If the FHR becomes irregular, a weak heart is suspected. Again, have the parturient change positions and see if that helps. Excessive, persistent irregularities in FHR that will not correct must be transported immediately unless birth is imminent.

In second stage, from about -3 to -0- station, check every few minutes for the possible development of adverse situations.

Anterior Lip

An anterior lip is one that has formed on the anterior (front) rim of the cervix. It resists the passage of the baby's head down and out of the uterus. Contractions are pushing the baby's head against this lip of the cervix and, though dilation may be near completion, it is very difficult for the baby's head to progress down the birth canal under this circumstance. Once there has been an anterior lip, it is apt to repeat in succeeding births. This dystocia may show up in the last part of first stage, prior to full dilation, or the mother may be fully dilated but the lip is preventing her pushes from moving the baby past the cervix. An unusual amount of pain may be felt low on the abdomen if an anterior lip is present.

The lip is usually somewhat thick, especially if it has been there long enough to have developed edema (swelling). The baby's head butting against the pubic bridge will cause this swelling. The force of contractions pushing the fetal head against the cervix can cause lacerations and that may certainly cause worse problems in future deliveries.

WHAT TO DO:

>Most anterior lips can be prevented by rimming the lip and watching the fetal head positions. It is best to catch the problem and begin to rim before swelling begins, but if you do not, the only solution is to hold the lip up the best you can with two or three fingers and let the fetal head slip under and through.

>For parturients with normal builds, 45 minutes is a good average time for a controlled second stage in home births. With primiparas, a longer period of time is safe and may be extended if the gravida has a slightly contracted or a narrow pelvis. If second stage is much shorter than 45 minutes, the baby is probably moving down the birth canal too quickly and in many cases the mother will tear.

Narrow Build

Most narrow pelvic builds will have opened quite a bit by term. During labor, however, the baby's head may take as long as six hours to **mold**[2] so that it is able to pass through the birth canal. A narrow build is not USUALLY a complication in an ultimate anterior vertex presentation; it simply requires patient waiting and close monitoring of the fetal heart tones. Frequent peripacs soaked in lobelia tea, mineral water, or comfrey tea help the parturient return to relaxation. Inferior symphysis pubis and sacral acupressures will greatly assist labor.

Having palpated early in labor (and also during prenatal exams), you will already be aware of this narrow build and will have prepared the mother for a longer labor. Reassure her that although her labor is slow, the birth is normal. She will not mind working hard and laboring long if she knows why, and if she knows that nothing abnormal is happening. If she is psychologically well prepared for a long labor, she will be pleasantly surprised when you say, "I can see the baby's hair!" REST BETWEEN CONTRACTIONS, AND NOURISHMENT, ARE VITAL TO THIS PARTURIENT.

Meconium Staining

When the baby is in stress for any reason, it will usually have a bowel movement. If this happens in utero before the baby's head is fully engaged, it may aspirate the expelled waste, which is called **meconium.** This can be dangerous. The amniotic fluid will be discolored (this is called **meconium staining**) to warn you of the degree of stress experienced. (Suctioning or stomach aspiration at birth may need to be done if heavy meconium staining is found.)

A bowel movement during the second stage of a cephalic (head-first) presentation is of little consequence if the head is past -0- station and birth is imminent.

If the baby has bowel movements 3 or 4 days before labor begins, it will be ingesting its own poisons and will be in serious trouble by the time it is born. If there has been this degree of meconium staining of the amniotic fluid, you will notice heavy discoloration of the fluid when the bag of waters breaks. You may even notice a greenish hue to vaginal discharge.

Second Stage of Labor   301

When there is a discoloration and birth is imminent, go ahead and deliver. If the staining of the fluid is dark, the baby can be in serious trouble. Suction carefully, but transport, because life-support systems need to be available. The baby can be born dead after a prolonged time in amniotic fluid with heavy meconium staining.

If the mother's water breaks before labor or at the onset of labor before the attendant is present, the mother should catch some of the water on a white towel or in a container so the midwife can inspect the fluid for meconium stainning when she arrives.

Eclampsia

If things have gone well during checkups late in pregnancy, it is unlikely that serious eclampsia will ensue before delivery--unlikely, but not impossible. The midwife must know the signs of PRE-ECLAMPSIA and know what to do about them in parturition (during childbirth). If birth is not imminent and signs are manifest, transport immediately. But suppose a midwife comes on the scene of a birth that is imminent and eclampsia is also evident. She must know how to protect the mother and baby while she completes the delivery.

Moving (transporting) an eclampsic parturient during the potentially dangerous delivery of a baby would be less wise than carefully carrying out the delivery. Getting the baby born is the only thing that will turn the tide of the mother's difficulties and let nature help her body to return to a normal state postpartum. This return to normal is more likely if fits (convulsions, seizures) are prevented.

Early signs of eclampsia in parturition are:

1. Greenish, earth-brown, meconium staining of the amniotic fluid. You may notice this staining when the bag of waters breaks, or it may even be noticeable in vaginal discharge. Blood pressure will be elevated.

2. Visual disturbances, such as headaches, dimming, milky appearance in the eyes, blurring, eyes rolling sideways or upward, and sharply elevated blood pressure.

3. Cyanosis (the body becomes blue or grey because of lack of oxygen), body edema, vomiting, pain in the abdomen.

The four stages of eclampsia are:

Premonitary stage or **stage of invasion** (lasts 10 to 20 seconds): restless behavior; twitches or unusual sensation around parturient's face or head; head drawn to one side; eyes rolled sideways or upwards.

Tonic stage or **stage of contraction** (lasts 10 to 20 seconds): body rigid, in state of muscular spasm; teeth clinched; eyes stare; she becomes cyanotic (blue).

Clonic stage or **stage of convulsion** (lasts from 60 to 90 seconds): violent contractions may throw parturient out of bed; face is congested and distorted; pulse full and pounding.

Stage of coma (lasts minutes or hours): it is possible that the parturient wil become extremely drowsy and go into a deep coma WITHOUT CONVULSIONS or convulsions may even occur without her regaining consciousness. Eclampsia often ends in death.

Second Stage of Labor   303

If fits can be PREVENTED, recovery is more likely.

At the FIRST EARLY SIGNS of ANY of these symptoms, you MUST take the following measures IMMEDIATELY:

1. Take the phone off the hook. (Have someone go to another phone, out of hearing distance, to summon the doctor.)

2. Do not drop ANYTHING.

3. Do not flush toilet or turn on taps.

4. Do not allow any doors to be opened, closed, or slammed.

5. Prevent door-knocking; quickly prevent unexpected visitors.

6. Whisper.

7. Allow no talking by others--tell them the mother needs quiet.

8. Have a calm, confident attitude.

9. Do not display any hurried or agitated movements.

10. Give the mother magnesia phosphorica homeopathic cell salts: 15 tabs each minute on her tongue, for 3 to 5 times. This may ward off a convulsion or prevent succeeding ones.

11. Darken the room so that the light is only sufficient to perform tasks. Do not let any light shine in the mother's face, and do not allow the light to be turned on and off.

12. Coach the mother with quiet encouragement.

If the mother convulses:

1. Have someone help you see that she does not fall from the bed by guiding her body, not by using restraint.

2. Have someone in the room (an assistant, the husband) place the index and median fingers of each hand through the spaces between the mother's great, second, and third toes of each foot. (Work from the bottom side of the feet.) Force, if possible, the feet to turn toward the knees, then hold this position until the convulsion stops. Doing this should bring the mother right out of the convulsion.

3. Do all you can to keep the baby from projecting from the vagina, as it sometimes does during a convulsion. If the baby is not born with the first contraction during a convulsive episode, the mother will likely quiet down until the next contraction. It may take several contractions to bring the baby out.

4. Have someone in the room hold the muscles at the top of the mother's shoulders and close to the neck, with a firm grip that DOES NOT HURT or cause injury.

5. Have everyone in the room remain quiet and still. All should speak softly if communication is needed.

6. You may suggest, without panic, a prayer or blessing for the mother and child, while you continue with your work. Ask in a matter-of-fact exercise of dependency on faith in Diety.

    As soon as the baby is born and taken care of, have an assistant care for it while you take the mother's blood pressure. (In most cases the fetus is stillborn or dies shortly after birth.) If within two hours after the birth the blood pressure goes no more than five points higher and stabilizes, then begins to fall back toward normal, the mother will be all right. If she is going to have additional problems, they will show up in those two hours after birth. If the blood pressure continues to rise, and the doctor has not arrived, transport her immediately or call the paramedics. Convulsions usually abate after delivery if the mother does not have a history of prepregnancy or prenatal toxemia. They may not develop at all if the mother has taken the precautions described in Chapter 8, Diagnosis of Pre-eclampsia.

Your back-up doctor should check the infant for any damage and help to assess the need for hospitalization of the mother or baby or both. When contacted, the doctor will want to know the current vital signs and the Apgar score of the infant. Be prepared to give these to him.

Excessive Bleeding

If at any time during first or second stage the mother begins to bleed excessively, one of two things may be happening:

1. THE PLACENTA MAY HAVE SEPARATED TOO SOON. (This is accidental and not related to anything the mother or attendants may have done.) This is called **abruptio placenta** and is very serious. The mother should be transported immediately, but before transporting you should give her cold shepherd's-purse tea with one-half teaspoon of cayenne (the tea should not be warm or hot). The mother should

be hospitalized (see also Chapter 11, Abruptio Placenta).

The mother's life is in the balance with a **complete premature separation** of the placenta any time during pregnancy or early labor. The baby will invariably die unless delivered by C-section within minutes. If there is only **partial separation,** the shepherd's-purse will likely stop the bleeding until the baby is born, providing labor is not prolonged. In this case, the baby can probably be saved.

The problem with abruptio placenta is that when the bleeding has stopped you still don't always know how much of the placenta has separated, or if brain damage has occurred. The shepherd's-purse is a safety measure for hemorrhage for both mother and child. Constant heart monitoring is essential, then, in guiding the decisions that have to be made, such as how long to allow labor to continue and whether to C-section the mother immediately.

2. THE MOTHER MAY HAVE TORN SEVERELY AT THE CERVIX, UTERINE WALL, OR VAGINAL FLOOR. Shepherd's-purse tea (with cayenne, as above) or HVC will stop the bleeding and give you time to transport or to deliver if birth is imminent, or to deliver while enroute.

Though not normal, slight bleeding during first or second stage is not considered serious. A few women bleed up to one-half a sanitary pad (1/3 cup) as the cervix dilates the first 2 or 3 centimeters. The bleeding is usually due to: (1) lack of elasticity of cervical tissue, (2) scar tissue from previous tears, etc., or (3) tension experienced by the mother in labor. One mother bled 1/2 to 2/3 cup over a period of hours in early labor with her first three or four children. By following the home birth program, she has not bled at all before third stage with the last three births.

If the mother has taken sitz baths regularly, has followed a good dietary program, and rimming has been carefully done during first stage, the cervix is unlikely to tear. However, the cervix sometimes tears slightly and the vaginal mucosa (tissue) may also tear in spite of good management.

Transverse Head Arrest

As the fetal head comes down the birth canal, it normally tilts and rotates internally, but if the baby's chin does not flex when the head reaches the ischial spines as it should, it can become wedged tightly and may not move on through the canal. With the strong contractions that introduce the fetal head into the smallest area it must go through to be born (-0- station), the chin should be forced down onto the upper chest in order for the crown of the head to move down first. This allows the little pointed head, if you will, to go through the tight spot first. If the crown does not go down first, the hard contractions could cause the head to get stuck, much like a square peg caught in a round hole. This is called **head arrest.**

If the natural pivoting of the crown is prevented, several things may happen. The head may arrest with the fetal brow (eyebrow/forehead area) facing either of the mother's hip sockets. If the chin does not flex properly and YET IT DOES pass through the canal without arresting, then expect that there may not be a normal rotation, perhaps even a posterior presentation (occiput posterior, face up). A brow or chin (face) presentation may result.

The fetal head has to adapt to all the diameters of the pelvis as it turns and tilts and moves through the various segments of the pelvis. Most of these movements are happening simultaneously. Nature usually maneuvers birth just as it should be done.

If you have noticed during prenatal or labor exams that the floor of the mother's vagina is flat, hot, and dry, then you should be especially alert to the transverse head arrest problem. A vagina that does not have the right curved incline cannot help the contractions to introduce the necessary flexion of the baby's head as easily.

Having discovered a flattened pelvic floor, you will be alerted to the possible head arrest, so you will be watchful as the strong contractions continue. If dilation has occured to a point where you can freely palpate the posterior fontanel (SMALLER soft spot at the crown of the head), there probably will be no problem. If, however, at full dilation you can feel only the sagittal suture across the cervix, then the head is still in a transverse lie: the forehead, as a contraction builds pressure, can be pushed forward (toward the baby's chest) to encourage flexion.

If there IS a transverse head arrest, have the mother get on her hands and knees and do three or four pelvic rocks. Doing this lifts the baby's own weight off its head and "sloshes" the baby back out of the pelvic inlet, giving it a chance to flex as it should. (Effective labor continues when you find the small fontanel progressing.

Second Stage of Labor   309

This is good. The head then smoothly leads the way for the fetal body to continue its course. The head crowns under the bony prominence of the pubic arch: it no longer recedes a little back and forth, but begins to open the vulva to start its external crowning.

However, if labor does not progress because of the head arrest, and if with a few more pelvic rocks the head does not disengage from the transverse arrest and you cannot encourage flexion of the head, you will need help. (As long as labor progresses, vaginal delivery is best.)

If the flexion of the head has not been accomplished but labor progresses, expect a malpresentation such as a brow or chin presentation (see Chapter 20, Face Presentations).

Shoulder Arrest

You might suspect a shoulder arrest when you see the head part the vulva at about +2, +3 station, then slide back repeatedly. Even in normal second stage labor the baby's head makes some progress, then regresses between contractions, but when it does this more than usual and reluctantly continues to progress to full crowning, begin to check some things out. Little boys sometimes have large shoulders, and in a shoulder dystocia, the baby's shoulder can become wedged between the mother's pubis and the sacral promontory, or behind the coccyx and the pubic arch, and it cannot turn and move smoothly through and out of the birth canal.

WHAT TO DO:

>Though it is uncomfortable for the mother, and a tight, stretched fit for the baby's neck,

you may have to reach inside the vagina with your fingers to free the baby's shoulders. Time is a factor, but caution is paramount. EXCESSIVE TRACTION (PULLING) ON THE BABY'S HEAD OR NECK CAN CAUSE SERIOUS INJURY. (Twisting the baby's head to move the baby will accomplish nothing but harm.)

The head is usually born, so first clear the mouth and nose, IF NEEDED. Then you must go in BEHIND the head and move the baby's shoulder toward its chest, and to the right or left, while at the same time you push GENTLY backward on the head (to allow more "give" for the shoulders).

Move the upper (anterior) shoulder away from the symphysis pubis, and the lower (posterior) shoulder away from the coccyx. If one shoulder won't move in either direction, try the other one. Sometimes it is possible to slip the posterior arm across the baby's chest and bring it out. Then rotate the shoulders slightly and deliver the anterior shoulder. Assistance from the abdominal side may be useful. The PARTURIENT may also roll to the left to help free the shoulder.

Cord Stress

It is normal for the head to move forward, then back a bit, two to three times with contractions as it moves through and past -0- station in second stage. However, if it continues to do this more than 3 or 4 times, and there does not prove to be a shoulder arrest, check the fetal heart rate again to see if there may be a cord stress. Consider what happens to a long, rubber balloon when it is stretched: it gets narrow. Like the balloon, the umbilical cord, when stretched, also gets narrow and restricts blood and oxygen flow through it. **Stress** is indicated by a rapid increase of 15 to 20 or more beats per minute above normal. After the increase, if the heart rate does not return to normal when the contraction subsides, serious problems are indicated. (This problem, though rare, can be responsible for a fetus not engaging sufficiently to dilate the cervix or to be born.)

An IRREGULAR heartbeat is serious and needs immediate attention. This condition is often a consequence of uncorrected **bradycardia** (abnormally SLOW heart rhythms) or **tachycardia** (abnormally FAST heart rhythms). If correction is not immediate, C-section is indicated.

Whenever the fetal circulatory system is in serious trouble, the fetal pulse goes high at first, because the heart pumps faster to compensate for the lack of circulation. Very soon, if the problem is not resolved, the pulse slows down and stops. So when the fetus has a slight lack of oxygen, the pulse rate and FHR will increase some. This is nature's way of saying, "Check things out!" or "Do something!"--before "stress" reaches "crisis."

Usually nature will take care of slight stresses from time to time without your interference. Your first obligation, however, is to know what is happening, then to observe to see whether nature is handling it adequately.

If the FHR alters without apparent recovery, you DON'T WAIT for nature; you ASSIST nature by doing the following:

WHAT TO DO:

1. Have the parturient turn to her left side. Turning may eliminate pressure to the cord if a shoulder or other body part is pressing against it. If the FHR does not recover or correct, and birth is imminent (the head is past -0- station), have the parturient bear down and give birth as soon as possible. The baby likely can be saved.

2. When the head is born under these circumstances--it may be very cyanotic ("blue," due to lack of oxygen)--check quickly to see if the cord is around the neck and perhaps under an arm or just going down the back. If the cord is extremely tight, and will not slip over the head, clamp it TWICE quickly at the easiest-to-reach portion of the cord and cut between the clamps. Unwind the cord and have the mother push the baby out; proceed with clearing the nose and mouth and helping the baby to breathe and cry.

3. If the baby's birth is not imminent and the FHR is persistently 20 beats or more high (or low), give the mother 800 units of Vitamin E (in capsules) and 1/2 teaspoon cayenne in cold water and transport.

4. If the FHR is not correcting, the baby's birth is not imminent, and/or there is bleeding in any amount, transport immediately. Under these circumstances, the placenta may be breaking loose (separating) prematurely because of the stress on the cord. Or, the FHR may be high and the cord is in good shape, but the placenta is separating for some other reason. In this case the mother's pulse rate will increase sharply, also.

Experience will tell you when and if to hurry or to transport. In one birth where the FHR had fallen to 90, and birth was imminent, we carried out birth quickly and found the cord wrapped around the baby's neck three times, under an arm and through the crotch. The rest of the cord was so short that the infant pivoted and huddled against the vaginal opening as if it would return to the womb at the first possible moment. When we unwound the cord, we found that it was quite short (16 inches) and could have posed a serious problem even if it had not been wrapped around the baby's neck.[3]

While CORDS AROUND FETAL NECKS ARE COMMON--up to five out of ten births--and seldom pose serious problems,[4] it is that unusual occurrence that a midwife must be prepared to handle adequately.

In another birth we found the cord so short that the fetus had to pivot around the placenta all during gestation. During delivery the FHR began to lower, but with birth imminent the safest thing to do was to get the baby born. So, we asked the mother to bear down hard. The baby was born, but as its body came out the cord was thin and white with no blood in its vessels and it broke immediately. The placenta end was caught, luckily, before it slipped back into the mother and the fetal end was clamped between finger and thumb. An assistant quickly clamped the two ends with forceps so attention could be turned to the infant. There was no bleeding, so the placenta had not been compromised, but then we saw the very short cord! (The cord length was measured after the placenta had presented and the total length was 8 inches.)

The infant was born with clubfeet, perhaps as a consequence of this extremely short cord. It is also possible that lack of proper nutrition throughout gestation may have contributed to the inadequacy of the cord. (Most clubfooted infants can be corrected within 12 months, if correction is begun the day of birth. It is no small miracle that this baby lived at all under the circumstances.)

Cord Knots

It is rare, but sometimes a cord comes out with a **true knot** in it. At some time (probably during early gestation) the baby slipped through its own looped cord. Because of the water environment of the uterus, the knot seldom cinches up tightly enough to shut off oxygen and nutrition to the fetus, so even rarer than the knot is a complication arising because of it.[5]

A **false knot** is one in which one or more of the vessels inside the amniotic sheath doubles back and causes a thick, peculiar-looking shape of the cord at that point (see Chapter 6, Figure 10). This does not usually cause problems.

Prolapsed Cord

ONE TYPE OF PROLAPSED CORD occurs when part of the cord finds its way down ahead of the presenting part, INSIDE the unruptured amniotic sac. A sausage-shaped protrusion can be felt pulsating inside the sac by palpating through the vagina or rectum.

ANOTHER PROLAPSED CORD is one that is flushed down and OUT of the amnion (bag of waters). This often occurs when the water breaks at a point close to the cervix. The cord will not usually prolapse with dribbles and small amounts of escaping fluid. However, when a real flush of water emits, check

Second Stage of Labor 315

for a prolapse, even though the gravida may not see the cord. This can occur BEFORE or DURING labor. Usually the rupture that occurs high in the amnion will allow continuous dribbles. Rupture nearer the cervix allows more of a flush of fluid, and the CORD CAN FLUSH DOWN AND OUT OF THE VAGINA.

Cord prolapses are rare in cephalic presentations. They happen more often in multiple births (horizontal lies) and some types of breech presentations—instances in which there isn't a solid body part blocking the cord from descending below the presenting part. If you should come across a cord prolapse, consider these ways of dealing with the situation:

WHAT TO DO:

Prolapse WITHIN the amnion:

WHEN THE MEMBRANE IS INTACT, but a knuckle of the cord protrudes (however slightly) and pulsates within it, IN FRONT OF THE PRESENTING PART, a knee-chest position will usually draw the fetus and cord back up into the uterus. Should the head be rather firmly engaged, it can be dislodged with one or two fingers in the vagina or rectum. After the cord has receded, the fetal head may be pressed into the pelvis and "fixed" to prevent another prolapse. Unless well into labor, keep the membrane intact if at all possible.

Prolapse OUTSIDE the amnion, prior to or in EARLY LABOR:

If a mother calls to say her water has broken and flushed rather profusely, the umbilical cord may have prolapsed. Have her IMMEDIATELY

GET DOWN INTO A KNEE-CHEST POSITION (knees and chest touching the floor or bed and buttocks high in the air) until you arrive (see Figure 41). This shifts the baby's head back away from the pelvic inlet, so that if there is a prolapse, the weight of the baby will not press against the cord, shutting off circulation. (Remember, the cord is the life line through which the baby gets oxygen until it is born.) The mother should do a few pelvic rocks, then resume the knee-chest position. This combination alone may encourage a prolapsed cord to withdraw inside the uterus.

THE MOTHER NEEDS TO BE CHECKED FOR CORD PROLAPSE after a FLUSH of amniotic fluid. If she is unable to reach you, or if you are unable to get to her within a short period of

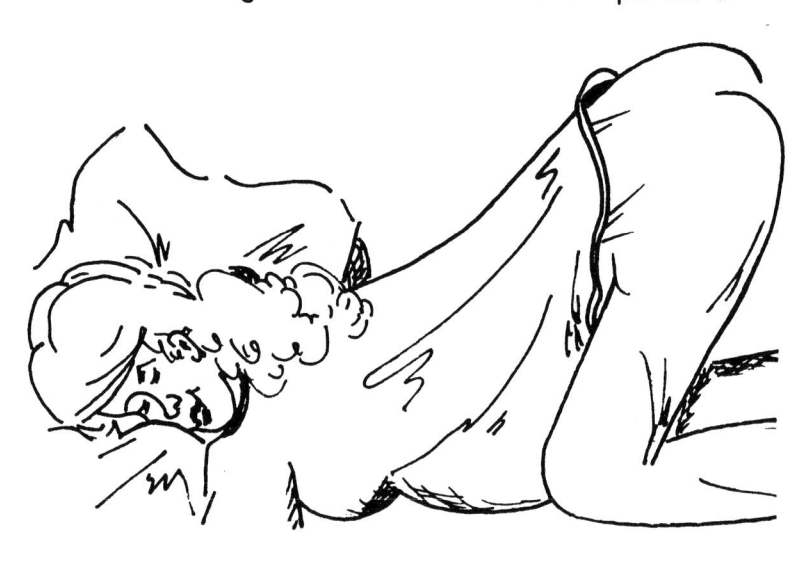

Figure 41. KNEE-CHEST POSITION. Chest is on the floor. Knees should be perpendicular (at right angles to the hips). Keep back as straight as possible.

time, she should be transported in a knee-chest position. If there has been a prolapse of the cord outside the vaginal cavity, the cord should be gathered back inside the vaginal cavity, if possible, to keep it moist and warm, or else the exposure will cause it to atrophy and occlude (close off).

If you are able to reach the mother quickly, and there has been a prolapse, you may be able to save the baby and avoid transporting. Scrub and rinse quickly and check the cord with WET hands (you don't want your hand to rob any moisture from the cord; the mother may lie down while you check). If the cord has stopped pulsating, the fetus may be dead already. If it has not stopped pulsating, it is probably because the mother has remained in the knee-chest position and prevented pressure from closing off circulation in the cord.

After you find the prolapse, have the mother once again move to a KNEE-CHEST POSITION while you try to work the cord back INTO THE UTERUS, NOT JUST BACK INTO THE VAGINAL CAVITY. You must get it back into the uterus, then BACK BEYOND THE FETAL HEAD. Work quickly: the cord must be replaced before it dries, and any stress to the baby's circulation must be alleviated. Reinsertion is not always easy, but it can be done.[6] There is a slight risk involved, that of **air embolism** (sudden blockage of a blood vessel by an air bubble),[7] but if no other recourse is at hand, this procedure may save the baby's life.

The mother will be uncomfortable while you work--your whole hand must reach inside to go far enough up to replace the cord, and you haven't much working room--but the mother will cooperate beautifully for you to be successful. You may work the cord back up a bit, then have her try a few pelvic rocks to see if that will help pull the cord further back inside.

Another thing you might use to assist with the reinsertion is a rubber or plastic catheter which has been prepared for this use (see Figure 42). The catheter has a hole in the side, near the top, and an open end at the bottom. Umbilical tape (cord, string) is doubled, then threaded through the tube and the loop comes out the opening. The umbilical cord is secured against the catheter by pulling the loop of tape over the funis and hooking it over the top of the catheter.

Hold the ends of the catheter tape securely but not tightly enough to occlude the cord, as you slide the catheter and cord into the

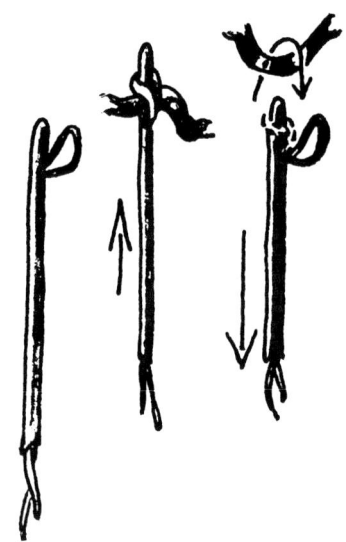

Figure 42. CATHETER FOR REINSERTING PROLAPSED CORD.

uterus and beyond the presenting part. If it meets resistance, gently turn the catheter from side to side, but DO NOT FORCE entry of the catheter (or pull the catheter backward--the loop will release the cord prematurely). When in place, release the tape ends, then gently turn and wiggle the catheter down and out. (With the tape ends released, opposition from the funis pulls the loop back over the top of the catheter, freeing the cord completely.) Cord replacement by hand is preferable, but use of the catheter may be called for. And, of course, great care must be taken.

IF THERE IS NOT ENOUGH DILATION OF THE CERVIX TO FACILITATE RETURNING THE CORD, simply hold your index and middle finger to each side of the cord where it comes out of and returns to the cervix to prevent pressure from the fetal head or cervical os from closing off the circulation coming through the cord (see Figure 43). The mother can indeed be transported in this position (and possibly on her left side, if pressure against the cord is lessened) while your fingers guard the cord at that site. Do not let anyone at the hospital talk you into letting go of the cord protection until doctors are completely ready to deal directly with the baby in utero.

Prolapse OUTSIDE the amnion, in LATE LABOR:

It is POSSIBLE that at the precise moment when the mother feels the strong, "uncontrollable" urge to bear down in second stage, that the amnion will rupture; the force of this bearing-down contraction and the flush of the amniotic fluid can move the cord and the biparietal diameter of the head into -0-

320 POLLY'S BIRTH BOOK

station together, wedging them in a tight fit! (The FHR will tell you so, if you are auscultating at this time.) Have the mother do about three pelvic rocks, QUICKLY, before the next contraction. While the mother is in knee-chest position, GIVE A SLIGHT PUSH ON THE BABY'S HEAD, BACK TOWARD THE FUNDUS, if possible, and return or protect the cord, unless birth can be accomplished relatively soon (less than about 10 minutes).

If prolapse occurs after the widest part of the presenting head (**biparietal diameter**) has passed -0- station, have the mother push and get that baby born as quickly as is safely possible.

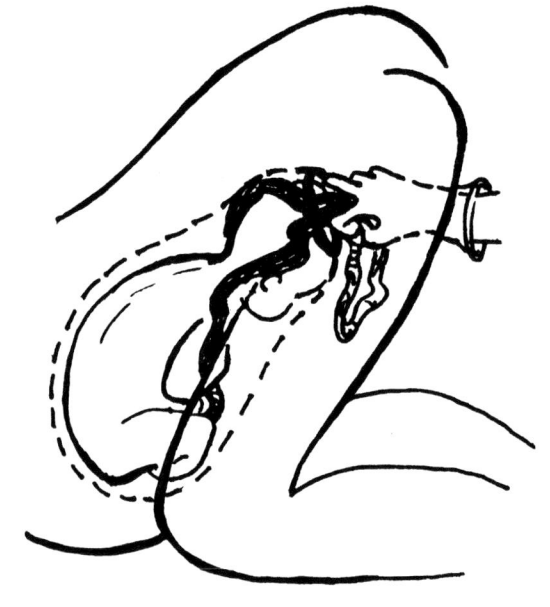

Figure 43. TRANSPORTING SUPPORT FOR PROLAPSED CORD. The knee-chest or lateral positions will lessen the pressure of the fetal head against the cervix, thereby allowing adequate hand protection of the cord while in transit.

DELIVERY POSITIONS FOR THE MOTHER

Position of the mother has a great deal of influence on the efficiency of contractions. Contractions work most effectively when the parturient is in a vertical position (standing, sitting, squatting, kneeling) instead of a supine or side-lying position: there is a better drive angle (see Chapter 15, Figure 34). The intensity of contractions increases, and discomfort decreases, if the parturient labors in a standing position. A delivery position that takes advantage of gravity and nature is obviously beneficial. (A birthing chair could indeed be advantageous.)

The reclining position for delivery is convenient only for the birth attendant, not for the parturient. The laboring mother should lie down only if she is too tired to sit up. Even then, she needs at least two to four pillows behind her back to keep her from working totally against gravity.

Outside American culture, one of the most common positions for delivery is squatting. DeLoy Johnson, an R.N., has delivered many migrant mothers at the L.D.S. Hospital in Rupert, Idaho. He observed an interesting phenomenon among these mothers.[8] He repeatedly found them getting off the delivery bed to assist their own labors and deliveries. They would rub their backs up and down on the wall or do squat knee bends to loosen the pelvis. They would squat in straddle fashion, do shallow breathing, chant or sing, and assist the contractions with their hands. They universally used the squatting position for delivery (see Figure 44). Furthermore, the separation of the afterbirth was clean and spontaneous in every instance.

Mr. Johnson reasoned that it seems only natural to squat for delivery, to allow for uniform pelvic flexion and adaptation. He said the squat position should be assumed only when the infant is "capping" (the head is parting the vulva). He felt that gravity helps to apply equal pressure on all of the birth canal so that it effaces and dilates uniformly, without episiotomy or traumatic tear.

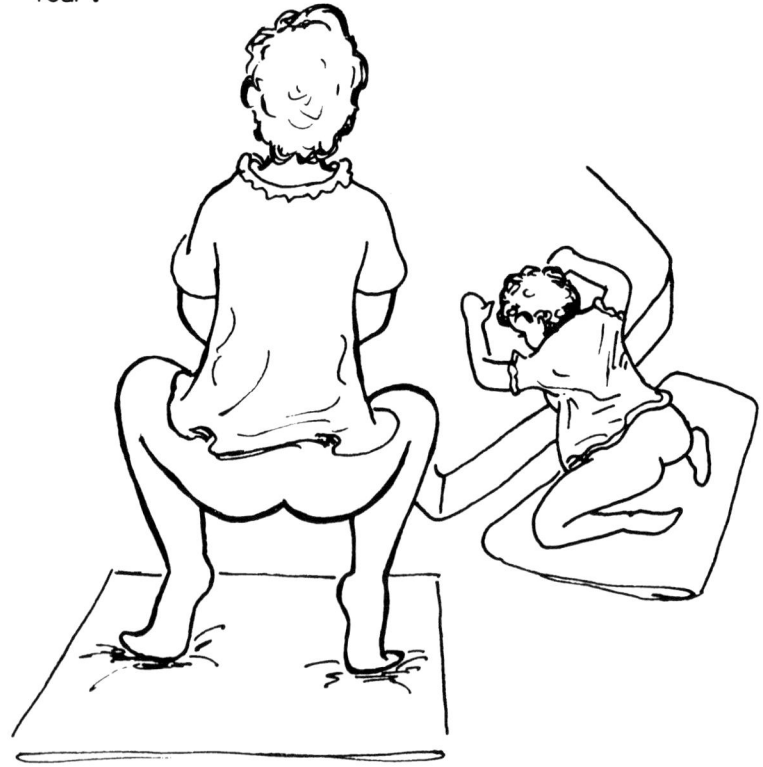

Figure 44. SQUAT POSITION IN PARTURITION. Squat position is taken AFTER full dilation, when the head is visible through the vulva. This position is conducive to any pelvic movement necessary, and also to a fully natural birth. An alternate method is kneeling or squatting at the edge of the bed.

Second Stage of Labor 323

He also suggested that the mother could limber the pelvis in early labor by rocking in a rocking chair, doing gentle knee bends against a wall, sitting tailor style (cross-legged or Indian sitting), or reclining at a 45° angle with thighs apart comfortably.[9]

Women often "just seem to know" when to squat or to do other things intuitively to assist their own birthing processes when given the opportunity.

Sometimes mothers prefer to lie on their left sides to deliver, especially if they have had long labors. This is fine (see Figure 45). The mother

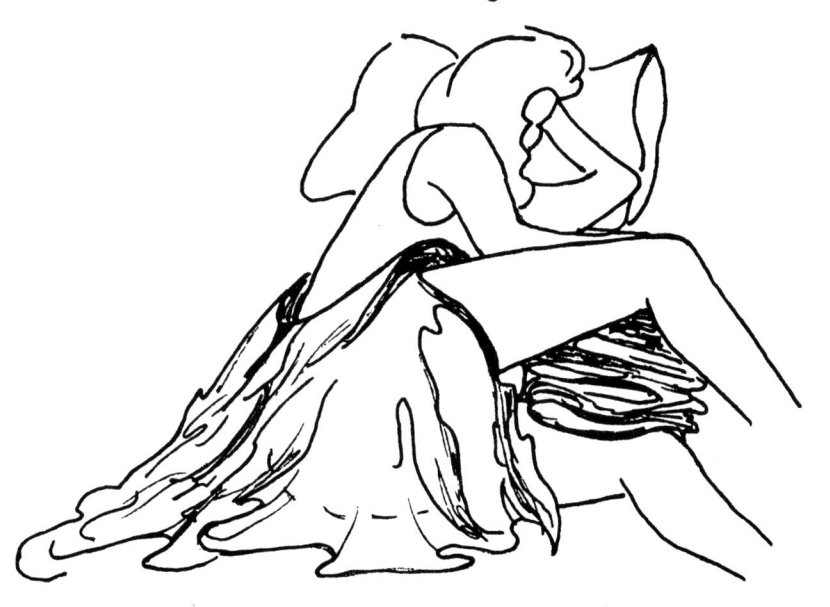

Figure 45. LEFT LATERAL POSITION IN PARTURITION. The left lateral position for delivery often corrects a labor dystocia or stress on the cord (manifested by an alteration in the fetal heart rate), and it more likely assures good placental/fetal circulation if the parturient has been reclining for long.

knows how she is most comfortable. She should be able to deliver in whatever position she pleases as long as problems do not demand attention from a position where the attendant can better observe and work. Resting on the left side lessens pressure on the major blood supply to the heart from the uterus and the lower extremities, improving maternal circulation and fetal oxygenation.

If a woman chooses an upright position for delivery, kneeling at the end or edge of the bed may give her support and be helpful for the attendant, and safer for the baby if it drops a little too fast. It also supports the mother and helps her keep her balance.

LATE SECOND STAGE

Pushing

After the cervix has dilated sufficiently to allow the baby's head to slip through, and it begins to travel through the birth canal, an entirely different set of sensations occur. The parturient feels a great pressure. It is as if her pelvis were a vise through which the head travels, but there is an absence of the sharp discomfort of late first stage. Remind her of this pleasant change. Help her to know she will soon be holding her baby. DO NOT PROMISE birth in two or three more pushes if you are not experienced enough to know—it may take two more hours. Nothing is so discouraging to a parturient than such miscalculations. (Time and experience will give most midwives a pretty sharp prediction quotient, but even the best practitioners are sometimes mistaken.)

During second stage, the primipara may have to push more than the multipara. However, do not hurry second stage. Some babies are literally breathed out, not pushed at all by the mother.

The contractions themselves can sometimes usher the fetus through the birth canal and out.

One woman may earnestly bear down for several hours to deliver, while another may need to bear down only two or three times. Still another may pant or breathe the baby out.

For those who need to push, warm peripacs, therapies for birth canal expansion, coaching, and bearing down with the contractions usually will help labor to proceed slowly enough to allow safe and adequate stretching, especially for those who have prepared the perineum for controlled crowning.

Coaching

The midwife judges whether the build of the birth canal warrants consistent pushing or bearing down, for how long, and when to do so. (The mother is often already aware of when she needs to push and when she needs to pant.) AT ANY POINT WHERE PROGRESS NEEDS DELAY, PANTING WILL PREVENT THE MOTHER FROM PUSHING.

1. Unless the para's build and the duration of labor to this point warrants the hard, sustained bearing down, a more controlled and safe alternative is favored. And this type of labor will more nearly assure a forty- to fifty-minute second stage. Try either "breathing down" or shorter duration bearing-down pushes—those that last only five or six seconds. The natural urge to bear down will in itself dictate the time and strength to be given to the pushing effort, and whether or not to hold the breath behind the push. It is said that fetal heart rates are not altered nearly so much and maternal blood pressure

does not lower as much when shorter pushes are carried out. A good position that supports the best drive angle (see Chapter 15, Figure 34), a normal pelvic build, and effective contractions work together beautifully to bring about birth.

2. If the para's build or the size of the baby indicates the need for more strenuous bearing-down efforts, or if for some reason it is imperative to get the baby out quickly, have the mother take advantage of the urge to push. Tell her to take two or three DEEP breaths as the urge develops, then to hold her breath through closed, quiet lips while she sustains long pushes.[9] SEVERAL SHORT PUSHES ARE INEFFECTIVE AND ACCOMPLISH NOTHING IN THE ABOVE CASES. If she needs to take a breath, have her SUSTAIN THE PUSH while she takes a quick, short breath, then have her hold her breath and push again until the urge or contraction abates. She should again take two or three DEEP breaths TO REPLENISH THE LUNGS WITH FRESH OXYGEN, then relax completely between contractions.

3. If she wants to, the parturient may:

Pull on her own thighs to draw them up with each contraction (but not back far enough to add stretch to the perineum, adding to the possibility of tearing).

Pull on someone's hands. The other person must assist her to pull equally toward 5 o'clock and 7 o'clock—not outward toward 3 o'clock and 9 o'clock. The direction of the pull is important so that she does not strain or damage her arm or abdominal muscles.

Rupturing the Amniotic Sac

One point of view is that the amniotic and chorionic membranes (which are as one membrane) should be allowed to rupture spontaneously (on their own). Some practitioners resist artificial rupture of the membranes because:

1. The baby is protected from infection, trauma, and uneven distribution of pressure by intact membranes.

2. The more even pressure on the placenta and cord results in better nutrition and oxygenation for the fetus during labor.

3. The baby has higher oxygen and pH levels, and lower carbon dioxide levels, when the membranes rupture spontaneously late in labor than when membranes are ruptured artifically early in labor.

4. Although artificial membrane rupture may slightly shorten the length of labor, shorter labor is not necessarily beneficial to the mother or baby; it may, in fact, be detrimental.

5. They hesitate to intervene unnecessarily in the natural process of birth.

I feel there are times when rupturing the membrane is helpful; in particular, to prevent a baby from being born with the membrane over its face, or when it is wise to hasten labor somewhat.

If you feel the need to artificially rupture the amniotic membrane, you should do so just BEFORE the fetal head BEGINS to crown at the vulva, seldom earlier. The baby is still several centimeters from the vaginal opening when the head begins to appear, say, at about +1 or +2 station. (On occasion, a prolonged labor will step up safely by rupturing the amnion as dilation is JUST COMPLETING.) Timing is important. Done at just the right time, the water will usher the head through that last bit of stretching without much discomfort. Done prematurely, it will cause more discomfort to both mother and baby as dilation completes.

I prefer to wait to rupture the membrane until I am sure the head is deeply engaged and any contraction has subsided, because a broken membrane's rush of water that has the thrust of a contraction behind it can flush out an umbilical cord or a little hand. Many times this is why the fetal head is born with a hand or two over the baby's ears or cheeks. This usually does not pose a problem, however.

As a contraction recedes, the membrane loosens a bit, allowing you to more easily catch a wrinkle of the membrane. If you are using scissors, they should be sharp/blunt—one tip is rounded, one is pointed (see Chapter 13, Figure 22).

Insert the scissors, holding CLOSED TIPS between your index and middle fingers. The tips must be closed and carefully guided and surrounded by your fingers so that you do not puncture any tissue but the amniotic membrane itself. Very slowly and carefully guide the closed scissors to the tip of the bulged membrane. The scissors must not under any condition wander in transit to the membrane.

When in place, the tips should be barely touching the membrane. Simply allowing them to touch the protruding bubble will usually do the job. If the membrane is unusually tough, open the tips ever so

Second Stage of Labor   329

slightly after you have captured a wrinkle of what you are SURE is the membrane, and rub the sharp tip carefully against it. Remember that the scalp of the baby is behind the membrane. It too will have a wrinkle from the collapsing of the skull as the head molds to travel through the pelvic area. (If aseptic care has been taken and gloves are not available, you can catch the membrane between two fingers and rupture it with a short fingernail.)[10]

When the membrane breaks, the amniotic fluid will rush out. Usually only a cup or two will spill out at this time. With succeeding contractions and when the baby is born, more fluid will follow.

About Tearing

A reliable, skillful midwife/herbalist reports that for eighteen months her mothers have not torn, or had real pain in childbirth. She attributes this success to a particular pattern of care in addition to the Good Program. Three to four weeks before labor, perineal rubs are given twice a day (not by the midwife) with warm olive oil, and an evening perineal rub is given with castor oil, all following warm ginger baths (3 T. ginger to the tub, or 1 1/2 T. to the sitz bath).

A lacerating birth is very likely if you find that the mother has an unhealthy vaginal floor. This type of tissue is porous and spongy instead of firm and smooth. Bumpy, lumpy tissue indicates multiple previous births, tearing in earlier births, or severe infections. Untreated yeast infections over long periods of time may have rendered the tissue high risk for laceration.

The mother seldom feels the tearing, since the fetal pressure obscures the sensation. All she is apt to notice is a stinging sensation if laceration occurs. There is no devastating awareness at all, unless there is uterine laceration. She should not fear the pain of a tear. The tenderness may occur later as healing takes place.

Even if the birth is managed well, an unhealthy floor could tear in various degrees, perhaps into the bowel, perhaps lacerating the anal sphincter. When this happens, it is called a **fourth-degree tear,** or a "blowout". Repair requires major surgery and suturing. After such an operation, drink teas of soaked flaxseed to heal the lower bowel and to keep the fecal matter soft and movable while repairs heal. Blowouts often occur with precipitous births. A **precipitous birth** is one in which dilation of the cervix, molding of the fetal head, and completion of second stage all happen within an hour and a half or less. Some precipitous births are concluded with just two or three bearing-down contractions. Unless suturing is correctly done, and possibly even then, the tissue will not hold the sutures in the bowel walls. If fecal matter is filtering into the vagina, prompt additional repairs will be needed.

Episiotomies

A small tear or two will, in spite of conflicting opinions, heal very nicely and is preferred over an episiotomy (which is usually extremely uncomfortable and may take weeks or months to heal). If multigravidas have been stitched too tightly from previous episiotomies, or primigravidas have not prepared themselves sufficiently (olive oil rubs, sitz baths, etc.), episiotomies might be deemed necessary. I have never performed an episiotomy (I was given a resounding ovation after this comment before a group of R.N.'s, C.N.M.'s, and practicing midwives), although, looking back, I perhaps ought to have done this on two or three

Second Stage of Labor 331

occasions only. When, in spite of all the mother and midwife do to control a crowning, there continues to be an all-encompassing blanching of the perineum at the sixth or seventh centimeters of dilation, the question arises as to whether an episiotomy would be kinder and safer than to chance traumatic laceration. This type of emergency first aid, though rarely needed, could hardly be deemed the practice of medicine. It falls under competent management of birth.

If the fetal head is exceptionally large or the fetal shoulders present a problem, you may deem it wise to perform an episiotomy. However, once you've learned how to do one, THE INCLINATION IS TO USE THE PROCEDURE MORE OFTEN. A good midwife will work toward preventing having to do it.

You can tell the size of the fetal head more accurately, and in time to incise (cut), by palpation during second stage, and more certainly when the head size bulges the perineum.

If all efforts to stretch the perineum do not keep it from widely blanching and you decide to do an episiotomy, do it as follows:

> As the fetal head stretches the perineum to about 6 centimeters, insert the tip of the blunt end of the sharp/blunt scissors between the perineum proper and the fetal head in a downward direction. Slip the palpating fingers inside the perineum between the fetal head and the scissors down as far as you need to cut. The fingers prevent any misguided cuts. Cut smoothly in one or two snips straight down at the median. Some choose a **mediolateral** cut (beginning at the median and angling toward one side), but this incision may be more tender during its healing.

If you wait until about 6 to 8 centimeters perineal dilation to do the episiotomy, the pressure of the baby's head against the perineum will prevent much bleeding. (The pressure also acts as a numbing agent so that anesthesia is not needed.) If you cut before this pressure is there, you'll have too much bleeding, and it will be difficult to see what you are doing. Cover the incision with a compress of gauze and complete the delivery.

You must be VERY CAREFUL not to cut closer than ONE INCH to the anal opening. ONCE YOU'VE CUT, THE PERINEUM TENDS TO LACERATE FURTHER, so support it with gauze and external pressure. Cutting too close or allowing laceration too close to the anal opening may damage the sphincter nerves. These nerves and muscles form a ring that prevent involuntary bowel movement. Injury to them may relinquish that control. The distance between the lower opening of the vagina and the anus differs from person to person. One person may have an area of 1 1/2 inches while another may have a 4- or 5-inch space with perineal stretching.

Some midwives want to use an anesthetic, such as Xylocaine, to numb the perineum before giving an episiotomy. One doctor told me that when anesthetics for episiotomies are given before the baby's head has crowned, the baby gets as much of the drug, if not more, as the mother does. The paradox here is that after the baby has crowned, there is no need for the drug!

CONTROLLED CROWNING AND DELIVERY

Crowning commonly refers to the stretching of the vaginal outlet and perineal tissues as the fetal head emerges. The actual moment of crowning per se occurs when the widest diameter of the presenting head is encircled by the vulvar opening.

As the baby's head comes through stations +1 to +3, control the crowning and the birth of the head as follows:

1. Pour about 2 tablespoons of olive oil into the vaginal cavity by letting it funnel down between your palpating fingers. If you do this at this point (NOT BEFORE -0- STATION), the fetal head pushes the oil back out and there is no danger of the baby aspirating it. Olive oil may be used with every other contraction or as needed until the perineum begins to stretch. Open the vulva and stretch the muscles there; work the perineum to keep it pink. (This can be done by bending your fingers and rubbing vigorously with the backs of your fingers.)

   Have the mother pant so that she cannot push if you are not ready for the head to crown. Together, both of you will slow the process of crowning in order to give the perineal tissue time to stretch easily.

   Blueing, then blanching (whitening) is a sign that the perineum is about to tear. If the mother feels stinging at the perineum, have her pant (not push) as you rim the perineum more to stretch it gently. (Stinging indicates that laceration is imminent or is already happening.)

2. Continue to rim (rub) outside the perineum gently, but quickly, so that circulation stays good and tearing is unlikely.

3. To deal with the oily surfaces, use gauze, a diaper, or a towel to support the lower perineum in a slight upward motion as the occiput (back of the head) tries to present first. Slight pressure at the top of the vulvar opening with the other hand will encourage the occiput forward (see Figure 46). This helps the smallest circumference of the baby's head to stretch the opening so that tearing is less likely.

4. When you can see that the crowning of the baby's head is almost complete (8 centimeters), put your hand on the perineum AND OVER THE ANAL OPENING and give a short, quick, firm press. The baby's head will pop out, and chances of tearing are almost nonexistent (see Figures 47 and 48).

   Another method used sucessfully is employed by cupping the hand under the crowning head with the small finger edge of the hand across the top of the perineum proper, and by pressing very firmly. The cupped edge of the hand encourages the perineum down over the fetal brow as it presents. Rarely will the tissue lacerate.

   Do not allow the baby to **project** or shoot out of the birth canal. The infant is wet and slippery and most certainly can project after it has reached a certain point. The infant's projection can be traumatic to the mother, and could pull on the cord and the placenta, causing the placenta to separate prematurely or the uterus to invert and pull out.

5. After the head is born, tell the mother not to push, if she feels another contraction, until you tell her to do so. Instead, have her pant

from the upper chest. You need time to check for the cord. Quickly feel at the back of its neck to see if the cord is around the neck. It could be hidden just inside the vaginal opening. If there is a cord there, slip it up and over the head quickly. (Do not force it if it does not give fairly easily. Instead, clamp it in two places and cut the cord between the clamps. Then unwind the cord.)

A fetal head that is born emitting bubbles through the nose is simply wiped or syringed. No hurrying of the birth is called for. The chest pressure will cause bubbling, but will also discourage any deep breathing. If the head is out, the baby can breathe if it has to do so. Do not hurry this stage of the birth, even though cyanosis (blueness, due to lack of oxygen) may be building. Wait for the next contraction to come after you have checked to see whether the cord is around the neck.

6. When the head is born, it usually makes restitution, or turns to align itself again with the rest of the body. (The baby will be on its side, with one shoulder above the other.) If the head does not turn to face one thigh or the other, gently assist it. This will allow one shoulder at a time to slip out more easily. (Usually the anterior shoulder delivers first.) Some physicians or midwives will have the mother push without the contraction. Others wait until the next contraction to begin maneuvering the shoulders and torso, thinking that the contraction opens and assists nature in a normal way to finish the birthing action. I prefer the latter. (The mother may even want to lift the infant out herself!)

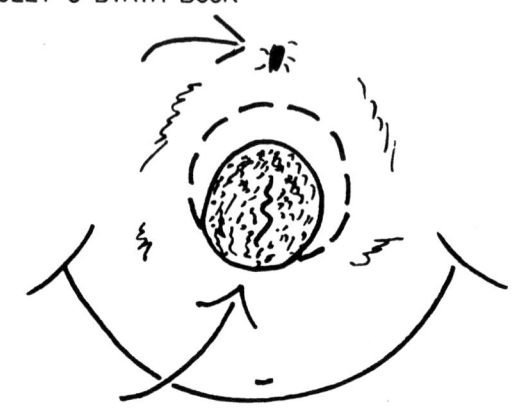

Figure 46. CONTROLLED CROWNING: PREVENTING PREMATURE EXTENSION. The occiput must slip under the pubic arch BEFORE the face begins "sweeping" over the internal perineum, so apply some resistance at where the top arrow points to accomplish this. Note that only half the crowning process has taken place at this point. (The bottom arrow points to the anus.)

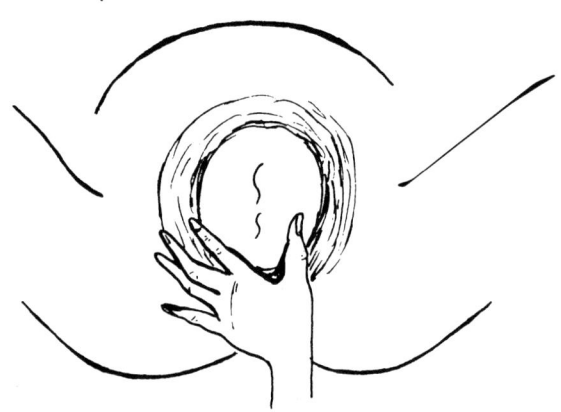

Figure 47. CONTROLLED CROWNING: ANAL PUSH TECHNIQUE. One way to prevent lacerations is to give a QUICK, FIRM push over the anus, with the palm of the hand, at about 8 cm dilation. This supports the perineum and "pops" the head out without lacerations occurring. (Use gauze or a towel between the hand and anus for cleanliness.)

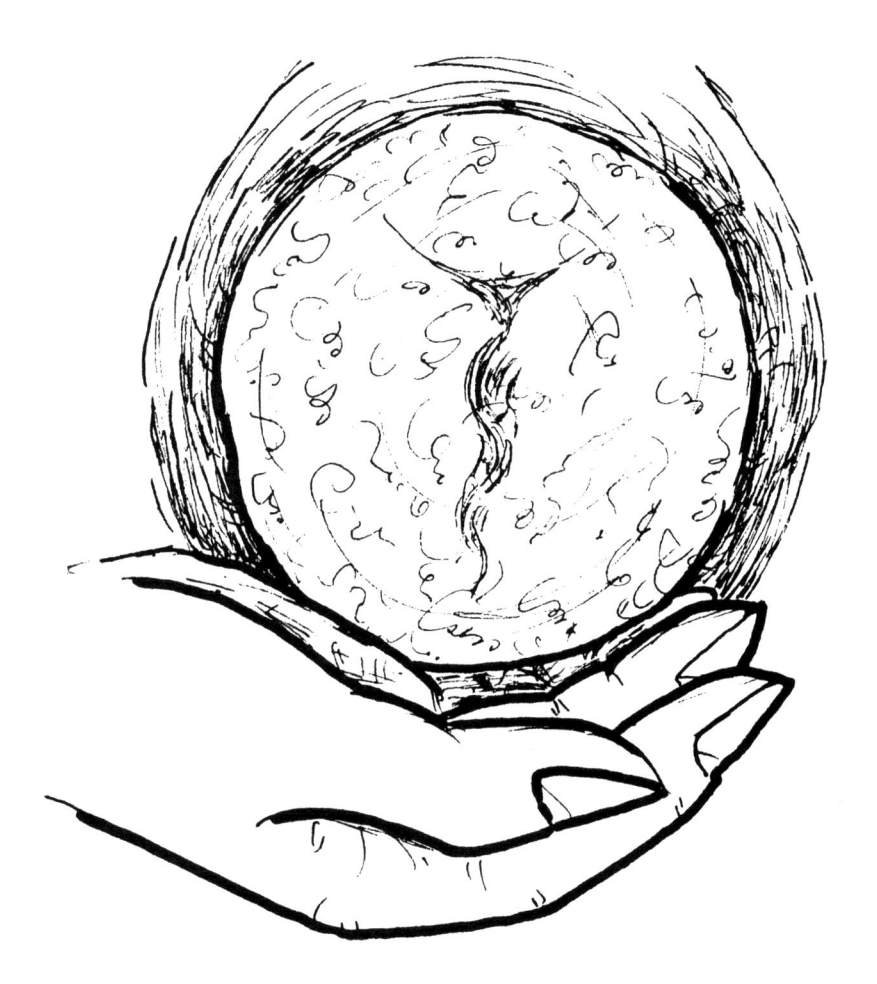

Figure 48. CONTROLLED CROWNING: PERINEAL PRESS TECHNIQUE. Controlled crowning can be accomplished in several ways. Here, the little-finger edge of the hand is placed FIRMLY against the perineum and pressed under the head as it crowns. This way, the perineum has been supported, a slight lift to complete extension is accomplished, and the occiput and face have been presented--without tears.

7. It is imperative at this point that you continue to observe carefully, even as you work with the baby, for the first signs of hemorrhage in the mother. (If bleeding should begin, your attention will turn to the mother at any point from then on, while some other trained person takes over the care of the newborn.) If, after having observed (1) the mother's prenatal hematocrit readings and the consistency of her finger-pricked blood sample, and (2) the type of second stage labor the mother has had (normal, traumatic, etc.), you expect possible excessive bleeding, have your assistant or the husband give mistletoe or shepherd's-purse to the parturient as soon as the baby's head is born. If there are no signs of hemorrhage and no previous indications that it may occur, but a strong prompting tells you to be prepared, make sure the mother gets the teas (see Chapter 17, Hemorrhage). Keep one eye on the vagina for bleeding and one on the care of the infant to make sure it begins to breathe properly.

8. Wipe out the baby's mouth with a gauze or syringe if it needs it. Also, wipe from the bridge of the nose in a downward stroke. (This may be done before or after the torso is born.)

9. Hold the baby's head with both hands. Place your index and middle fingers on each side of the neck. This will prevent uneven tension on the neck. Gently move the head downward to allow the top shoulder joint out; then carefully lift the baby's head to allow the lower shoulder joint through; then allow the baby's body to slip right out onto the towel below. If the parturient is squatting, you won't drop the baby if you take a towel over your hands

and hold one hand under the side and back of the head and neck, and let the baby's back slip onto the palm of the other hand (which is also covered by the towel).

NOTES

[1] Remember the story in **A Superior Alternative** about the girl who sang "Popcorn Popping on the Apricot Tree" while she was being sutured? There were too many voices saying "push" too loudly for her to hear instructions from the one in charge. She had three small tears she need not have had.

[2] Molding is a natural, partial collapsing or overlapping of the fetal skull to allow passage through the pelvis. Evidence of this is the wrinkle in the scalp as the occiput bulges open the vulva in birth. With the birth of the head, cranium plates relax and are back to normal in a day or two. Anterior presentations usually result in round, beautifully-shaped skulls, with the apex in the occipital/parietal area. (These people are the dominant, "doing" individuals in life.) Posterior births usually result in the prominence of the frontal lobes. (These are the "thinkers," the "dreamers" in life.)

[3] The cord may be too short to accommodate birth. The average length of a cord is 55 centimeters, or almost 22 inches. Medical books give the "usual range" of cord lengths as being from 30 to 100 centimeters (from about 12" to just over 39"), with abnormal variations from the baby's abdomen being in contact with the placenta (1/2 cm) to about 78 inches (198 cm). They mention that high placenta implantation requires a cord length of about 35 cm (about 14") and a low implantation must have about 20 cm (8"). A "long" cord may be wound about the baby, leaving the relative cord length too short. (Obviously, the longer the length of the cord, the greater the likelihood that it will entwine the fetus.) Cords looped around the neck as many as three times are usually in excess of 27 1/2 inches long (70 cm), in contrast to the 16-inch cord of this baby.

[4] Fetal death due to cords about the neck is unusual. According to **Williams Obstetrics** (14th ed., p. 597), "It is clear that the lethal role assigned to [coiling of the cord around the neck] has been exaggerated."

[5] Only about 1 percent of the time do true knots occur, and in only about 6 percent of these case does the knot cause death. Death due to cord knots or loops of the cord around the neck is a freak accident.

[6] When I was lecturing in St. George in 1978, a woman in the audience said that this was exactly what her old-fashioned doctor had done for her three months before. Afterward she went on into labor and delivered a fine and healthy baby.

[7] When the mother is in the knee-chest position, her internal organs and vaginal opening are in such a position that a sort of vacuum may be created inside the uterus. This vacuum can draw air into the uterus. If an air bubble gains access to the maternal or fetal circulation (through the uteroplacental circulation), it can be carried by the blood current to where it forms an **embolus**, or plug, blocking a blood vessel. This obstruction can cause serious, or even fatal, results. Also, especially if most of the amniotic fluid has escaped, there might be a problem with the baby inhaling air before it has a continued access to air.

[8] DeLoy Johnson, R.N., report on squat delivery (1980).

[9] During the bearing-down stage, pressure on the anus from the vaginal floor will sometimes cause hemorrhoids to develop, or, if they are present, to protrude. The midwife or the mother should push them, postpartum, back into the opening with a lubricant. They will stay in, shrink, and heal if the mother replaces them for a few days and continues taking cayenne and the sitz therapy.

[10] Once a hospital-oriented midwife raised her eyebrows and gasped in horror while telling me that another midwife had actually used "kitchen scissors" to rupture a membrane. I asked her simply, without sharing her horror, "Were they clean?" This is the important thing. There is more than one way to skin a cat safely, and there are times and places when unorthodox but very reasonable alternatives can suffice very nicely and very safely. Cleanliness and skill in the use of any instrument are imperative.

CHAPTER 17

THIRD STAGE OF LABOR: BEGINS WITH THE BIRTH OF THE BABY AND ENDS WITH DELIVERY OF THE PLACENTA

EARLY THIRD STAGE

After the baby is born:

1. Suction the baby, ONLY if necessary.
2. Note the baby's Apgar score.
3. Assist the baby to establish respiration, if necessary.
4. Cut the umbilical cord.
5. Encourage bonding.

Suctioning the Baby

When the baby is born, it may need to be suctioned:

SUCTION ONLY IF NEEDED. If bubbles are coming out of the mouth AFTER WIPING, or if the wiped-out material is stringy and difficult to get, then suctioning is called for. If you must suction, do it quickly. Expel the air from a small, 2-ounce syringe before inserting it into the baby's mouth.[1] Usually mucus will withdraw from the throat if you suction toward the back of the cheek or beside the back of the tongue. Be careful not to draw the baby's breath back out if it seems to have inhaled. This can also be done with a DeLee suctioning device. Timing is important. Withdrawing air that is filling the lungs can bring the fetal heartbeat dangerously low. Crying is a healthy sign that the lungs are being filled more completely with air.

Apgar Evaluation

The **Apgar Scoring System** is the standard measure for evaluating the newborn (see Figure 49). Practice will soon help you to make this evaluation quickly at one minute after birth and again at five minutes after birth. The Apgar checks for five things, rating each a 0, 1, or 2: (1) **color**, (2) **respiratory effort**, (3) **heart rate**, (4) **muscle tone**, and (5) **reflex irritability**.

If the newborn's Apgar score is at or under 3 at the first minute, notify the baby's pediatrician. If the score is under 6 at five minutes, notify the pediatrician. A score of 10 is perfect.

Establishing Respiration

The baby should breathe in less than a minute. Gently rub along the right side of the UPPER SPINE (there are nerves that stimulate the lung area here) to stimulate and assist the baby to

APGAR SCORING SYSTEM

RESPONSE	SCORE
COLOR:	
pale, blue	0
body pink, limbs blue	1
completely pink	2
RESPIRATION:	
absent	0
slow, irregular, weak cry	1
good, strong cry	2
HEART RATE:	
absent	0
slow, less than 100	1
over 100	2
MUSCLE TONE:	
limp, flaccid	0
some flexion of limbs	1
active movement	2
REFLEX IRRITABILITY (response to stimuli):	
absent, no response	0
facial grimace, cry	1
strong cry	2

APGAR SCALE

Apgar score of 10-8: no asphyxia
7-5: mild asphyxia
4-3: moderate asphyxia
2-0: severe asphyxia

Figure 49. APGAR SCORING SYSTEM. At ONE and at FIVE minutes following birth, five physical responses of the newborn are evaluated and each given a score from 0 to 2. The COMPOSITE score, the Apgar score, provides an objective indicator of the baby's condition. A SCORE OF 10 AT ONE OR FIVE MINUTES IS PERFECT. IF THE SCORE IS 3 OR LESS AT ONE MINUTE, OR 6 OR LESS AT FIVE MINUTES, NOTIFY THE PEDIATRICIAN.

breathe (see Figure 50). I have found that doing this and talking to the infant in a soft, happy, reassuring way is all that is usually needed. Some babies come out letting the whole world know they are here as soon as the head is born. Others open their eyes and look around to see who is there to greet them, and still others cry two or three times—as if to say, "My, that smarts just a bit!"--while the lungs are filling, then look around. (It would be my judgment that about 90% of home-birthed babies do the latter. I would also estimate that their average Apgar score is about 8 at the first minute and 9 to 10 the fifth minute.)

If the baby fails to breathe right away, DO NOT STRIKE IT ANYWHERE! A flip of the finger on the bottoms of the feet may help. Or, hold the baby securely up in the air, then lower it suddenly, ten or twelve inches ONLY. This sudden drop may cause it to inhale quickly and initiate breathing.

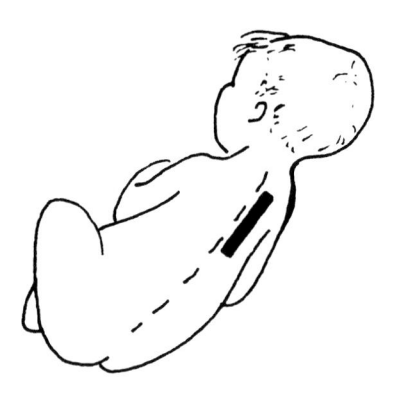

Figure 50. ESTABLISHING RESPIRATION: THORAX RUB. Rubbing along the RIGHT side of the upper spine stimulates nerves that go to the infant's lungs. This is the first (and usually the only) gentle assistance rendered in establishing respiration.

Talk to the baby, prompt it to respond to your call. A healthy cry or two should be encouraged because crying, however brief, does ensure a more complete filling of the lungs. A desperate or prolonged cry is not necessary.

If the baby is not breathing in a few seconds:

1. Clear the passageway again, lift the baby's chin, cover both the nose and the mouth with your mouth and blow ONLY SMALL PUFFS--not even cheeks full--of air into the baby two or three times. MORE THAN GENTLE PUFFS AT A TIME COULD RUPTURE THE BABY'S LUNGS.

2. If breathing is accompanied by a grimace and a grunt with each breath:

    a. Speak softly to it; snuggle it warmly.
    b. Soothe and calm it by stroking it lovingly.
    c. Put it to the mother's breast.

    Usually these procedures will remedy the problem. If the grunting does not lessen within 10 to 15 minutes, or if it gets worse, transport immediately. There may be a mechanical problem: the lungs are insufficiently expanded or incapable of expanding. This, coupled with pain and emotional distress, is demonstrated in the baby's facial contortions. Grunting usually lessens soon.

3. If there is deep retraction of the stomach muscles, showing the rib cage clearly, and the baby seems to be frantically searching for air, do the above numbers 1 and 2 while you transport.

If there is no place to transport to and no other help, begin warm, moist-air humidifying, and keep the baby warm and calm. Speak reassuringly to the infant.

4. Vitamin E always helps with cyanosis by distributing available oxygen through the system, but it cannot be administered through the mouth in large amounts or the baby might aspirate it (inhale it into the lungs). Instead, administer 100 IU's of vitamin E a drop or two at a time onto the baby's tongue every few seconds until it is all swallowed. The vitamin E moistens the tongue and throat, aiding in respiration, and penetrates to the circulatory system, where it aids in the distribution of oxygen.

5. A prayer and a blessing are always appropriate if the baby is in stress. However, the midwife continues her work quietly while blessings are being administered.

To PREVENT breathing problems, the mother should have taken 400 to 600 IU's of vitamin E with lecithin per day all during pregnancy. (The baby's **lecithin-sphingomyelin ratio** must be 2 to 1 in order to assure good lung development; **sphingomyelin** is a natural substance of the secretory system found in the amniotic fluid.)

INFANT CPR

Cardiopulmonary resuscitation (CPR) is of value at times if the newborn is not breathing, but it must be emphasized that training is essential. I recommend that midwives and mothers (indeed, couples together) take the Red Cross Advanced First Aid Course as well as the CPR training by itself. The latter takes only eight hours of your

Third Stage of Labor 347

time, and it is well spent. Remember in administering CPR to infants that: (1) ONLY SMALL PUFFS OF AIR are blown into the infant's oral and nasal orifices, NEVER full breaths of air, and (2) ONLY TWO FINGERS are used to depress the sternum over the heart, NEVER the whole hand or the two hands that are used in adult resuscitation. And remember that never is mouth-to-mouth administered until the air passages are cleared as much as is possible. Two or three puffs of air will usually do the trick for the baby.

I like **Byrd's Method of Resuscitation** just as well, if not better. Administered properly, it works very nicely for the **apneic** (suspended respiration) infant. Hold the infant by the ankles or under the knees and at the back of the neck while supporting the head (see Figure 51). The idea is not to sandwich the lower extremities and the chest, but to roll these parts within a reasonable proximity, then to lay the infant open in a reclining position, then to return him to the closed position. Folding the infant to where his legs touch his chest would be to invite damage (laceration of the liver, by the ribs). What you want to acomplish is to "close the lungs," then to open the posture to "draw air" into the lungs.

STILLBORN INFANTS

I have only worked with one stillborn baby, and in that instance all ended well. I was assisting a physician in a home birth, and both of us worked simultaneously for at least a half-hour or more before the baby began to breathe. (Within an hour, the baby's early signs of brain damage had disappeared and the baby recovered completely.) A brief summary of what we did follows, and a more complete account can be found in **A Superior Alternative,** pages 178-81.

348 POLLY'S BIRTH BOOK

We did not force oxygenation. Instead, we worked together to "prime" the heart and lungs with numerous techniques. The initial objective in a situation where there is no breathing (or even no pulse) is to clear the airways and keep them clear. We cleared the nose, mouth, and throat at different stages of our work. We gave mouth-to-mouth, did Byrd's Method of Resuscitation, and kept the infant's body very warm by working with it in warm water. (We kept the head above the water, and the water was changed every few minutes.) We kept manual circulation constant by vigorously massaging the entire body, constantly turning the baby from side to side, and so on, until the heart could take over and circulate the vascular system on its own.

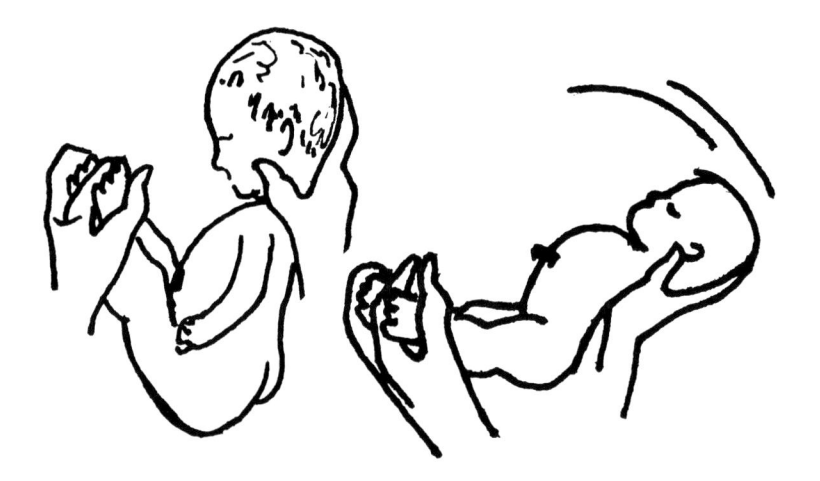

Figure 51. ESTABLISHING RESPIRATION: BYRD'S METHOD. The lower extremities are "rolled" TOWARD--not TO--the chest, to close the lungs. The lungs draw in air as the infant is "opened" to a reclining position. Air is expelled when the infant is returned to the "closed" position. Repeat to simulate (and stimulate) breathing.

After the first inhalations and coughs, oxygen was administered for a few seconds. At that point the baby was wrapped in a towel and held near an oven door. Turning the baby, gentle massage, and verbal communication were continued. Then 550 IU's of vitamin E were dropped onto her tongue a few drops at a time. (Nothing should be given by mouth until after a baby has begun to breathe on its own--DO NOT give anyone who is unconscious anything orally.[2]) The new little one was rubbed with warm olive oil, dressed snuggly, and given to the mother.

Cutting the Umbilical Cord

Hematologists have found that early clamping of the cord,[3] before breathing is established, may be a factor in causing **respiratory distress syndrome ("hyaline membrane disease")**, a fairly common complication in the hospital-delivered newborn.

Never cut the umbilical cord until the baby is breathing properly unless:

1. A cord is too tightly wound around the baby's neck for the baby to be born, or the cord is so short that it would create stress on the placenta, uterus, or navel.

2. The cord is in a tightly-drawn true knot and is not giving the baby oxygen anyway.

3. You must work with a distressed infant (in a warm water bath, resuscitating, etc.) and the attached cord would too seriously hamper your efforts, or the cord is deteriorated.

When the baby is breathing nicely, turn your attention to the cord. Several things need to be done at this point:

1. COVER THE BABY'S BODY AND THE TOP OF HIS HEAD WHILE YOU HOLD THE CORD ACROSS THE FINGERS OF YOUR LEFT HAND.

   Baby's thermostat does not work for a few days, and he loses body heat quickly-- especially when he is wet. The birthing room should be warm (75 to 80° F) and there should be warm blankets ready to wrap the baby in. As soon as the cord is cut, the baby can be warmed by the mother's body heat. However, in cold weather a diaper or receiving blanket should cover any exposed portion of the baby. Heat loss occurs quickly through the HEAD and FEET of an infant. (A too rapid heat loss causes a lactic acid build-up in the muscles, which in turn throws the pH balance in the body so far off that depression and even loss of life can result.) Keep the baby warm during this time.

   The pulsing of the umbilical cord is magnified when the cord is laid across the palm and fingers of a cupped hand. The flow of blood in the cord runs completely across the hand, which leaves no doubt about when the pulsation stops. Over the years I have noticed that when the cord pulsates for a long time (3 to 5 minutes) the placenta is very likely to delay separation. If pulsation ceases almost immediately, the placenta will separate quickly. Any effort to hasten cessation of the cord pulse may result in denying the baby the extra iron that particular baby may need very much. The blood which comes from the cord belongs to the baby, and he should have it.

2. WHEN THE CORD CEASES TO PULSATE, IMMEDIATELY STRIP THE RESIDUAL BLOOD FROM THE CORD INTO THE NEWBORN.

Third Stage of Labor   351

Strip the cord while the newborn lies BELOW THE LEVEL OF THE PLACENTA, which is still in utero at this time. (Many midwives and doctors like to lift the newborn onto the mother's abdomen as soon as it is born, prior to cutting the cord; I do not, for the above reason and also to prevent undue stress on the cord or the placenta or the placental site.) Hold the cord close to the mother's vaginal opening, to prevent any tugging on the cord, and with the other hand strip all the way down the cord almost to the baby's navel. This gives the baby 60 to 100 ml of blood, containing 50 to 80 mg of iron; however, do not worry if you do not get every drop of blood into the navel. (The extra iron reduces the possibility of iron-deficiency anemia later in infancy.) Do this quickly so as to not allow a clot to be formed and introduced into the baby. When the pulsating stops, the blood coagulates because the sheath and the suspending Wharton's jelly have begun to atrophy. The umbilical cord atrophies rather quickly with exposure to air.

3. CHOOSE A PLACE ON THE CORD ABOUT THREE INCHES FROM THE BABY'S NAVEL TO CLAMP THE CORD.

This allows extra room for reclamping if for some reason you should need to. This can be done with umbilical tape (which looks much like hem binding and can be purchased with obstetrical supplies), a plastic clamp, or the stainless steel clamp (clamps can be bought in bulk). Of course, the smallest, thinnest shoestring or slightly heavy wrapping cord may be used. Do not use wet strings.[4] When they dry they loosen and may allow serious bleeding. Thin string may cut the cord and allow bleeding.

Some attendants do not use any **ligation** (tying off or clamping the umbilical cord). I prefer to do so in case there is a delay in the natural occlusion of the umbilical vessels of the infant, or the infant cries, or some other thing happens to cause the blood vessels to open again and the infant to bleed. Normally, expansion of the lungs as the newborn begins to breathe and the clamping of the cord cause changes in the infant's circulation which result in the collapse of the umbilical vessels, since they are no longer needed (see Figure 52). However, the timing for these vessels to atrophy and for related circulatory closures to become permanent may differ from baby to baby. Not all umbilical stumps dry quickly enough to prevent reopening, and I prefer to be cautious. Blood loss in ANY amount is dangerous to the newborn.

4. NOW CHOOSE ANOTHER SPOT ON THE CORD--TOWARD THE MOTHER AND ABOUT TWO INCHES FROM THE BABY'S LIGATURE--AND CLAMP THAT OFF.

    This side can be clamped with one of your hemostats or forceps, because when the placenta has presented there is no longer danger of the mother hemorrhaging through the cord; your forceps can be removed, washed, and put away with the rest of your instruments. You need to tie the cord off in TWO places, with clamps or whatever.

5. CUT BETWEEN THE CLAMPS (see Figure 53).

    The one clamp will prevent the baby from hemorrhaging, the other will prevent the mother from bleeding through the cord. It is usually a big thrill for fathers to be able to make the severance.

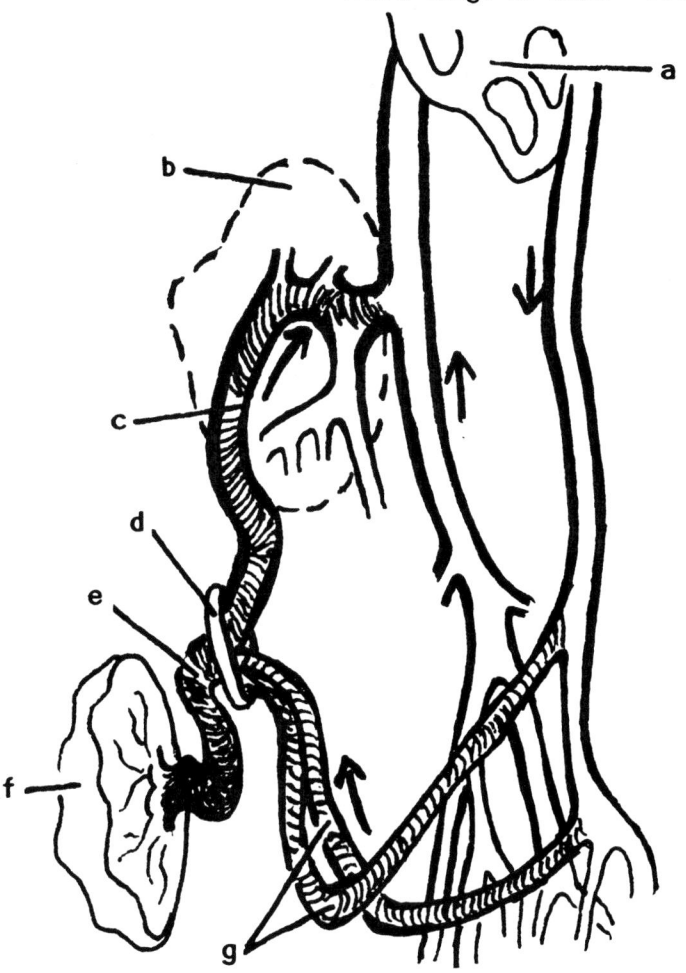

Figure 52. FETAL CIRCULATION. (a) fetal heart, (b) liver, (c) the umbilical VEIN, which carries oxygen and nutrients INTO the fetal circulatory system from the placenta, atrophies by the fourth to sixth day following birth; (d) navel (umbilicus), (e) umbilical cord, (f) placenta, (g) the umbilical ARTERIES, which return wastes FROM the baby to the placenta, SHOULD close off when the cord is clamped, obliterating within three to four days after birth.

354 POLLY'S BIRTH BOOK

6. LOOK CAREFULLY AT THE CORD TO SEE IF THERE ARE THREE VESSELS IN IT--TWO ARTERIES AND ONE VEIN.

   If not, the baby may have a congenital defect, perhaps a heart defect. Let the parents examine the cord with you. It is reassuring to them.

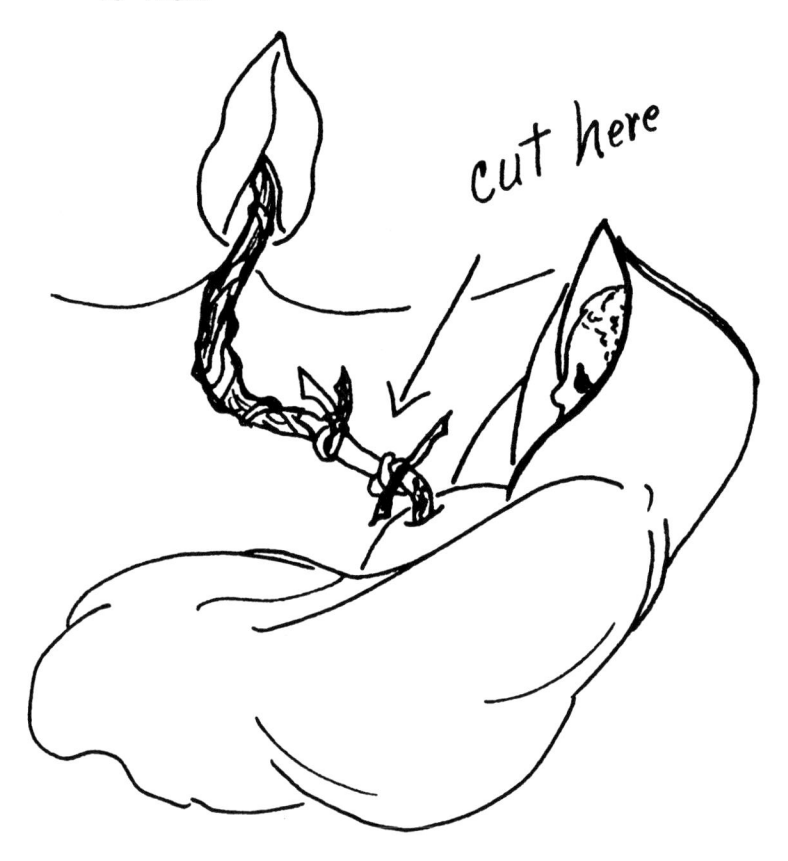

Figure 53. CUTTING THE UMBILICAL CORD. Clamp the cord twice: on the maternal side with forceps, and on the fetal side with an umbilical clamp or umbilical tape. Cut between the ligatures.

Bonding

Put the baby to the mother's breast for a most important "first half-hour" of bonding. Nursing helps the placenta to separate and uterine contractions to persist and to prevent bleeding. The baby can be cleaned and dressed after the placenta has been presented. I call this bonding a "birth of natural affection," a time when love, comfort, security, and trust are physically and emotionally welded between people. Many psychological benefits come with this intimate welcoming of the newborn. The presence or absence of such opportunities taking place within the first half-hour of life is manifest clearly in levels of individual security. It is at this time that emotional crises begin to build for the mother who has aborted her offspring. She never gets to bring her procreative process to a warm and natural conclusion, despite her presence of mind and decisions made to this point.

DELIVERING THE PLACENTA

While attending to the baby during the first few moments after birth, keep your eyes on the vaginal opening to watch for blood. As soon as the cord has been clamped and cut and the baby is high in its mother's arms and at her breast, your full attention turns to the placental separation.

THE MOST COMMON MISMANAGEMENT OF THIRD STAGE OF LABOR INVOLVES THE ATTEMPT TO HASTEN IT! Being very observant at this point--when everyone else is excited about the newborn--may be difficult, but it will pay dividends and is a critical time in your responsibility zone. The midwife's job is NOT YET finished.

First, watch for a small amount of blood to issue forth (about 1/2 cup, probably less if the mother has taken the Polly-Jean Five-Week Antenatal Formula). When the placenta separates, the uterus changes shape: it becomes more globelike. The bleeding begins, the umbilical cord descends a little, and the fundus rises. A palms-on palpation of the abdomen during a number of separations will help you become familiar with these changes in the uterus. A slight prominence appears just above the symphysis pubis, the cord slips out more, and the fundus rises and becomes **mobile** to one side or the other, usually the right (see Figure 54). If you notice this, the placenta has probably already separated and may be sitting just inside the vaginal opening.

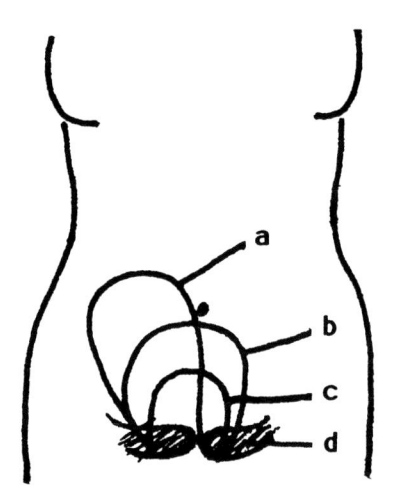

Figure 54. FUNDAL MOBILITY. (a) At third stage, the fundus lifts and becomes "mobile" following separation of the placenta; (b) before placental separation, the uterus remains upright; (c) following delivery of the placenta, the fundus should be low and the uterus the size of a grapefruit; (d) pubic arch.

Third Stage of Labor 357

If you do not observe this, there are several things you can do to determine the progress of this third stage of labor:

1. Wrap the cord around your fingers twice or so (it will be wet and slippery) and pull it just enough to make it slightly taut. With your other hand on the mother's abdomen (over the fundus), watch and feel--DO NOT KNEAD. Ask the mother if she is having or has had another contraction, but do not pull hard on the cord or knead the fundus. If you disturb the fundus too much at this point and the placenta has separated, you will prevent the open blood vessels in the uterus from closing off naturally by themselves. If there has been no noticeable contraction, wait.

2. When the parturient says she feels a contraction coming on, have her bear down with it. Actually, the uterus should never have stopped contracting, but Mom is so excited about the baby that she may not notice these milder contractions. When she feels a healthy contraction, the placenta usually separates. With your hand lightly palpating the fundus from the abdominal side, you may feel the placenta slip down. If you don't feel it slip down, see if you notice the fundus slide under your palm to the mother's right side. We call this "becoming **mobile**"--the fundus moves. If you find it moveable, the placenta has separated and slipped down into the vaginal cavity and is sitting there ready to be lifted out.

3. If you cannot be sure what you are feeling, use cord tension to do a **fundal lift**. Watch a given spot on the cord just outside the perineum and pull on the cord gently to make

it taut. Then, place one hand on the abdomen on the bottom side of the fundus while holding onto the cord with your other hand; push the fundus an inch or so toward the mother's heart and see if the cord pulls back into the vagina with it. If it DOES pull up, then the placenta has not separated. If the cord does not move in the least with the fundal lift, the placenta is probably sitting in the birth canal waiting to be lifted out or for the mother to push it out.

4. If you believe that the placenta has separated and is sitting in the vaginal cavity, simply palpate inside the vagina about an inch or two and you'll be able to feel it. It is an easily-felt, solid mass. Then have the mother bear down as you lift the placenta out by the cord. As you lift it out, TURN THE WHOLE PLACENTA CLOCKWISE ONCE OR TWICE and let the membrane very gently peel off and out. Turning the placenta puts equal torsion against the residual membrane so that it is more likely to peel away without leaving fragments.

Second Placenta. Occasionally a second placenta develops. The second placenta can be just as big as the first one, but it is usually a smaller lobe. There are many variations. (Sometimes the extra placenta sustained a twin that was miscarried early in the pregnancy.) It is important to watch for this irregularity so that if only one placenta has presented, you will know that another should be expelled.

If a placenta has presented and you notice large blood vessels feeding out from the placenta through the membrane, suspect another placenta (see Figure 55). These large blood vessels will be found on the fetal side of the placenta and can be easily seen traveling off into the membrane tissue. There may be a hole in the membrane at the site where the second placenta was attached to it, if the placenta retained. You can see why it is important to turn the placenta as it presents, since even tension on the membrane helps the additional placenta to separate cleanly.

If you determine that a second placenta has been partially retained, expect profuse bleeding. Employ the measures to treat retention of the placenta (described next) to get this second placenta to present: false unicorn, shepherd's-purse, and mistletoe, with manual separation.

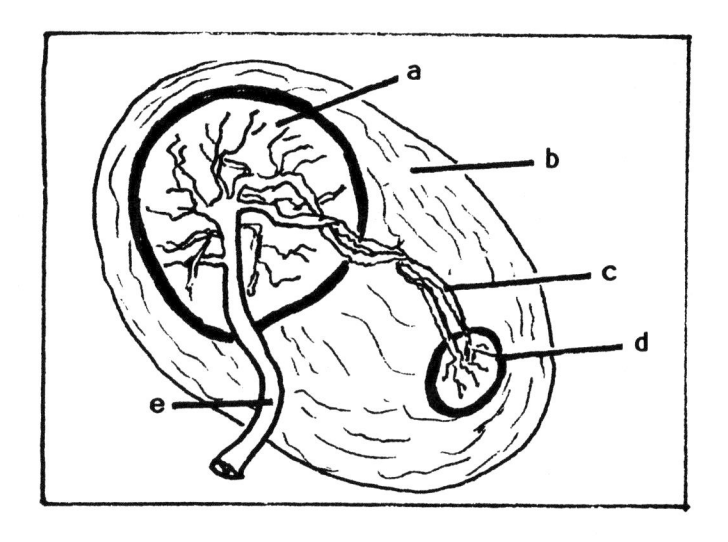

Figure 55. PLACENTAL ABNORMALITY. Heavy blood vessels (c) that branch away from the placenta (a) into the membrane (b) indicate the presence of another, probably smaller, placenta (d) which must come out. These blood vessels precipitate hemorrhage if broken or unduly disturbed in the separation process. (e) umbilical cord.

POSSIBLE THIRD STAGE COMPLICATIONS

Retained Placenta

If the placenta has not separated after about half an hour, have the parturient cough about five times or have her sit up on the toilet or squat. These techniques may do the trick. Should there be severe bleeding you may need to FOLLOW THE CORD INTO THE UTERUS TO THE ADHERING SPOT and peel it away gently, but quickly, using the tips of your fingers (see Figure 56).

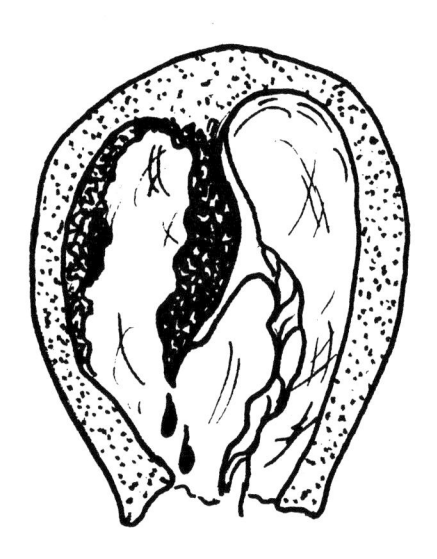

Figure 56. RETAINED PLACENTA. This incomplete placental separation (**partially retained placenta**) requires manual separation before the hemorrhage can be stopped. A **completely retained placenta** (NO part has separated) does not bleed until it is separated.

Never separate the placenta by pulling hard on the cord. Tearing the placenta from the uterine wall is dangerous, because doing so may tear the uterus or break the placenta into pieces, leaving parts of it attached while the rest sloughs off. Pulling the placenta out may even invert the uterus altogether.

One midwife encountered a placenta problem that could only be handled in the operating room. Her parturient retained a nine-pound placenta. The back-up doctor had to remove it from the uterus surgically because it was so large it would not present. Had the midwife tried to remove this placenta manually, the uterus would have been inverted (pulled outside). The mother continued to hemorrhage during the operation, but an IV was set up to replace lost body fluids. A curettage cleaned away any fragments and the mother recovered nicely.

Fragments of the placenta or membrane that are left behind on the uterine wall will cause two things: (1) hemorrhage, and (2) continued uterine contractions (not to be confused with the afterpains of the multipara). Nature knows that something has not been completed, so it works to get rid of the pieces left and contracts at regular intervals, just as in the first stage of labor. Also, blood vessels do not close off as they should and they continue bleeding.

Any retained portion of a placenta is more dangerous than a retained portion of a membrane, because the placenta is more deeply "embedded" into the uterus; and when the amnion is no longer a protection, blood vessels will then hemorrhage. Retained placenta is also a predisposing cause of **puerperal infection** (infection associated with childbirth, "childbed fever"--temperature will rise when infection mounts).

Retained placenta fragments or lobes must have immediate attention because of the potential hemorrage. Heavy bleeding must be halted and fragments can be manually separated. Otherwise they must be removed by surgical cleanup. Do not be afraid to insert a gloved hand through an already dilated cervix and feel for any remaining "blobs" of material—or for any lacerations—along the uterine wall.

With complete retention of the placenta there will be no bleeding until you separate it manually. Any lobe or fragment that retains will bleed profusely from the time that it is separated from the main body of the placenta. Because bleeding is already happening or is inevitable, give the mother shepherd's-purse, mistletoe, and false unicorn. In emergencies, tinctures of these herbs (1/2 tsp. of each in two or three ounces of water) will more quickly curb the bleeding.

Plantain, shepherd's-purse, bayberry, cayenne, and others will stop hemorrhage, but will not initiate uterine contractions as mistletoe does. These herbs can be taken WITH THE MISTLETOE or alternately in doses of 1/2 cup to 1 cup at a time. Use 1/2 cup herb, or herbal combination, to 2 cups of boiling water: steep, strain, and cool.

Mistletoe, especially, and nursing will cause the contractions to continue. Contractions are vital because they help crowd out the afterbirth (placenta and any fragments) and they are the means of stopping bleeding from the placental site. (Give mistletoe to the parturient in strong doses only as needed; however, even smaller doses are not to be continued longer than a day or two.)

The strong dose consists of 1/3 cup powdered mistletoe (or the leaves) to 8 ounces of boiling water. The tea is steeped, strained, and cooled. (Emergency herbal supplies should be prepared and cooled beforehand.) In emergencies, put the herb in water, stir, and have her drink it all down.

In spite of your turning the placenta in your hand to put equal "pull" on the membrane, sometimes a strip of it will tear away and remain attached to the uterus. Use your keyhole forceps to very gently peel that fragment out. If you meet firm resistance, don't force the strip to separate. Instead, clip the membrane (if very long) so only about an inch or two protrudes from the vaginal opening and leave it. False unicorn and St. Johnswort (two capsules of each, three or four times a day) will cause it to separate on its own in a day or two. If not, the uterine environment will certainly have been so affected by the herbs that by then the fragment can be peeled away very easily. There is not the danger of bleeding or infection from retained fragments of membrane as there is from retained fragments of placenta--unless heavy toxemia or meconium staining has been present. In that case, add two capsules of goldenseal-echinacea mix to the false unicorn and St. Johnswort, and watch her temperature closely.

Uterine Retraction Ring

If you are sure there is no internal bleeding,[5] there is usually no harm done if the placenta (intact) retains for several hours. There is no possibility of hemorrhage as long as no part of it has separated. However, past the first hour you run the risk of the **retraction ring** closing (see Figure 57). Caution is the watchword.

When a placenta is retained, and there IS bleeding, you have to palpate internally to see what is happening. Sometimes this stimulation of the uterus will cause the retraction ring, a ridge of muscle between the upper and lower uterine segments, to constrict, trapping the placenta inside the uterus and possibly trapping your hand! Other things such as ergot preparations or a stimulus such as turning a fetus in utero or palpating too firmly may also trigger the clamping action. If the parturient has had a long, hard labor (24 hours or longer), the retraction ring can clamp shut on its own, though this is rare. Sometimes the placenta begins to move down and out of the uterus and the retraction ring contracts, leaving the placenta partially in and partially out of the uterus! This constriction can remain for some time. (This problem is sometimes called **midring constriction,** because the retraction ring is found just above the isthmus; see Figure 58).

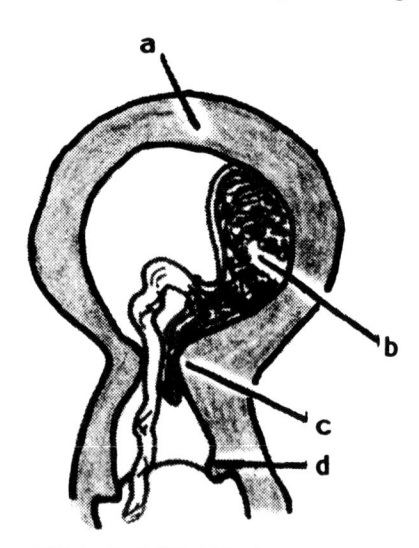

Figure 57. UTERINE RETRACTION RING. (a) fundus, (b) completely retained placenta, (c) the retraction ring has trapped the placenta; (d) the external os is still dilated from birth.

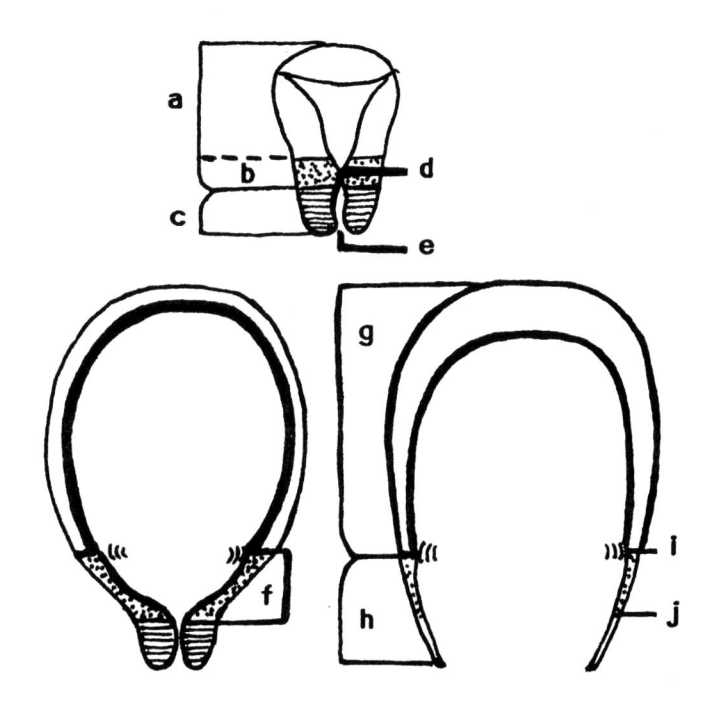

Figure 58. UTERINE ACTIVITY IN PARTURITION. **Nonpregnant uterus:** (a) body, (b) isthmus, (c) cervix, (d) internal os, (e) external os. **Pregnant uterus at term:** (f) The fetal head causes the isthmus to thin; it becomes the lower uterine segment. **Uterus in labor:** (g) The upper uterine segment is the actively contracting portion, becoming THICKER as labor progresses; (h) the lower uterine segment and cervix are more passive, THINNING as labor progresses; (i) the retraction ring is a ridge that forms between the different-acting upper and lower uterine segments; (j) the internal os is obliterated by dilation and effacement of the cervix.

The lesson here is that THE FUNDUS MUST NOT BE UNDULY STIMULATED BEFORE THE PLACENTA HAS SEPARATED if you can at all avoid it. On its own, the fundus begins to thicken as the fetus moves down and out of the birth canal. Kneading it or even placing the new baby on the mother's tummy, too low on the abdomen, can possibly cause the retraction ring to constrict. **Ergonovine** (an ergot alkaloid[6]), given in the hospital for bleeding, is believed to be the main cause of midring constriction. I have never known mistletoe to trigger this constriction; rather, it promotes normal contraction of the uterus.

IF RESTRICTION HAPPENS, the mother will know something is wrong, especially if your hand is caught! She may go into shock, so watch for the signs and employ first aid measures if needed: drop 3 to 5 drops of antispasmodic tincture on her tongue as a first step. You can help make any crisis like this one less traumatic if you behave matter-of-factly or even laugh. If you don't ACT upset, she won't BECOME upset. You're not keeping anything from her, but you're also not panicking. Something is happening, but you know what it is and you know what to do about it.

If your hand is caught, do not pull it out. If you do, you will damage tissue and will probably pull the whole uterus out. You want the retraction ring to relax. You do not, however, want the fundus to relax so much that once the placenta has separated, it will not contract again as it should. If your hand is caught (constriction has occurred), saturate a cotton ball with antispasmodic tincture and slip it up beside the caught hand with keyhole (ring) forceps and apply the tincture to the constricted area. If your hand is not caught, use a speculum to hold the vagina open (the external os, or cervix, is already opened), then locally apply the antispasmodic by inserting a saturated, folded, sanitary napkin (turned so the plastic is inside). (Ring forceps can also be used in this case.) About 3 to 5 seconds of contact with the rigid tissue should relax it, and it will release its hold on the placenta or your hand. Then withdraw the forceps and the placenta.

If you do not have any tincture available, you may have to put the mother into a (sterilized) tub of warm—not too hot—water. This will relax her. If you cannot deal with this problem at home, you will have to transport.

Adhered Placenta

You may have to deal with an adhering placenta, though this is rare. An **adhered placenta (placenta accreta)** occurs when the conceptus implants in the "wall" of the uterus and the placenta builds from that area, becoming "part of the uterus." This occurs when there is little or no formation of decidua at the implantation site. It is important that you be able to recognize this unpredictable problem so you will not lacerate the uterus by trying to separate an adhered placenta. This, of course, will cause additional bleeding. A RETAINED placenta can be peeled off with little effort; an ADHERED placenta will not peel away (it may adhere only partially or totally). You will have to transport.

HEMORRHAGE

Women can lose a fair amount of blood before they go into shock, but this does not mean you can treat any excess bleeding lightly. Never "wait to see" if the mother is going to bleed just a little bit. Anything over the initial amount emitted from the placental separation is too much; 1/3 to 1/2 cup is the usual, unharmful amount.[7] Individuals are different. Their abilities to tolerate bleeding vary greatly. Only experience will refine your judgment about when to transport and when to deal with a bleeding problem yourself.

Remember, THERE ARE PRIMARILY THREE CAUSES OF POSTPARTUM BLEEDING: (1) defective functioning of the uterine muscles--**inertia** or **atony,** (2) deep tears in the birth canal, and (3) retention of a partially separated placenta or of placental fragments.

Normally you can expect shock after a woman has lost a pint of blood. Shock occurs when loss of fluids causes a change in the body's pH balance. Only a very slight change to acidity can cause the pulse rate to increase sharply. Then acidosis sets in, the pulse rates drops, and death occurs (see Appendix B, Shock: Symptoms and Treatment).

The pulse is the best clue to the parturient's condition. If any problem arises, keep a finger on the pulse (at the wrist, in the groin, in the neck). It should range between 60 and 70 beats per minute, and the blood pressure about 110/76 to 130/82. Use as a rule of thumb that something should be done to alter a steadily rising pulse (20+ beats above normal) or blood pressure (15+ mm Hg diastolic and 30+ mm Hg systolic above normal). Then you have time to act and to prevent the situation from getting out of hand. Just ASSUME THAT THE MOTHER IS HEMORRHAGING AND GOING INTO SHOCK. The treacherous thing is that there will not be EXAGGERATED ELEVATIONS in blood pressure or pulse rates until it is probably too late!

Normally the parturient's skin is dry (except during second stage when she perspires) and warm

Third Stage of Labor 369

and her color is pinkish. If she begins to pale, it is serious. Paling is not only a sign of hemorrhage, it can also be a result of severe exhaustion, shock, or even cardiac failure. Without panic, just be observant and do your work when it should be done. PREVENTION is the watchword. You CAN do a good job if you learn well and do what needs to be done.[8]

Avoiding Hemorrhage: Points to Memorize

An unfortunate feature of postpartum hemorrhage is the failure of the pulse and blood pressure to undergo more than moderate alterations UNTIL LARGE AMOUNTS OF BLOOD HAVE BEEN LOST, so NEVER "wait to see" how much a person can tolerate before shock symptoms appear.

Every midwife should memorize the following things to AVOID during labor and delivery in order to decrease the chance of hemorrhage.

1. PREVENT HEMORRHAGE WITH GOOD PRENATAL CARE AND GOOD LABOR MANAGEMENT.

2. SEE THAT THE GRAVIDA GETS LIQUIDS, NOURISHMENT, AND REST DURING LABOR.

3. DO NOT ALLOW OR ENCOURAGE THE MOTHER TO BEAR DOWN BEFORE SHE IS FULLY DILATED. This can lacerate the cervix.

4. CHECK FOR THE DEVELOPMENT OR PRESENCE OF AN ANTERIOR LIP OF THE CERVIX, especially when there is pain in the lower abdomen. Bearing down vigorously under such a condition without proper support to the cervical lip could result in laceration and bleeding. Rim to prevent anterior lips, especially if there is a history of previous ones.

5. DO NOT FORCE SECOND STAGE LABOR. Let it proceed naturally and with control. In the event of a situation which requires a more rapid conclusion to the birth, control is still essential.

6. DO NOT PULL THE PLACENTA OUT AFTER THE BABY IS BORN. It must separate on its own if possible. You lift it out after it has separated unless the mother wants to push it out and unless there is bleeding above normal. (In the latter case, place the PALM OF THE HAND ONLY over the fundus and bear down towards the vagina. DO NOT SQUEEZE the fundus.)

7. DO NOT KNEAD THE FUNDUS UNTIL THE PLACENTA HAS PRESENTED. Why? As the placenta breaks from its mooring, thousands of blood vessels break open. Nature designed the vessels so that they close off and heal shortly. This is a normal physiological mechanism of placental detachment. If the attendant disturbs this process needlessly, she may not only cause the blood vessels to reopen and bleed, but she may also increase the chance that the weight and bulk of the placenta will be at a disadvantage to separate uniformly from the uterine wall and will therefore fragment. When fragments are left behind, nature works to separate them and bleeding continues.

Kinds and Causes of Bleeding

Basically, there are two types of bleeding associated with childbirth. Being able to identify kinds of hemorrhage will assist the midwife in drawing out of her mental files the appropriate action when she encounters a bleeding problem.

The first kind of bleeding is the slow, bright-colored, CONTINUOUS flow that fills pad after pad. Some call it "the silent killer." This kind of hemorrhage usually starts immediately after the birth of the baby. It is usually caused by deep lacerations of the cervix or the vaginal floor or walls or the perineum, or lacerations near the clitoris on the vulva, as may occur in a posterior birth. A placenta embedded in the lower uterine segment may cause serious bleeding. Also, the cervix tears more frequently than most attendants suspect. Tears occur most often in precipitous or forced births or with women who have not prepared themselves properly during pregnancy. Some stretches and tears are not severe enough to bring on much bleeding; others are. The slow, steady flow can also accompany **uterine atony** (no muscle tone or action) following birth. This bleeding CAN BECOME heavier and pulsating or spurting.

If you notice a little bleeding during dilation, the cervix has likely torn slightly somewhere. If the cervix was rigid enough to tear, the other anatomy may also tear, so be aware of this possibility and watch for it.

WHAT TO DO:

> To treat this kind of bleeding following third stage, give the parturient cold shepherd's-purse tea with 1/4 to 1/2 teaspoon capsicum and pack just the VAGINA with sanitary pads saturated with calendula tincture. When bleeding has stopped--within minutes--very gently remove the pads and suture the vaginal floor or perineal lacerations (you should not try to suture CERVICAL lacerations, a physician does this). If there are blood clots in the VAGINAL cavity, you will need to remove them and clean the laceration(s) before

you suture. It is hoped that the placenta has presented. If it has not, wait for it to do so if at all possible, or your repair work is apt to be interrupted.

OXYTOCIN (PITOCIN) WILL NOT STOP BLEEDING FROM LACERATIONS. It causes uterine contractions and therefore curbs bleeding from that source (the uterus).

PERINEAL COMPRESSION, HERBAL AIDS, and SUTURING will stop hemorrhage from lacerations.

If the steady bleeding BEGINS later after the birth, ALWAYS CHECK THE FIRMNESS OF THE UTERUS BEFORE YOU DO ANYTHING ELSE. If the uterus is soft, it must be kneaded before it becomes the second kind of bleeding. Administer additional mistletoe and shepherd's-purse. (Even ordinary nutmeg found on the kitchen shelf will contract the uterus and help stop bleeding.)

The second kind of bleeding is the SPURTING flow. This bleeding is placenta-oriented. This kind of hemorrhage may be hidden at first if a blood clot is blocking the cervical opening and preventing the blood from coming out of the uterus. You may suspect this internal bleeding if the mother's pulse rate rises SHARPLY and her ABDOMEN BEGINS TO FILL. The clot may soon give way to a spurting action synchronized with her pulse rate.

If you see bleeding or suspect internal (obscured) bleeding, quickly check the expelled placenta and see if it is complete. If some pieces are missing, they are probably still in the uterus and are causing the problem. Also, the incomplete placental separation gives rise to this hemorrhage.

WHAT TO DO:

To treat this problem, you will have to remove the clots and employ the first aid for bleeding from the uterus.

If the parturient is bleeding in spurts and it seems the placenta has not completed its separation, DO NOT pull the placenta out. If the mother does not feel an urge to bear down, feel just inside the vagina to see if the placenta is there waiting to be lifted out. If it is, lift the placenta out quickly and knead the fundus immediately. If the placenta is NOT there, introduce a gloved hand into the uterus and follow the cord into the uterus and peel the placenta, or retained part, away carefully AT THE EDGES. This includes removing polyps and blood clots. If you have reason to believe the uterus has ruptured in any degree, give first aid and transport immediately.

If you have had the mother on a good herbal and nutritional program throughout pregnancy, her placenta will be healthy and will separate as it should, not fragmenting. You will rarely have to go in after a placenta. However, you may find yourself helping a mother who has not been on your preventive program, so your skills must include being able to manage any eventuality.

Summary: Kinds and Causes of Bleeding

IMMEDIATE, STEADY FLOW MEANS THERE HAVE BEEN LACERATIONS IN SOME PART OF THE REPRODUCTIVE CANAL.

WHAT TO DO:

1. Give shepherd's-purse and capsicum; pack the vagina for 2 to 10 minutes (as needed) with calendula tincture or other astringent on 1 or 2 sanitary napkins.

2. Unpack; suture, if possible, AFTER placental delivery.

NOT IMMEDIATE, BUT **HEAVY OR SPURTING FLOW** IS USUALLY RELATED TO PLACENTAL/UTERINE PROBLEMS. (Remember, it is POSSIBLE that BOTH kinds of hemorrhage can run simultaneously.)

WHAT TO DO:

If the placenta HAS SEPARATED and delivered:

1. Give mistletoe with shepherd's-purse.

2. Remove clots from the vagina or uterus.

3. Knead the uterus to a hard ball.

4. If needed, pack with calendula tincture, give bimanual compression, etc.

WHAT TO DO:

If placenta HAS NOT SEPARATED completely:

1. Put the baby to the mother's breast.

2. Give mistletoe with shepherd's-purse and capsicum AGAIN.

3. Remove clots.

4. Go up after the placenta.

5. If the placenta is ADHERED AT ANY POINT, pack with calendula tincture, give HVC, and transport.

WHAT TO DO:

To PREVENT bleeding (if possible):

Shepherd's-purse can be given as early as +2 station, if the parturient is not nauseous. If she is, then give mistletoe and shepherd's-purse as soon as the head is born.

Controlling Postpartum Hemorrhage: Points to Memorize

My emergency childbirth and midwifery class tests call for memorizing first aid management of hemorrhage. If students make these points second nature, they can adequately handle 99 percent of all hemorrhages without having to transport, by administering the appropriate first aid in the moment.

Hemorrhages can be handled very well if you have determined the cause and know you can deal with it without panic. You have, according to the physical tolerance of the parturient, 10 minutes to one hour to completely control a hemorrhage. This leaves an additional half-hour to transport if that becomes necessary. Unless heavy uterine lacerations are involved (these are almost unheard-of in home births where Pitocin is not used), almost any home birth hemorrhage can be managed in 5 to 15 minutes. Memorize the emergency techniques, use whatever technique is called for, and always be prepared with the equipment and supplies you may need. As early as first stage, you should evaluate the possiblity of hemorrhage and begin gathering the ice cubes, hot water bottles, blankets, teas, etc., that you may need. Do this as a matter of routine so that you do not alarm the mother.

Memorize the following things to do to control hemorrhage:

1. GIVE ORALLY ANY ONE OR TWO OF THE FOLLOWING TEAS, following the birth of the fetal head: MISTLETOE (a must), SHEPHERD'S-PURSE, CAPSICUM (in cold water), BAYBERRY, PLANTAIN. These teas can be administered several times, about 2 to 3 minutes apart. The teas should be strong concotions. You can continue to give these teas as you think they are necessary. (The herbs CAN be given before fetal head presents if needed. Mistletoe probably should not be given before the fetal head reaches -0- station.)

   These teas are a blessing for several reasons: (1) they stop the bleeding, (2) they give nourishment, (3) they replenish lost fluids, and (4) they prevent shock. While hospital-administered oxytocin (Pitocin) acts quickly, it wears off quickly. Herbs are slower to act, but they sustain longer.

2. PUT THE BABY TO BREAST. If this cannot be done, have the father stimulate the mother's breasts. (He may have to suckle her breasts in order to be effective.) This is a life-saving measure, because it stimulates the production of the oxytocin in her own body, which causes the uterus to contract and clamp down on open blood vessels.

3. APPLY FOUR POUNDS PRESSURE WITH AN 8"-X-8" COMPRESS TO THE ENTIRE BIRTH OPENING.

Although this is not the actual site of the bleeding, IMMEDIATE pressure often PREVENTS additional bleeding. Hold the compress firmly for three minutes. Peel back one side of the compress to see if the bleeding has ceased. IT WILL USUALLY STOP WITHIN TWO TO THREE MINUTES, but if it does not, quickly proceed to other measures.

4. REMOVE ANY BLOOD CLOTS IN THE UTERUS; these will prevent the fundus from putting pressure on open blood vessels. To do this, you must go into the uterus with a gloved hand and remove clots that may have formed as blood has coagulated. The fundus cannot contract effectively if it is full of clots. You MUST scoop the clots out, even if blood flow is still heavy. Then immediately knead the fundus externally. See that the uterus knots into a grapefruit-sized ball and stays that size and hardness.

5. HAVE THE MOTHER USE HER MIND TO CONTROL HER BODY (biofeedback).[9] Both the midwife and the parturient should know that the mother has much more control over her body and body parts than either may realize. But the mother must allow her body to follow directions; she cannot "tell" the perineum to stretch and relax, for instance, and at the same time be afraid for it to do so. This concept may be new to some, but mind over matter can be effective in many cases.

6. ASK THE FATHER (OR SOMEONE) TO PRAY, even silently, or a priesthood holder present to give a priesthood blessing[10] while you continue to administer emergency techniques. I have seen hemorrhages stop instantly with blessings.

7. HAVE SOMEONE ELEVATE THE MOTHER'S HIPS AND FEET 8 TO 10 INCHES.

8. PLACE COLD PACKS ON THE MOTHER'S LOWER ABDOMEN AND BOTTLES OF HOT WATER AT HER FEET AND ALONGSIDE HER LEGS. This draws the blood away from the heavy uterine blood supply while stemming against shock.

By now the above measures will probably have worked to stop the bleeding. If not, proceed to the next steps:

9. IF THE PLACENTA IS RETAINED, SEPARATE IT. Follow the umbilical cord up and into the placenta site, then follow the placental body to its edge. Gently, but quickly, peel away whatever portion of the placenta is still attached to the uterine wall with your finger tips. When the placenta slips into your hand, withdraw the placenta by the cord, being careful not to allow the uterus to also come out. The fundus may then be kneaded into a firm ball.

10. USE TINCTURES TO PACK JUST THE VAGINA IF BLEEDING PERSISTS FOLLOWING PLACENTAL PRESENTATION. (Packing the UTERUS would take a volume almost as large as the baby). Sufficient tincture applied to the adjoining tissue is needed--and will work. Saturate the absorbent side of two sanitary napkins with calendula tincture, fold them in half so that the plastic sheathing is inside, and slip them into the vagina only. (Rarely will you need more than two napkins.) Bleeding usually stops quickly after the napkins are in place. Calendula is an astringent, so it causes blood vessels to contract. It is also an

antiseptic, so it arrests the growth and multiplication of microorganisms.

The minerals in herbal preparations are as effective as the hot, sterile, saline douche used in years past to completely stop hemorrhage (following placental separation).

11. USE BIMANUAL COMPRESSION IF THE ABOVE DOES NOT WORK. One hand is inserted into the vaginal cavity, then fisted, while the second hand works from the abdominal side to push the fundus firmly against either the fist or the pubic arch. Hold until bleeding has completely ceased. Then gently remove the fisted hand and treat for shock. The need for some of these actions is unheard-of where the Good Program and herbs are used during pregnancy.

12. COMPRESS THE ABDOMINAL AORTA by placing two hands--one flat hand over the other--exactly over the fundus, and pressing them hard against the backbone until bleeding stops. The parturient must, of course, be on her back in order for the midwife to obtain effective pressure. This closes off the major source of blood supply to the uterus. Hold this until oral aid is effective or the paramedics arrive.

13. TRANSPORT IF AN ADHERING PLACENTA IS FOUND (one that has PARTIALLY grown to the uterine wall and will not separate). Give shepherd's-purse and capsicum orally before transporting. Bleeding will have probably ceased before you arrive at the hospital. (A COMPLETELY ADHERING PLACENTA OR A TOTALLY UNSEPARATED PLACENTA WILL NOT BLEED.)

For bleeding from the inert uterus, and to help keep the situation in hand after hemorrhage has been controlled:

14. KNEAD THE FUNDUS FROM THE ABDOMINAL SIDE (if the placenta HAS SEPARATED). It is imperative that the fundus remain firm; otherwise, bleeding will continue. Even after the fundus has been kneaded into a grapefruit-sized ball, it must be watched constantly. Almost instantly, the fundus can become flaccid, and have to be "looked for" and gathered back into a hard ball. IF THE PARTURIENT HAS UTERINE INERTIA, THE FUNDUS WILL DEMAND CONSTANT ATTENTION. Sometimes an abdominal band pinned tightly over a rolled hand towel or washcloth will be stimulus enough. However, be diligent in checking the fundal rigidity every 5 to 10 minutes after serious bleeding seems to be arrested. This must be watched for 24 to 48 hours.

15. BIND THE ABDOMEN. Get a towel that will go all the way around the mother's torso. Fold it (for extra strength) lengthwise and wrap it around her abdomen; then pin it very tightly. Take a small towel or two washcloths, roll them, and slip this wad under the pinned towel. Put it directly over the fundus. This "knot" over the fundus acts as a continuous stimulus to keep the uterus contracted and to prevent bleeding from an inert uterus. It feels very good to the mother to have her abdomen firmly fitted against her following its long distention. Continue, as a safety measure, to check the mother's sanitary pad for excessive bleeding. (Binding of the abdomen may be done profitably even when no abnormal bleeding has occurred.)

Transporting

If there is a hospital within reasonable distance (10 to 15 minutes), there is usually time to transport persistent cases of hemorrhage. Paramedics should be called to do the transporting if they are available. They carry blood, so you should know the mother's blood type in case she needs a transfusion.

However, TRANSPORTING IS NOT ALWAYS THE SAFEST THING TO DO IN A HEMORRHAGE CRISIS. The midwife must be able to diagnose the CAUSE OF THE BLEEDING in order to determine whether transporting is called for or whether MANAGING THE BLEEDING IMMEDIATELY IS SAFER. Your skills may be just what the mother needs, or she may need surgery immediately, as in the case of an adhering placenta or anything greater than second degree lacerations.

Your decision about whether to transport must take into account the degree of bleeding, the kind (cause) of bleeding, and the distance to the nearest hospital.

If you must transport, remember that hospital emergency rooms are notorious for delays. You can minimize that delay by telling the hospital by phone that you are coming. Give the mother's name and blood type, tell WHY you are coming in and who the back-up doctor is. If you are able to use the services of the ambulance team, you still want this information readily available.

Treatment Following Postpartum Hemorrhage

A mother who has hemorrhaged seriously may need to be hospitalized for transfusion after the crisis is over. (This will depend on her overall physical condition, whether she was already anemic, and her general tolerance for blood loss.) If hospitalization is not possible, you must know how to build blood and replace electrolytes quickly: give HVC, orange juice, or grape juice immediately. Follow daily with blood-building foods, herbs, and drinks.

Potassium is especially essential to replace. This can be accomplished by giving the mother homeopathic cell salts: potassium phosphate, calcium, and the bleeding-prevention formula. These potassium sources should be in the mother's storage supply as well.

Restoration of the blood needs to be accomplished before the mother begins activity. If she has lost a lot of blood (in excess of 1 1/2 cups) and she does not allow her blood to restore before she is up and around, she may become light-headed and fall and injure herself or the baby if she is holding him at the time. Some bodies are able to replace their blood supplies within the hour; others will need days (see Chapter 10, Anemia, Other Deficiencies, for blood-building foods and herbs).

EVALUATING THE PLACENTA AND MEMBRANE

Earlier, you should have quickly assessed the afterbirth as it presented. Now, a better look will tell you several things (see Figure 59).

> Normally, a placenta weighs about 1 pound and is 1- to 2-inches thick at the center. Women who smoke have smaller, less adequate placentas.

The color of the placenta should be dark bluish red.

The placenta should have a shiny membrane on the fetal side and be raw on the maternal side where it has broken away from the wall of the uterus.

The placenta should be firm. A mushy or porous placenta is unhealthy.[11]

When the placenta is intact, all the **cotyledons** (lobelike areas separated by furrows or "valleys") should be present and fit together when cupped in your palms.

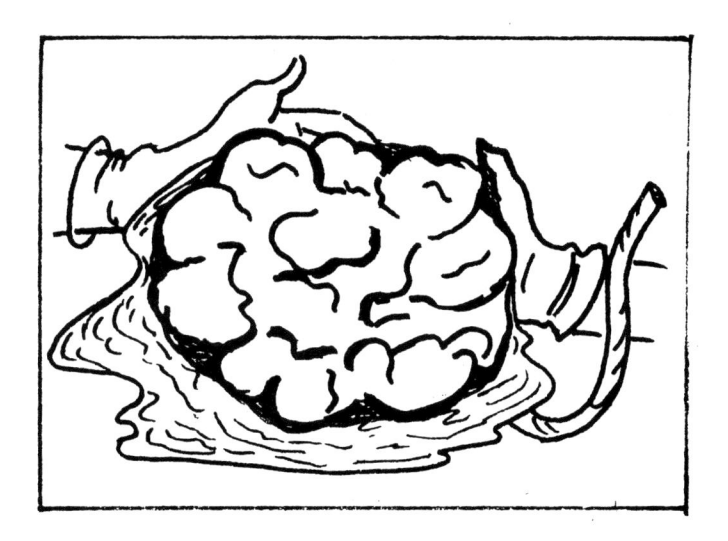

Figure 59. EXAMINING THE AFTERBIRTH. Examine the maternal side of the placenta for missing portions (lobes or fragments) and for abnormalities, and the membrane for missing (retained) pieces.

Whitish areas may be found on the placenta, on either side, but usually on the maternal side. They are about the size of quarters or fifty-cent pieces and feel much like cartilage. Their presence indicates death of tissue in that area, and placental insufficiency is the result.

Calcium deposits on the placenta are normal. They look like thick, white taste buds or bumps and feel almost like coarse-grained sandpaper. These textured areas are associated with normal degeneration of the placenta at term.

Any blood clots attached to the placenta indicate areas where premature separation took place. The clots should be saved with the other blood emitted to evaluate the amount of blood lost at birth.

If at any time the membrane has ruptured, then healed, scar tissue can be found at the site. Rupture at term may or may not be the hole through which the baby leaves the sac in birth. Some membranes are "paper thin" (only translucent, though); others are a little thicker. When the placenta is held up by the cord, the membrane will drape down from it. This may help you examine it better for missing strips or portions.

Large blood vessels may lead away from the placenta (on the fetal side) into the membrane, indicating a second placenta. If this did not present, it will have to be retrieved.

If the mother had edema or was Rh-negative, the placenta will be large and pale and may have water oozing from it.

Third Stage of Labor 385

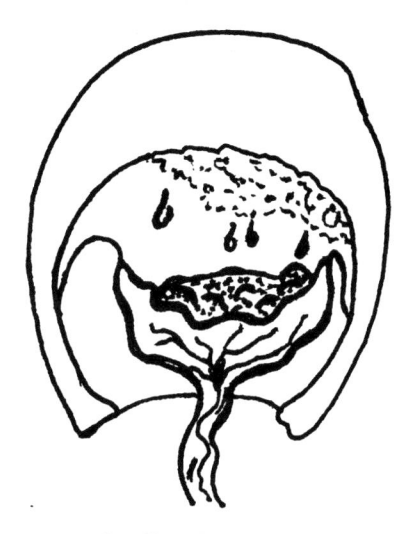

Figure 60. "SHINY" SCHULTZE PLACENTAL SEPARATION. The fetal (membrane-covered, "shiny") side of the placenta follows the cord out.

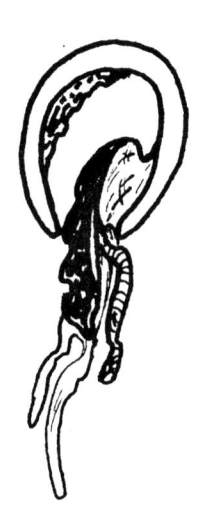

Figure 61. "DIRTY" DUNCAN PLACENTAL SEPARATION. Part or all of the maternal side of the placenta presents first, more likely leaving fragments of placenta and strips of membrane behind.

If the mother you are attending had a **"Shiny" Schultze presentation** (see Figure 60), be glad. This is normal. If her placenta came in a torn, broken, or fragmented way, with part of the raw (maternal) side presenting, this is a **"Dirty" Duncan presentation** (see Figure 61) and demands care to see that all parts are removed from the uterus.

NOTES

[1] Larger syringes are almost impossible to handle with wet hands, and will withdraw needed oxygen. Also, if the mother does not have her own unused bulb and you must use one of yours, leave it with the mother. This will keep you from accidentally using it again on another infant.

[2] An exception to this rule is dropping 1 to 3 drops of antispasmodic tincture inside the lip, by the gums, of a person who is in a seizure or who has lockjaw.

[3] Research indicates that delayed clamping of the cord does not increase hyperbilirubinemia (jaundice). Also, some researchers feel that if the cord is severed before it has completed its function--it is delivering oxygen and nutrients to the baby as long as it is still pulsating--that the baby suffers emotionally and physically, even to the extent that the experience remains subliminally as a fear of suffocation.

[4] Umbilical ties which are sterilized in alcohol must be soaked for at least an hour--a wipe, dip, or splash, or even soaking for a few minutes, WILL NOT ELIMINATE GERMS. If you must sterilize and use ties which have not had time to dry sufficiently, strip out all the moisture you can (with a sterile towel) before you use them, and then keep a close eye on the ligature. In an emergency, strips of cloth (from a petticoat, blouse, shirt, etc.) will suffice.

[5] Internal bleeding can be detected in two ways: (1) the abdomen will begin to fill, and (2) facial pallor is seen and maternal pulse rate rises sharply above its normal rate.

[6] Some ergot alkaloids are very effective in emergency situations. They contract the uterus and stop bleeding well. It must be noted here that large doses of preparations that contain ergot (a fungus that grows on cereal grains) would rapidly increase the pulse rate and cause vomiting and even convulsions. Continued intake of ergot can be harmful because capillaries and blood vessels are closed off, curbing natural distribution of body

fluids. Animals that get into molded grain will actually have tails and hind legs atrophy and fall off.

[7]Women do not really need to bleed at birth, though we are taught that birth is a bloody affair. A healthy woman who has been on the five-week formula need only bleed a couple of tablespoonfuls or less with placental separation. Lochia need not be heavy or remain long in healthy women.

[8]Sometimes what you need to do in a difficult situation has been revealed to you already. I don't believe I have ever talked with a midwife who has not "delivered babies" in her dreams. It is as if she were being prepared for and trained to handle a particular birthing situation, because the very same problems she ENCOUNTERS AND SOLVES in her subconscious state arise within a few days or weeks in reality. Indeed, she recognizes the identical situation and goes through it, on the job, as if she were role-playing her dream.

[9]Recent studies conclude that mental directions to the body can influence even the autonomic nervous system, and they offer a number of techniques to accomplish this direction. For example, fear or tension can decrease the secretion of natural oxytocin needed to contract the uterus. Remove the cause of fear or tension, or deliberately calm the mind, and the body will step up the output of oxytocin sufficiently to prevent hemorrhage from possible uterine inertia. Researchers refer to this phenomenon as **psychophysiological intervention**, others call it **biofeedback**, or more simply, the effects of mind over matter. Practitioners witness this marvel with some regularity. The unfortunate trend, however, is to impose a similar outcome with the use of drugs.

[10]In the LDS Church, adult male members usually hold the Melchizedek Priesthood. One of its functions is to bless members of the family by the laying on of hands and through prayer, in times of need.

[11]One mother told me she had eaten a good diet and had taken herbs during pregnancy. (She had consumed many gallons of red raspberry leaf tea, especially.) She delivered in the hospital and was amazed and amused when she saw her obstetrician-gynecologist running all through the hospital demanding that his colleagues see what a good, healthy placenta should look like. It was the healthiest one he had seen in many years. He asked her what she had done and she told him about the red raspberry leaf tea. His response was, "I should have known."

CHAPTER 18

FOURTH STAGE OF PARTURITION

The fourth stage of parturition begins after the placenta has presented and ends within about two hours after that.

The primary focus during this period is on the care of the fundus to prevent hemorrhage and the suturing (if necessary) of either lacerations or an episiotomy. IF HEMORRHAGE IS GOING TO OCCUR, IT IS MOST LIKELY TO OCCUR WITHIN THE FIRST TWO HOURS POSTPARTUM AND/OR ON THE TENTH DAY. Your secondary focus is on the giving of instructions to the parents about the mother's care of herself and the care of the newborn.

KEEPING THE FUNDUS HARD

You must emphasize to both parents that checking, irritating, and gathering the fundus into the hard, grapefruit-sized ball must be done every few minutes during the first 12 to 24 hours after birth. This is a must. You should be present for at least two hours postpartum, so you and your assistant(s) can teach the mother to watch the fundus for at least that amount of time. This can be done by asking her every 5 to 10 minutes if she has checked it. Even if the mother is sleeping later on, she must learn to be awake enough to check the fundus. Or, her husband might be able to do this for her. Usually the fundus will begin to remain firm within the first two to three hours after birth, but don't count on it. Often a binder made of a large towel (folded the long way) pinned tightly around the abdomen will provide the needed stimulus to keep the uterus contracting if a hand towel is rolled and placed underneath the band (over the fundus).

If ever you notice that the mother is bleeding more than she should be, as a rule of thumb, the fundus has softened and should be kneaded (assuming that any tears have been sutured and are not bleeding).

Within the first two hours postpartum, a maximum of three saturated sanitary napkins is allowed. The normal amount of **lochia** (blood-stained discharge) runs from 1 teaspoonful to 1 1/2 napkinfuls the first hour following home birth. After that, a slight menses-type flow is normal.

When the mother turns over in bed or gets up, a small amount of blood that has collected in the vaginal cavity may spill. It should not, however, be a continous flow. (With nursing and activity, a little bit of additional flow is normal from time to time.) If it should continue to flow more than normally expected, she should lie back down and check the fundus for firmness.

LACERATIONS

Lacerations range from superficial breaks in tissue inside the labia to what some term fifth-degree "blowouts" involving deep vaginal lacerations and extensive tears into the rectum. To simplify, let's describe tears of the vagina and perineum in degrees of depth.

First-degree tears involve the uppermost and outermost layers of tissue: the vaginal mucous membrane (**mucosa**) and the perineal skin. They do not involve muscle tissue. Superficial tears, usually 1/2-inch to 1-inch in length and of practically no depth, cause little, if any, bleeding. They need not be sutured and heal nicely on their own. Tears which run deeper into the mucosa or **subcutaneous** (beneath the skin) layers may be sutured if the length and location suggest problems of discomfort or infection.

Second-degree lacerations are longer and deeper; they go through the mucosa into the muscle tissue of the perineal body, but do not involve the rectal sphincter or the rectum. ANY WOUND DEEPER THAN SECOND-DEGREE REQUIRES MUCH SKILL AND SHOULD NOT BE ATTEMPTED BY THE MIDWIFE. In extreme cases of emergency where sphincter and bowel involvment has occurred, suturing must be done within a few hours, preferably within a half-hour, for best healing results and to keep feces from contaminating the wounded area.

Tears that cause excessive bleeding should be sutured quickly. If vitamin K is plentiful in the mother's blood and her iron level is good, the blood will coagulate and bleeding will shortly stop, but larger blood vessels tend to lose a lot of blood quickly, before coagulation can take place. This kind of tear should be sutured.

SUTURING

Suture, as a noun, refers to: (1) the seam formed in sewing up a wound or incision, (2) the line or seam where two bones join, especially in the skull, or (3) the material used in the act of sewing surgically, such as thread, gut, or wire. As a verb, **suture** refers to the act of sewing up a wound, incision, etc.

A woman who has just given birth (**puerpera**) may have, in spite of your best efforts, tears (lacerations) or an emergency episiotomy which needs suturing. Immediate outside help may be unavailable or impractical. If you are skilled at suturing, you may be able to render invaluable or perhaps even life-saving assistance.

Check with the laws of your state to determine when suturing or carrying any form of drug or medication is considered the practice of medicine. However, I believe one or more persons in each family should understand suturing techniques that can be used for bleeding wounds. Suturing, butterfly bandages, and practical first aids for bleeding should be learned for emergency use.

To practice suturing, use a wet poly sponge, foam rubber, or other similar material. I recommend the following book for detailed instruction in suturing: **Manual for Suturing Knots,** Bashir A. Zikria, M.D., FACS Co., Ethicon Suturing Practice Kit. (Check the catalogue of your medical supply outlet.)

Suturing Materials

You will need needles, thread, needle holder (suturing forceps), scissors, ring forceps, and cotton or gauze.

Needles. Check supply catalogs for various sizes and styles of needles and needle points. For most suturing needs, I prefer half-circle, precision point or taper point needles. These do not have cutting edges.

Suturing Threads. Suturing threads come either attached to the needle (**thread-bonded**) or separately. If you want to thread your own needles, 18- to 30-inch strands are adequate. Bonded needles usually have 27- to 30-inch strands.

Absorbable material should be used for suturing inner layers, and black, **nonabsorbable** sutures (to be easily seen and removed) are used on outer layers. Sizes and tensile strengths for suture materials are standardized by government regulations. Size denotes the diameter of the material. The more zeros (0's) in the number, the smaller the size of the strand. I like a number 3-0 (000) strand.

Braided nylon multifilament strands (nonabsorbable) are treated for **noncapillarity** (they will not act as a small blood vessel, or wick, to carry infection into the tissue). Use it DRY so it won't lose tensile strength. **Surgical cotton thread** (a nonsynthetic material) is strongest when wet and is moistened prior to use.

Surgical gut aborbs easily. **Chromic** gut has been treated in a chromium salt solution. This helps the gut resist body enzymes that dissolve it, prolonging the absorption time. This resistance is useful for tissue that heals relatively slowly and that needs support for a longer period of time. Chromium-treated gut is less irritating and causes less tissue reaction.

Suturing Techniques

Anesthetics. A good selection of equipment, used with skill, usually precludes the need for an anesthetic. If you suture soon after the baby is born (within 1/2 hour), the perineum is usually still numb from the stretching and pressure it has experienced. Some midwives carry Xylocaine or other local anesthetics to deaden tissue before they suture. I do not carry any anesthetic and prefer not to use any medication in childbirth. An ice cube rubbed over the affected area prior to suturing works nicely if you keep the rest of the mother very warm.

Do not handle your needles with hemostats or other sharp-toothed instruments (only the needle holder), nor grip the needle close to the point when pulling it through the tissue. This will dull or scar the needle and make it more traumatizing to the tissue in which it is used.

To suture, do the following:

1. Place a firm pillow or padding under the mother's hips to elevate the work area. A folded blanket works nicely. Good lighting is a must.

2. Cover the mother's legs and torso with blankets to make sure she stays warm (she will cool off quickly after birth is completed).

3. Use forceps (or hemostats) to hold gauze or cotton balls to clean the wound with mineral water or an herbal astringent, and to absorb lochia above the suture site while you suture. This will prevent your work area from being hidden by blood which occasionally will drain from the uterus. Blood, clots, etc., must be removed from the wound before suturing is done. You may need to use a speculum to hold the vagina open while you suture some internal tears.

4. Look for tissues that look alike and tears that match when held together. Tissue to be sutured must be handled gently, not bruised, stretched, pinched, or sutured tightly.

5. If a tear is second-degree or deeper, suture each layer of laceration separately, beginning with the deepest layer. This prevents bulges or excessive scar tissue, infection pockets, and more painful recovery. (To prevent strain on the sutures, the mother should hold her legs together when she sits, stands, or moves until healing is done.)

6. For tears at the perineum or on the labia, begin suturing at the edge where the tear began. This assures a clean, ordered repair at the edge of the vaginal opening. Other stitches should be spaced evenly, in alternate fashion.

7. When suturing, if you do not make sure the needle point goes completely underneath the wound, it may not close properly, leaving a pocket for infection.

8. You may use an **uninterrupted stitch** pattern, which is continuous, one stitch after the other, before you knot the suture (see Figure 62). Or you may use the **interrupted stitch** pattern, where you knot the suture after each stitch, using a square knot. Do not use extra knots "just to make sure." Avoid unnecessary bulk.

Some doctors urge the use of interrupted rather than continuous sutures, reasoning that if there was infection, bacteria would travel along the length of a CONTINUOUS suture line, infecting the entire area. An INTERRUPTED suture helps lessen the chance of infection, and leaves less foreign material (surgical thread) in the wound. Also, if an interrupted suture should break or come loose, the remaining sutures may still hold the wound together.

They take a bit longer to do, but, I prefer the interrupted stitches, except when suturing deeper layers.

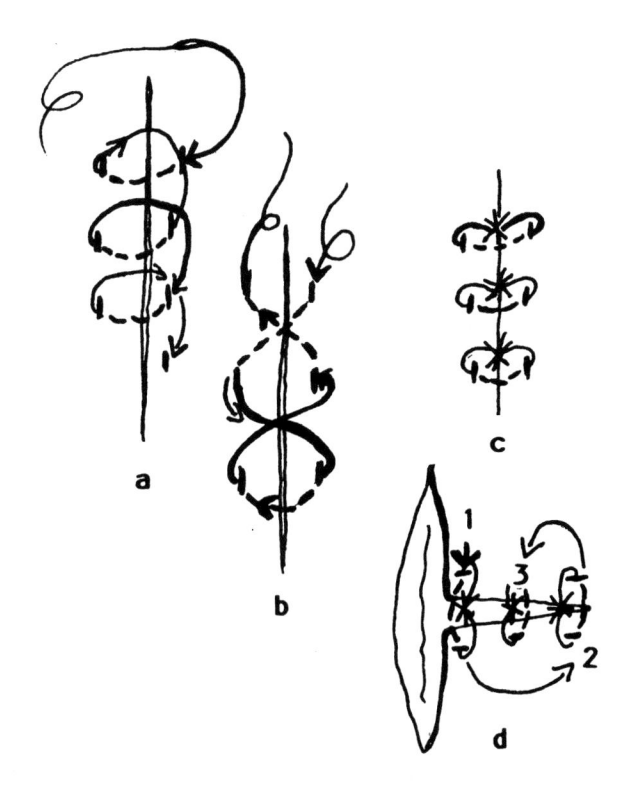

Figure 62. SUTURING TECHNIQUES. A **continuous stitch** BEGINS in a deep layer (**a**) and a figure 8 is made on the RETURN (**b**), then the ends are tied. Top layers are tied separately with **interrupted stitches** (**c, d**). Puckers and uneven repairs of the vulva (**d**) and perineum are avoided when stitches are placed in alternate fashion: (1) stitch first where the tear began, (2) next slip to the end of the tear, (3) then return to the center.

9. Never cinch up a stitch tightly. Simply draw the severed tissue together snugly and knot the suture, or continue to stitch succeeding areas, depending on which type of stitch you are using. Stitches placed about 1/4- to 3/8-inch apart will close tears nicely.

If your clients wince, jump, or ask you repeatedly how many more stitches you'll have to make, you are probably using a needle that is too large or too dull, and you may be using the needle as if you were penetrating a quilt that is too full of batting. Short pushes are forbidden. QUICK, WELL-DIRECTED, SINGLE-MOVEMENT PENETRATIONS THROUGH ONE LAYER OR PORTION OF TISSUE AT A TIME GO ALMOST UNNOTICED.

The secret of good suturing is in the twist of the wrist. One quick movement does the trick. You need practice and better needles if you create a lot of pain when you suture.

Wound Healing

Normal body defenses restore and give strength to tissues that have been torn or incised. Healing by **primary union** (union of the wound surfaces, with little scar tissue) follows suturing of an aseptic, accurately closed wound (tissues have been well matched and well joined).

The first 4 to 6 days following suturing, tissue fluids, new cells, and an increased blood supply accumulate at the wound site, and adhesion of the cells holds the wound edges together. Enzymes are produced by the body to dissolve and remove damaged or foreign tissue. This is known as the **lag phase** of healing. During the **healing phase** (days 6 to 14), cells which create fibrous tissue multiply rapidly to knit the surfaces together and to increase **tensile strength** (amount of tension or force it can withstand before tearing apart) of the wound.

The **maturation phase** (days 14 to 21) brings about a more solid healing of the wound by means of **scar tissue (fibrous connective tissue)** formation. The connective pattern of the **collagen** fibers in the scar tissue becomes stronger over a period of six months, or more, further increasing the tensile strength of the wound and decreasing its pliability. (Anytime after about 10 to 14 days, application of vitamin E may aid this process by dispersing collagen fiber patterns evenly and softening the growing rigidity so that tearing is less likely the next time that tissue is stretched to capacity.)

The speed and efficiency of the healing process depends upon the individual (age, nutritional status, physical condition, etc.), the kind of wound and where it is found, and whether environmental and other factors promote healing. Healing generally is faster when there is a good supply of blood and of oxygen to the wound. Usually an itching sensation tells you that the nerves are mending and healing is nearly done.

USE OF ASEPTIC TECHNIQUE TO PREVENT INFECTION, AND MINIMAL TRAUMA TO THE TISSUE ARE IMPORTANT TO SUCCESSFUL HEALING BY PRIMARY UNION. Too many sutures, or sutures tied too tightly cause **tissue strangulation** and **necrosis** (death of the tissue), delaying healing.

Pericare

For pericare to tender, sore, torn, or sutured areas, the following are helpful:

1. Saline solution applied to the painful area. Use 1 teaspoon salt in 1 quart warm water.

2. Jewelweed, comfrey, swamp balsam, or any astringent or nervine herb in a poultice or sitz bath. Ten-minute sitz baths are soothing and, in most cases, will not dissolve the stitches. If they do, it is better to remain clean and have a stitch dissolve prematurely (this is unlikely) than to court infection.

3. Fill a **peri bottle** (a CLEAN, plastic, squirt bottle) with 1/2 mineral water and 1/2 warm tap water. Squirt it slowly over the affected area after each trip to the bathroom--for cleanliness--and whenever additional relief is desired. You are fortunate if you have a mineral spring nearby. Fill your sitz with mineral water or squirt it slowly over the affected area.

    Even if the stitched or torn area is kept clean, infection can occur and this will prevent wound healing. Mothers should be instructed to watch for exaggerated soreness, pus, spreading redness, and elevated temperature.

4. The warmth of light directed to this area 10 minutes at a time is beneficial.

Removing Stitches

Stitches, if absorbable, begin to dissolve under the closed tissue about the seventh day. Any part of the stitches outside or above the tissue will not usually dissolve and should be removed after that. To remove them, you may or may not need to clip the thread(s). Use thumb forceps to pull the undissolved pieces out. This may tickle, but it should not hurt. Nonabsorbable stitches can be removed then, also, if desired.

CARE OF THE MOTHER

When the baby has been put to breast, the placenta has presented, the fundus is firm and in place, and any suturing has been taken care of, do the following:

1. Clean the mother's perineum, buttocks, and legs with sterile water and disinfectant. Freshen her face, chest, back, and underarms, as well. Comb her hair, if needed.

2. Pad her with a sanitary napkin and dress her in clean clothes.

3. Remove the soiled birthing linens, and change the sheets, if necessary.

    To do this without having to make the mother get up (she usually wants to rest and she should not have to get up for a while), roll the soiled linens up against the mother and tuck them underneath her, so she can easily roll over the lump. If you need to put on clean sheets, put them on after rolling the dirty linens against the mother. Tuck the clean bottom sheet in on one side, and slide the rest up against the mother, alongside the soiled linens, and have her roll over the whole bulk. When the mother has rolled over the dirty and clean linens, the dirty ones are removed, and the rest of the bed can be made.

4. The mother may now want something to eat while you jot down particular instructions she might forget later, particularly if she is a first-time mother. Keep track of her lochia and

observe her general condition as you go on to other duties.

CARE OF THE BABY

Weighing and Measuring the Baby

Weighing the baby. This may be done prior to dressing the baby. The newborn, wrapped in a receiving blanket, is placed on the scale adjusted to zero. After weighing the baby, deduct the weight of the blanket when you are through dressing the baby.

While newborn weights are fun and interesting, they may also be helpful in cases of prematurity, sickness, and the like, since they give an indication of regression or progression. When a mother is with her infant day in and day out, she may not quickly notice a stationary weight or a loss of weight. This information serves as a good barometer for the baby's current health progress.

There are several reasons why the baby may be light (5 1/2 to 6 1/2 pounds), even though he is full term: heredity, parents who smoked, a maternal history of short-gestation pregnancies. Check other signs that indicate **prematurity**: heavy, white, waxy substance on his body (**vernix**); slight breast tissue; ears flat against his head; scrotum small and tight and smooth, or labia and clitoris visible when legs are held together; hair bushy; soft hair (**lanugo**) on shoulders and elsewhere on the baby's body. Signs of **postmaturity** (overdue) include: thick, pale skin; creases on the bottom of the feet with smooth heels (the deeper the wrinkles, the more overdue); and flat, silky hair that's already beginning to give way to new hair.

Measuring the length. This is done by putting the baby on a flat surface and stretching the feet, momentarily, while using a tape or yardstick, or marking with a pencil on a paper towel or counter under the length of the baby. Measure from the top of the head to the bottom of the heel.

Examining and Dressing the Baby

The following is to be done within reach or eyesight of the mother. NEVER LEAVE THE ROOM WITH THE BABY. It is the mother's, not yours. All that you do with and for the baby must be done in her presence. This way she can ask questions or make suggestions to you about the care or dressing of her newborn.

In home birth, we don't bathe the baby with water. Use warm olive oil, temperature-tested at the wrist, with gauze to cleanse every nook and corner, fold and crease. Take care to use soft cotton tips, dipped in oil, to go around the ears and, on little girls, the vulva. Do not remove the white material in the vulva. This is protective and will absorb in a short while. In fact, use oil to encourage the absorption of the seen and unseen (clear) **vernix caseosa** all over the body. (Most home birth babies have little, if any, waxy vernix on their bodies, whether pre- or post-mature.)

Perform a brief examination as you clean and dress the newborn. (This, coupled with the infant's Apgar evaluation and a more thorough examination later on, will allow a good assessment of the infant's condition and whether specialized care is needed.) You probably will develop a routine for this:

1. Begin at the head. Saturate the head with olive oil and leave it to soak bits of blood

and mucus, etc., while you clean the face, neck, ears, and arms. (Of paramount importance is to KEEP THE BABY WARM. COVER ALL OF THE BABY BUT THE FACE AND THE AREA BEING CLEANSED.)

2. Check the roof of the mouth for cleft palate or any other irregularity (see Chapter 21, Cleft Palate and Lip).

3. Check the eyes for a milky appearance.

4. Check fingers and hands as you clean them.

5. Blot away the excess oil and don undershirt and gown. (If you can work quickly and keep the baby warm enough, oil the entire body, then dress the infant.) Check the spine for dimples or openings. Any abnormal growth anywhere on the baby (especially along the spine) should be covered with sterile, moist gauze and referred immediately to a doctor.

6. Clean below the waist. The vulva or male genitalia will probably be a little swollen. Check the anus for imperformation. If there is no opening through the anal structure, lubricate your little finger and insert it very carefully to the second joint. Sometimes only a membrane obstructs. If the obstruction does not yield, report it to a physician within three to six hours following birth.

7. Check one leg at a time. Check for webbed toes or clubfootedness (inturned feet). Clubfeet can usually be corrected if treatment is begun right away (within 24 hours of birth).

8. Diaper and either swaddle the infant or wrap him in a receiving blanket. Babies love to be swaddled (see Figure 63) the first few days.

Fourth Stage of Parturition   403

However, in order for their postures to begin to ready for walking and for their hip joints to begin to assume proper alignment for the same reason, they should not be swaddled for long. Swaddling may be good transitional care for assisting baby from the **fetal curl** to being handled in the supine and many other positions.

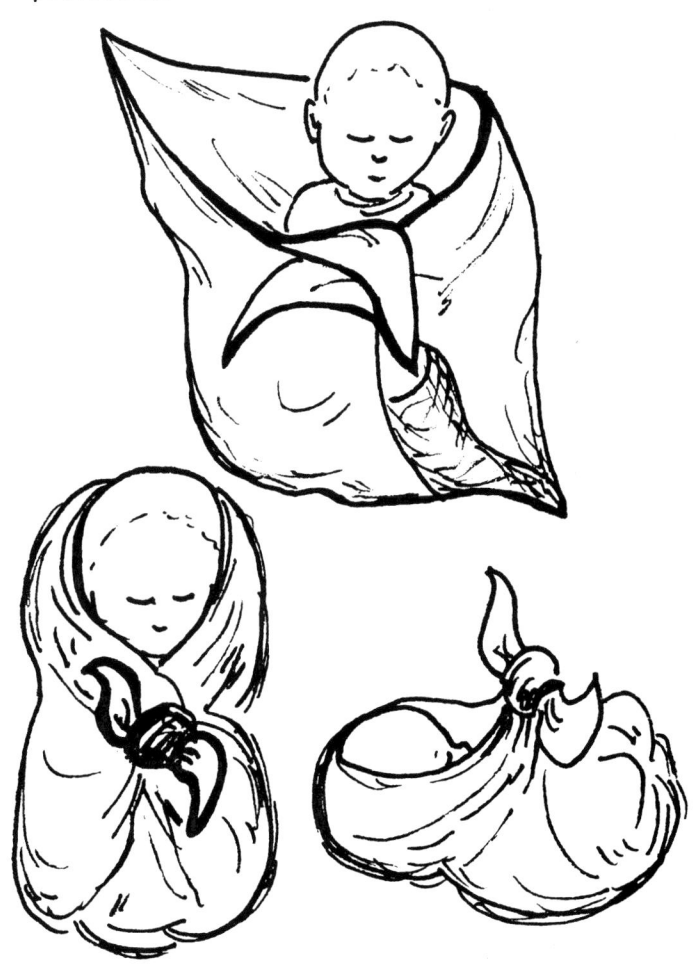

Figure 63.   SWADDLING.

Swaddling is done by laying the baby on an open receiving blanket, the baby's head cradled between two corners. Then opposite (diagonal) corners are brought together and tied securely in the center of the baby's body. Baby is lifted by the knots. Newborn's head is supported and he is curled again in the fetal position. Blanket size has to be folded to adapt to baby size and needs.

Now that Baby Dear must have his lungs open to draw in needed oxygen, the fetal curl position does not particularly contribute to lung-filling. For this reason I would not hold the baby in a curled-up position for long periods of time. On his own, he will assume the snuggle position to his liking. At any rate, blankets (even a light one in the summer) are appropriate until the baby's warmth is stable.

9. You are ready now to go back to the head. Hold the baby under the left arm (if you are right-handed), cradled between the elbow and your waist (much as you would carry a football!), with the newborn's head—face up at first—to your front (see Figure 64). Use a clean comb to draw any material away from the scalp; turn the baby's face down to clean the back of the head. The baby loves this attention.

A gently vigorous scrubbing with gauze and warm oil will render the hair and scalp clean. Remove excess oil. This head care will prevent a build-up of **cradle cap,** if the mother will continue to keep the head clean thereafter. A little hair may rub off as the scrubbing is done, but be assured that a healthy head of hair will appear in a few weeks or months, depending on genetics. Comb

Fourth Stage of Parturition 405

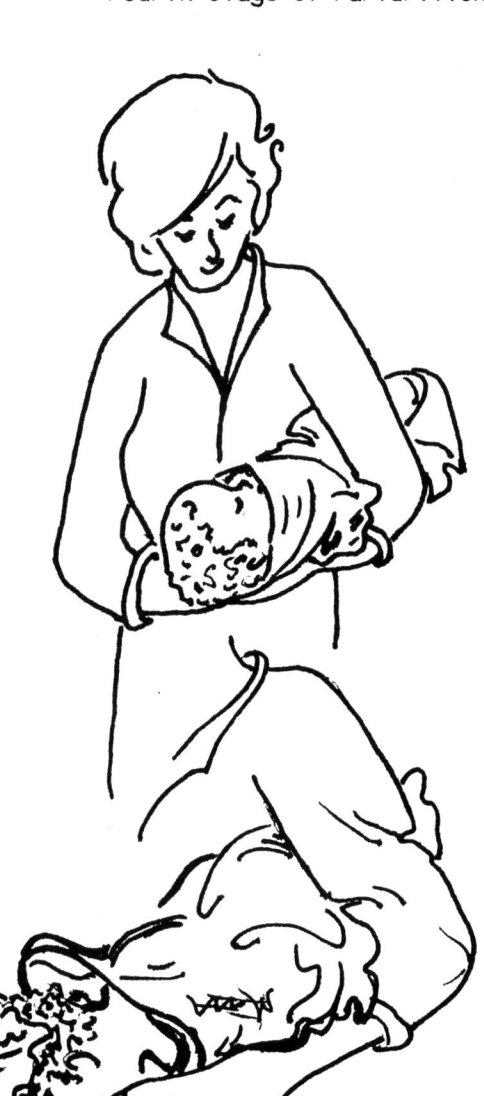

Figure 64. CARE OF THE NEWBORN'S SCALP.

the hair nicely; ribbon (with tape?) the
little girl if you wish. Parents love having
dimpled, coiffeured darlings handed to them in
sweet, clean clothing.

10. Now is the time to put **Argyrol** (or another
antibiotic preparation, in accordance with
state law) into the eyes. Put one drop into
the inner canthus, and let it run out the
other side of the eye. Then IMMEDIATELY wipe
over the closed eye two or three times with a
"dripping wet" cotton ball, from under a warm
tap, until no sign of the Argyrol is evident.
(Argyrol stings the eye a bit.) Repeat in the
other eye. (Remember that the baby's eyes do
not form tears yet, so they cannot fight eye
irritation or infection.[1])

Argyrol, a mild silver proteinate, is a nonprescription, stabilized preparation that can
be used, then stored for future use. When
dilute silver nitrate is used, care must be
taken to assure that it is a 1 **percent
solution**. Rinse with water or a saline
solution (1/2 tsp. salt to 1 cup sterile
water).[2]

11. Now Baby Dear is ready to be handed to Mother
or Father. On occasion, Mother will reach for
the baby, and you will observe a tender
moment. She delights in presenting a bit of
posterity to her husband: "Here is your son."
"I give you a daughter."

On other occasions I have witnessed fathers
giving their offspring their first fatherly
advice: "Your mother has gone through a lot
to get you here. Always respect and love her
for it." Others will say, "Welcome, Little
One. You made it fine. We have waited for

you so long, and we have loved you all the time. Now come meet your sister and brother. Son, here are Josie and Mike."

Sometimes even I get into the act later: "Baby Dear (in front of the older siblings), if you will watch them closely, your big brothers and sisters will show you how to walk and run and talk and lots of things. They love you. You are theirs . . ."

12. Be sure the baby nurses at least every four hours for the first three days TO PREVENT HYPOGLYCEMIA IN THE BABY[3] and to bring in the mother's milk. (Breast-feeding also helps the baby eliminate any remaining meconium, and it stimulates uterine contractions in the mother, helping her uterus to return to its normal size.) DON'T LET MORE THAN FOUR HOURS GO BETWEEN FEEDINGS THE FIRST THREE DAYS.

13. Babies are nose breathers--they choke if they have to breathe through their mouths--so check to be sure the baby can breathe as he sucks. The mother may need to press down the portion of the breast in front of the baby's nose. If there is any problem, be sure he is relaxed. (Babies who have had a face presentation will have brow, lip, and nasal edema, but with calming they can usually breathe all right.) Stroke the baby, reassure him, and humidify the air.

To shake down any mucous blockages not readily removed by suction, hold the baby with his face down, cup your hand, and tap it on his chest. If he cries, you're helping. (Also see Appendix D, Mucus-Cutting Formula.)

After the mother and baby have been cared for, if their vital signs are good[4] and if you have given the parents all the immediate instructions needed, you may leave after the second hour postpartum. You will want to allow the mother and baby and family to rest for 6 to 12 hours, then to return to give futher instructions and to evaluate the newborn in more detail.

NEWBORN EVALUATION

Evaluation of the general health and welfare of the infant can be done after everyone has had a rest, but this matter must be attended to. The baby is breathing. Looks happy. Seems well enough—but is he? Check the baby in the parent's presence, or you tell them what to do and have them evaluate:

1. Feel the front fontanel. It should be open and pulsating. A bulging fontanel at three to four days signals danger (probably **sepsis,** or infection in the blood stream). Have it checked by a pediatrician.

2. Check the baby's sucking response by putting your finger in his mouth. The best sign of health is how well he suckles. Also check the gag response. If both are strong, the baby is probably healthy. Little white mucous pearls on the baby's gums are normal and will go away with time.

3. Use a penlight 12-inches away from the baby's eyes to check vision. Babies can see, though they may not know what they're looking at. (Remember, they've never seen a hand, a face, or a toy before in this life, so treat their sight gently.) There should be a red reflex (called the **cat's reflex**) seen through the

Fourth Stage of Parturition 409

pupil. If the area is white, the baby may be blind, and an ophthalmologist should see the child. (Milky, pussy, green mucus in the baby's eyes is a sign of gonorrhea, which can cause blindness in three to six days if not treated.) If the baby squints or his eyes turn in, don't worry—eye movement deviations (**strabismus**) are normal. The baby has to learn how to use his eyes together and to develop the eye muscles. Observe the eyes again at six weeks, at three months, and at six months. If strabismus is still there, take the baby to an ophthalmologist.

4. If there has been no urination within six hours, check the urethra at the vulva or penis. The physician may have to examine for internal obstructions. Palpate the abdomen to check for masses or a distended bladder. If found, they should be reported. If help is not readily available, catheterization may be necessary to relieve the urine. If this cannot safely be carried out, get help. An operation may be necessary.

5. Check the face for abnormal facial features. Oriental features, a short upper lip and thick, fissured tongue, stubby fingers and clear **simian lines** (deep horizontal lines) on the palms indicate **Down's syndrome**. A receding chin, broad nose, and low-set ears[5] may indicate a congenital kidney immaturity. Check also for facial paralysis, which may have occurred because of pressure from the pelvis on a nerve during delivery. This will probably disappear within a few days.

6. Check for hip dislocation. It rarely occurs, but to check, hold the **lesser** and **greater trochanters** (processes on the inside and

outside of the upper part of the **femur**, or thigh bone, next to the hip socket) and shift the hip joint (see Figure 65). If there is a dislocation, have the mother put a triple-thick diaper on the baby for a while (about three to six weeks) to secure his legs open.

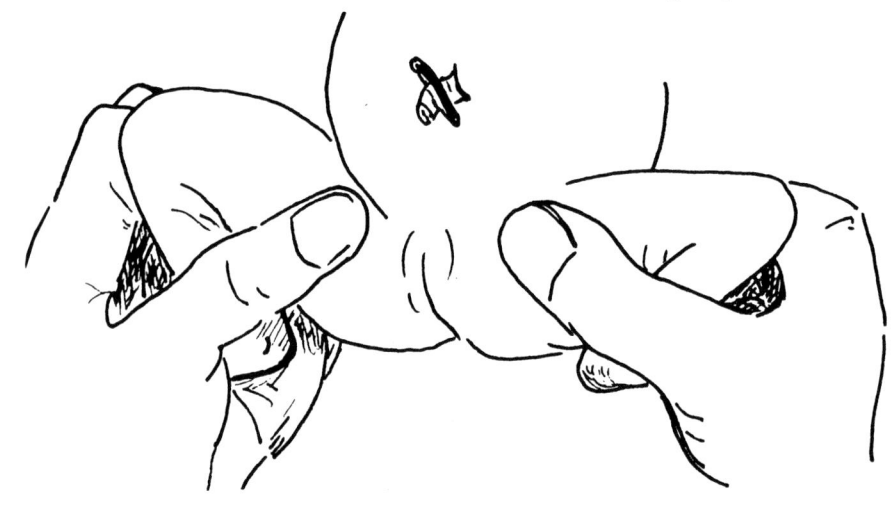

Figure 65. HIP DISLOCATION. Abduct (spread outward) the thighs and lift SLIGHTLY from behind. (Thumbs are on both sides of the pubic arch, in the creases of the legs, and middle fingers are at the outside bend of each thigh, on the process where the femur extends into the hip socket. If this movement causes a "clunk," the hip is dislocated. (No clunk, no dislocation.)

NOTES

[1] The best of all treatments for eye irritation or inflammation is a drop of mother's milk into the infected eye several times a day.

[2] "There seems to be a lack of agreement regarding the eye rinse to use after $AgNO_3$ [silver nitrate] instillation. Some nurseries employ saline because it forms a precipitate (silver chloride), which more quickly inactivates the irritating $Ag O_3$.

Fourth Stage of Parturition   411

Others consider the precipitate itself to be irritating and prefer to use water." (A. Joy Ingals and M. Constance Salerno, **Maternal & Child Health Nursing**, 3rd ed. [St. Louis: The C. V. Mosby Company, 1975], p. 180n.)

[3]Dr. Camilla S. Wood, nurse physiologist and director of a graduate program in nursing at BYU, conducted a pilot study which revealed that infants who fasted (were not nursed or fed) for 10 hours following birth continued to have blood glucose decreases (lowered blood sugar levels) for as long as 24 hours after birth. Dr. Wood believes the nerve tissue must have glucose: "Without it, I believe the brain could be affected." She also suspects that the long-range effects of this early glucose depletion are learning disabilities in children. She contrasts infants with adults, explaining that babies are in an entirely different situation. They come from just having had all their caloric requirements met by their mothers, and they have very small amounts of glucose reserves to call upon in times of need.

[4]MATERNAL VITAL SIGNS at norm are: temperature, 98.6 degrees F; **pulse rate,** 60 to 70 beats per minute; blood **pressure** 113/78 to 125/90 mm Hg; **respiration,** 14 to 18 breaths per minute. (You will know the mother's INDIVIDUAL norms from your prenatal records and from your labor log.)

NEWBORN VITAL SIGNS. A newborn's temperature is about 1 degree higher than the mother's at birth, but rapidly drops outside the womb. With warm blankets, contact with the mother's skin, etc., it reaches a normal 98.6 degrees F within 8 to 12 hours. Unless bedded by the mother or dressed warmly, if the temperature is cool, care should be taken to maintain room temperature at 75 to 80 degrees F, with the humidity below 50 percent. The pulse of the newborn is VERY difficult to take, so all readings must be taken with a stethoscope over the heart region (through the chest or back). The pulse will be the same as the baby's normal fetal heart tone was. The respirations of the newborn are "normally" irregular. They come from the abdomen or diaphragm and range from 30 to 50 breaths per minute, depending on the baby's activity. A PERSISTENT 50 count or more per minute is too fast, and ANY TIME retractions over the sternum or chest wall, caused by sucking in air, occur, they indicate respiratory distress. Evaluation by the physician should be done immediately. (The blood pressure of an infant has to be taken with a 1-inch-wide cuff. It usually averages 80/46 mm Hg, but is almost inaudible and DIFFICULT to take.) One should remember that as a person grows older, pulse and respiratory rates DECREASE and blood pressure readings RISE.

[5]A broad nose, receding chin, or low-set ears are not of themselves abnormal, but according to medical records certain CLUSTERS of features seem indicative of abnormalities.

CHAPTER 19

POSTPARTUM

After everyone involved with the birth of the baby has rested, you may want to instruct the mother about things to expect **postpartum** (after delivery). Tell her things she should watch for in the next several days, and things she should do.

POSTPARTUM INSTRUCTIONS

1. If the mother is Rh-negative, she must have a **RhoGAM** shot within 72 hours of birth to prevent **Rh sensitization** (see Chapter 12, Rh Factor and Hemolytic Disease).

2. A **PKU** test for the baby needs to be done within 48 hours after the mother's milk (not colostrum) comes in, to determine whether the baby has **phenylketonuria** (an inborn defect in the body's ability to metabolize **phenylalanine**), which results in retardation if not detected and treated early enough. (Some physicians will wait several days following milk flow for this test.)

3. A birth certificate should be registered within the limits of the law in your state.

4. An antibiotic preparation should have been used in the infant's eyes following birth (this is usually required by law) to prevent V.D.-caused blindness. (If a mother has gonorrhea, her baby's eyes are frequently infected as it passes through the vagina.) A number of states still require the use of **silver nitrate,** but health professionals are working to remove such restrictive legislation, since other effective products are available. (The silver nitrate solution causes chemical irritation of the eyes, and it can cause blindness if it is not dilute enough.) (See Chapter 18, Examining and Dressing the Baby.)

5. The newborn should sleep on his right side with his head down three inches below the hips for 24 hours, especially if he is mucusy. (A brick under the foot of the crib will do nicely.)

6. The mother should keep a two-ounce ear syringe in the crib or at the head of her bed if the infant is sleeping with her, for easy access in case she needs to suction mucus from the infant's nose and mouth.

7. The baby should urinate within the first six to eight hours after birth. If he does not, have the pediatrician check this. A colored paper tissue placed in the diaper will reveal the presence of moisture.

8. The midwife should discuss the newborn evaluation with the parents.

9. The midwife should warn the mother to be especially watchful for hemorrhage during the 6th to 11th days after birth. It seems that

about this time mothers begin to feel much better and begin household duties more quickly than they should. Hemorrhage becomes likely because of this excess activity too soon after birth. When the mother notices extra bleeding, she should reduce her activity and rest more. (Tending only herself and the baby for about two to three weeks is making use of common sense.)

Also at about this period, a disruption in **involution** (the process by which the uterus returns to its original proportions), particularly at the placental site—perhaps because of an undetected, retained placenta fragment—may cause hemorrhage. This needs immediate attention by the physician, as does any other condition which causes profuse bleeding.

10. Intercourse should not occur for six weeks—after healing has had time to take place and internal organs have had time to return to their normal places and sizes. Conception can take place before the mother's strength and energies have replenished. With the extra burden of nursing her newborn, her body needs time to rebuild while she is getting back into the role of caring for the rest of the family as well. Becoming pregnant immediately can give rise to numerous problems.

LOCHIA

Midwives must be knowledgeable about postpartum lochia and be able to answer questions about it. **Lochia** is the blood-stained vaginal discharge following birth. An average pattern for lochia flow is as follows:

1. The bright redness turns darker the first 2 to 3 days.

2. In 3 to 4 days, the color turns pale.

3. After about the 10th day, the color turns whitish or yellowish, and then lochia should discontinue.

If brownish red lochia passes, it indicates that a little fresh bleeding took place, stopped, and is now old and passing. If the lochia at any time has an unusually foul odor, there is probably an infection. This odorous condition sometimes is an indication that the uterus has tipped abnormally, trapping old lochia (see Chapter 21, Anteflected Uterus).

When a mother thinks her lochia has ceased after about 8 to 12 days, she may find perhaps a third of a pad of fresh, new blood, and then the flow may cease again, only to return similarly in perhaps three days. This is sometimes caused by nursing, which stimulates the uterus. She may want to take 1 or 2 capsules of ginseng and sarsaparilla daily. This increases progesterone, which curbs the bleeding.

AFTERPAINS

Afterpains accompany lochia the first one to five days postpartum. These are contractions that assist the fundus to remain firm and to return to its normal size. The cramps usually can be relieved by drinking St. Johnswort tea, a glassful ten minutes before nursing. If afterpains are very uncomfortable, the mother may take 2 or 3 capsules of St. Johnswort, as needed. (The TEA made from St. Johnswort gets into the system more quickly.)

One chiropractor found a consistent distortion of lower back alignment in a group of women suffering with afterpains. In each case, the fifth lumbar vertebra had rotated posteriorly on the right side and the sacrum had rotated posteriorly and inferiorly on the left side, interfering with proper neurological functioning of the uterus. A chiropractic manipulation, sometimes called a **lumbar roll**, was used to correct this distortion (see Chapter 15, Back Adjustments). Approximately 20% of the women had relief from their afterpains following this adjustment. The remaining 80% required additional therapy.

One therapy found to be very helpful was stimulation of the **Neuro-Vascular Dynamic reflex points**[1] for the uterus. To do this, the husband (or attendant) presses the area just to the side of the spine in the lower back with the finger tips of one hand, while the other hand holds finger tip pressure on a point approximately one inch above the middle of the pubic arch (see Figure 66). These contacts are simply held with a steady pressure (3 to 5 lbs.) until a slight pulsation is felt in the finger tips at both points.

Some women reported that if these contact points were held while they nursed, the afterpains would reduce, then fade away. Often, repetition was necessary to cause complete cessation of the afterpains.

At every turn we are continuing to see the value of holistic health care. We have recognized the benefits of chiropractic and other physical therapy care during pregnancy. Now it seems that such care is helpful following birth.

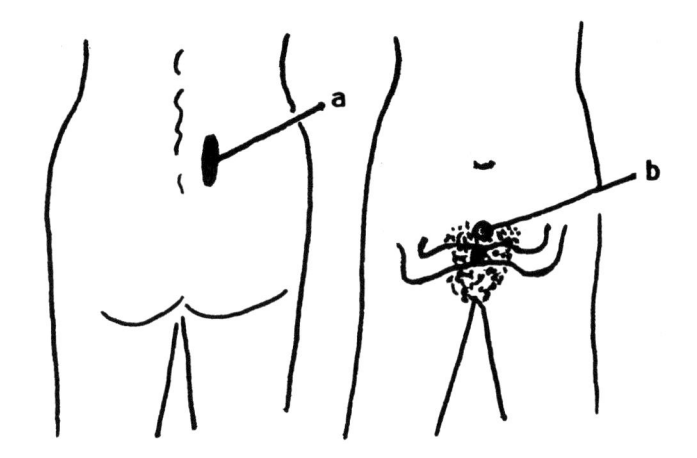

Figure 66. UTERINE REFLEX POINTS (NEURO-VASCULAR DYNAMICS). Simultaneously hold the sacral dimples (**a**) and a point one inch above the symphysis pubis (**b**) to lessen the discomfort of afterpains postpartum.

BREAST-FEEDING

When I gave birth to my last child in the hospital (I was converted to home birth too late for my own children), my roommate was an R.N. She had given birth to a boy. After two or three days of unsuccessfully trying to nurse her infant, she became desperate. It was obvious to me that the baby had been fed between nursing times and so did not make much effort to nurse.

This baby was the first child of my roommate, and nursing was a new experience for her. Finally, she turned to me in tears and asked me what she should do. I would have offered help sooner, but I thought R.N.'s knew everything--literally, everything. I suggested to her that while her infant was in utero, everything he had touched or had had in his mouth was the same temperature and about the same texture and density—the thumb, the cord, the toe. He could not recognize her nipple as anything distinctive.

I suggested that she hold her breast above the colored portion, between her forefinger and middle finger, so that it presented a firm object to her baby, something he could latch onto and recognize as something different from what he had felt before. I told her to hold the nipple and keep it firm until he began to nurse. After two tries, my friend began to cry again, but this time for joy, because the baby was nursing beautifully.

You can be sure that your baby "has read the same book you have!" He knows how to nurse. For best results, though, nothing extra should be given the newborn--he should be fed just what nature intended.[2] Let him nurse on demand until he sets his own schedule and "supply demand" within a few days after mother's milk comes in.

A newborn should be fed within the first half hour after birth and at least every four hours during the first week, in order to prevent hypoglycemia. Feedings every two to three hours are fine if the demand is there, but do not let the baby go a full four hours without feeding him.

In the home birth setting, mother's milk (not colostrum) comes in within 18 to 30 hours, as opposed to 3 to 5 days in the hospital. This is because at home no drugs have been used and there has been less trauma; nursing occurs on demand. In the hospital, the baby is usually not fed on demand, and medication slows the milk.

A word of caution should be added here. The nursing mother must still be wary of her use of drugs or medication, which are passed to the infant through the milk. At least one drug-- **thiouracil**, used in treating hyperthyroidism-- becomes MORE CONCENTRATED in mother's milk and may affect the baby SEVERELY.

LAXATIVES will go through the mother's milk and physic the infant, especially such things as milk of magnesia, Epsom salts, cascara, and Ex-lax. (Also, some "strong" vegetables, such as asparagus or cabbage, or other foods or spices, will distress some infants. The baby's individual tolerances and needs will guide dietary decisions.)

With a few exceptions (catnip-fennel tea for abdominal distress, lemon water for jaundice, drinks of water, etc.), infants need ONLY mother's milk for about six months, because certain digestive juices are not available to the infant until later. Mother's milk is rich and contains all the essential nutrients in the right proportions. It may not look like it because, unlike colostrum, which is thick and rich, mother's milk looks thin and a little clear. (Blonde mothers tend to have a greenish cast to their milk. Other mothers may have a bluish-colored milk.)

Milk Loss

At about the third, seventh, and eleventh weeks the baby is growing especially fast, and his demand for milk rises. You may THINK you are losing your milk at these times. THAT'S PROBABLY NOT THE CASE AT ALL. It's just that the baby is growing and needs an additional ounce or two. To bring supply up to demand, let him nurse a little more frequently, since this stimulates the supply to increase. Activity that is refreshing, but not tiresome, and sufficient rest also help. Be sure to get plenty of liquids (juice, teas, water--drinking milk does not make milk, and it may cause congestion in the baby).

When your supply is plentiful, you can prepare for the leaner times by pumping some milk and freezing it in sterile containers. Breast pumps can be purchased at the drugstore, or milk can be accumulated in breast cups that are fitted into the bra.

A mother can also bring in an ample supply of good, rich milk by drinking 2 to 4 cups of tea per day made from a combination of red raspberry leaf, marsh mallow root, and blessed (holy) thistle. The marsh mallow root (a rich source of zinc) soothes tender breasts while supplying nutrients. Red raspberry leaf, the woman's herb, provides nutrients and antacid qualities. Blessed thistle helps produce good milk, as do dill and other herbs.

Do not become discouraged about nursing. Many mothers nurse and are usually very willing to give you some helpful tips. All over the United States members of the La Leche League can give nursing mothers valuable help. I encourage mothers to take advantage of their services if they have any questions about nursing.

Excess Milk

When the *primigravida* gives birth, she is likely to have a rather full enlargement of her breasts when her milk comes in. She may think her breasts are engorged. It will be uncomfortable because her mammary glands have never been filled to this extent before. WITH SUCCEEDING PREGNANCIES, her breasts will fill only enough to meet the demand. If this filling of the breasts becomes too uncomfortable and she spills or drips milk profusely, she should reduce her intake of all liquids. She can stand under a warm shower to allow the excess milk to empty from the breasts without distress. This will relieve her greatly.

Let-Down Reflex

It is important that mother and baby have quietness and contentment at nursing time. A mother who has been under emotional stress of any kind, because of quarrels or tensions, will hold her milk back involuntarily and upset her baby.

The mother must learn to think in terms of relaxing and of letting her milk down. Emotional upsets curb this normal **let-down reflex**, which allows the milk to flow freely. As nursing routine is being established, a glass of water, tea, or juice just before nursing will assist the let-down reflex.

Mastitis

Following birth, especially, when milk first comes in and the supply increases, a little hard knot(s) will sometimes develop in the breast, perhaps because of a clogged milk duct or a "back-up" of milk. It swells, then spreads and impacts other areas. One of the most soothing remedies for inflammation or infection of the breast (**mastitis**) is to let warm water from a shower beat down on the breasts to break down the impacted areas, and to allow them TO EMPTY WITHOUT FURTHER STIMULATION TO PRODUCE MORE MILK. If a shower is not available, the following will help:

1. Poultices of comfrey (fresh leaves with enough warm water to blend well) applied to the sore breast. (Support the breasts with a good foundation garment.)

2. Marsh mallow root powder made into a paste with a little mineral water and applied to the breast with cheesecloth or flannel (keep the nipple dry); place plastic over that. This should be applied between feedings. Gentle rubs with warm comfrey oil or olive oil help.

3. Poultices of pokeroot leaves that have been bruised or blended can help. The roots, when roasted and powdered, then applied are as good as the tops for this malady.

4. Have the baby nurse frequently on the affected side. (DO NOT STOP NURSING.) When the hard lumps go away, the problem is gone.

Sore Nipples

Before and after feedings, nipples should be kept clean and dry. If nipples become sore, you can still let the baby nurse, even though he may get a little blood. If the nipple is INFECTED, don't let the baby nurse from that breast until the infection is gone (express and discard the milk). Continue to let him nurse from the other breast. BF & C Ointment (bone, flesh, and cartilage ointment) is reported to be superb for breast care. Any preparation that will not harm the baby, but which effects nursing comfort, can be used.

Illness

If you have a fever, it will depend on what is causing it whether you should continue to nurse the baby. A debilitating, infectious disease, such as hepatitis or tuberculosis, would preclude nursing. If the baby has a fever, he probably needs teas and water more than milk.

Weaning

When it comes time to wean the baby, drink sage or parsley tea and rub wild alumroot tea over the breast to gradually dry up the milk. Normally, a minimum of a year of nursing gives the baby a good start. (Cow's milk given to infants is associated with allergy problems and with anemia.)

SUGGESTIONS FOR THE NEWBORN'S CARE AND COMFORT

Circumcision

Seldom is there a real need for this operation to the newborn male. Dr. Richard C. Hochberger, an osteopathic physician, states:

> Although considered a minor surgical procedure, reported complications of neonatal circumcision include infection, hemorrhage, loss of penile skin, laceration of penile and scrotal skin, injury to the glans, urethral fistula, urinary retention, staphylococcal scalded skin syndrome, concealed penis, necrotizing fasciitis, Fournier's syndrome and sepsis. . . .
>
> Elective newborn circumcision is a cruel procedure. . . . The beliefs that infants "do not feel pain" or "won't remember it anyway" reflect concepts which cannot be substantiated and are barbaric. . . . Marked flushing frequently occurs during circumcision and a propensity of newborn infants to wail and vomit under the stress of circumcision is well appreciated by nursery personnel. The alteration in pitch, the intensity of cry when the first crush and clamp is applied to the foreskin is unmistakable. . . .
>
> . . . Questionable potential benefits including the facilitation of penile hygiene and diminution in the risk of cancer seem to be outweighed by the risks of hemorrhage, life threatening infection, and lack of cost effectiveness. The neglect of the operator to obtain informed consent and [to] perform a needlessly radical technique with apparent disregard for pain needs to be abandoned.[3]

Sometimes the exercise of patience and simple care will solve the problem of a tight foreskin. At each bathing time (and this begins with the oil baths prior to the dropping off of the umbilical stump), application of olive oil to the glans penis and a gentle but firm effort to pull the foreskin back will yield a solution within a few days. It may take the application of oil to a cotton-tipped swab and carefully inserting it under the foreskin fold at each bath time to help it stretch. Care must be taken not to introduce bacteria under the foreskin, but within a few days to a month or so there will be good results.

When the foreskin does slip back completely, do not leave it in that position. Quickly oil and wash the area and bring the foreskin back to cover the glans. Good hygiene calls for pulling the foreskin back, washing, and replacing it at each bathtime throughout life, anyway. It is the matter-of-fact way that this is expeditiously attended to that prevents undue curiosity or the development of sensations that would be unwise for a youngster to be overanxious about at tender ages. The same can be said for the female infant and child. Attitudes develop healthy or unhealthy attention to bodies and their functions.

Care of the Umbilical Stump

It is imperative that the mother be instructed to use a cleaning and drying agent of some kind on the umbilical stump to promote: (1) the discouragement of bacterial build-up, and (2) the drying of the stump as rapidly as possible. Alcohol is a good agent to use if the mother will remember not to bathe the whole abdomen with it. Saturating the cord stump with alcohol has been standard procedure for a long time. However, the tendency to saturate the abdomen as well causes actual intoxication of the newborn (the alcohol is absorbed into the system through the skin).

There are other preparations that work better, and if they are used correctly they will dry and assist the separation of the stump as quickly. Myrrh gum and goldenseal powder have been used successfully, although they tend to discolor the clothing and skin. Mineral water works extremely well to dry and to keep down infection while it hurries atrophy and separation. Saturate the stump with mineral water, then place a rolled piece of dry gauze around the stump before diapering the baby. The snug diaper will hold the gauze in place until the next diaper change. The mineral water will in no way harm the baby's system.

IT IS VERY IMPORTANT TO KEEP THE STUMP CLEAN OF URINE AND DRY. With EACH diaper change THE STUMP MUST BE CLEANSED TO ACCOMPLISH THE DRYING AND TO KEEP INFECTION DOWN. If a powdered agent is used, DO NOT allow this to be breathed by the baby. The stump will usually atrophy and fall off within three to five days. Apply hydrogen peroxide to the rather raw area for a day or so until signs of healing are evident.

Jaundice

The newborn infant's liver sometimes has difficulty disposing of dead red blood cells, leaving his **bilirubin count**[4] high and his color yellowed (**jaundiced**).

Expose the baby (with only a diaper on) to INDIRECT sunlight and fresh air for half an hour a day the first three or four days after birth. The room should be warm. Lay the baby on his stomach, to protect the eyes. The baby's bilirubin count can go high in a dark room, so he needs this light.

Early jaundicing (during the first 12 to 36 hours) is usually Rh-related (the Rh-negative mother has formed antibodies which attack and destroy the Rh-positive baby's red blood cells, creating toxic bilirubin levels). The baby will need a lab test done every two hours to keep track of bilirubin.

Jaundice which appears three to five days after birth is not too unusual, and is considered "normal." Fetal blood loss in any degree, even the pricking of the heel for the PKU test or the bruising of the fetal scalp during labor, can cause this jaundicing.

ANY jaundicing, however, should be watched carefully to see that it does not reach the deeper yellow or orange color proportions. In either case of jaundicing, the baby will need the extra sunlight (the light helps detoxify the bilirubin), plus increased liquid in the form of 3 drops of lemon juice in two ounces of water, twenty minutes or more before nursing, two or three times a day.

Onset of jaundice can be detected by pressing the pad of your finger against the frontal bones of the baby's skull (just above and between his eyes) or on the chin or the end of the nose. If the skin is yellow when the finger is lifted, the treatment noted above should be enlisted. The mother should continue to nurse the baby.

Crying

If the baby cries constantly, watch him for a while. Try turning him upside down. He may like that better (he's probably been that way almost all of his life, so far).

Before the mother's milk comes in, the baby may become hungry because there is not enough colostrum at the feedings. Or, as the mother's milk comes in plentifully, the baby may drink too fast and get a stomachache. These two distresses can be relieved by giving the baby 1 to 2 ounces of warm catnip tea prepared with boiled water and steeped with six fennel seeds. In the second instance, where the baby is already full, wait 40 minutes or so before giving him the tea. The catnip-fennel tea soothes the tummy, moves the gas, and lulls the baby to sleep.

A baby that is snuggly warm, comfortable, dry, fed, and loved seldom cries. However, a normal birth can be somewhat traumatic to some babies. Soft, slow music or the "Lullaby of the Womb" cassette (uterine sounds, maternal heartbeats, etc.) can be helpful when played for the baby. Nervine teas coming through the milk, or catnip tea directly to the baby will also help. If pediatric exams clear any pathologies, any of the above will help calm the crying infant.

Colic

Colic usually comes during the latter part of the day and in early evening hours. It is seldom seen in the breast-fed baby, but infants exposed to wind or drafts will swallow air and get colic.

Catnip and fennel tea can be given to the colicky baby. One-half teaspoon catnip and six fennel seeds steeped in one cup boiling water, covered and then cooled, works wonders to promote relief and sleep. These herbs carry off accumulated air, alleviate cramps in the bowels, and help the baby to sleep comfortably. One ounce or more will do the trick.

How do you know the baby has colic? When fed, the baby thinks he is still hungry and will cry and fret. This is usually accompanied with severe stomach cramps that cause the infant to curl up, just as an adult does when faced with abdominal pain. The warm tea, given by drops to newborns, or by bottle, and a snuggly warm blanket will solve the problem. The persistently crying baby may benefit from the use of the mucus-cutting formula for the stools (see Appendix D, Mucus-Cutting Formula, Stools).

Solid Foods

Do not feed the baby solid foods. He will not begin to secrete saliva until he is about three months old, or to produce certain digestive juices until much later, so he needs little or no supplement to mother's milk until six to nine months. What little iron is found in mother's milk is very easily digested and utilized by the baby.

When solid food is introduced, it should be pureed food from the table. Given small amounts, one kind at a time for a few days; vegetables can be given first, then fruits. Certain foods will bring loose bowels, hives, etc., quickly. Discontinue those until a much later time. I do not agree that babies need animal protein (meat).

Constipation

Since the stools of breast-fed babies are soft, they are rarely constipated (even when bowel evacuations are days apart). Mothers, most of whom have great intuitive or maternal instincts, will sense when bowels need to move and are not

Postpartum 429

doing so. It is seldom necessary to give enemas to infants, but on occasion a simple thing such as environmental tension, emotional stress in the mother who nurses her baby, etc., will cause constipation.

At such times, a glycerine suppository, or the small, gloved finger (cut the nails) that is salved with petroleum jelly, inserted through the anus just past the sphincter muscles, will stimulate the baby's peristaltic nerves to evacuate, pushing it out. The stool will follow. If it does not, after inserting the finger or suppository two or three times, and holding it there for a few minutes, a cup of tepid water enema will do the trick. Do not worry if the water does not come out immediately. Diaper the baby and give him some TLC and it will soon pass.

Diarrhea

Watery, loose, greenish stools, lethargy, dehydration, unstable temperature, loss of appetite, and loss of weight are symptoms of a contagious diarrhea. Infants cannot handle this condition for long without serious consequences. (Strict hand-washing must be followed by those who handle infants to prevent passing these pathogenic **colon bacilli** to the baby.)

Extreme care must be given to halt the diarrhea and to replace body fluids and electrolytes, and to gradually return to normal feedings. Immediate help is recommended when the above symptoms appear.

Unusual Baby Odors

If the baby gives off any unusual odor, he should be watched carefully and possibly hospitalized. Protein intolerance gives off a musty, mousy odor.

Inability to metabolize one of the amino acids, **leucine,** gives off a sweaty-feet odor. The fishy or rancid butter odors, and the cooked or rotten cabbage odors sometimes are followed by irritability, progressive drowsiness, convulsions, and hemorrhage in the one- or two-month-old baby.

Umbilical Hernia

If ever a rather mobile lump bulges under the skin at or near the navel, it may need attention. An **umbilical hernia** (protrusion of the bowel), if very large, can be helped somewhat by placing a soft pad over it, then covering this with an abdominal band until it can be seen by the doctor. Small-to-medium herniated lumps can be contained in this fashion and some seem never to be a cause for concern. (We continue to find the application of a few old practices very sensible--for instance, the use of abdominal bands for both mother and baby.)

Short gestational cords, especially, are responsible for some umbilical hernias. Small hernias usually disappear in a few weeks unless the infant cries vigorously or for long periods. Adhesive tape (applied to pinches of skin) across the hernia helps, but if the skin is irritated by the tape, place a clean copper penny over the hernia and hold it in place with an abdominal binder. These can be made with two or three layers of unbleached domestic (muslin) or flannel. Abdominal bands must be kept clean and dry.

Yeast Infection (Thrush)

Occasionally yeast infection will persist in the vagina and the fetus picks up the infection during birth. The newborn will then develop **thrush:** cankerous sores in the mouth, on the face, and in the diaper area. This can become fatal when the infection spreads into the nose, mouth, throat, and throughout the alimentary canal. Different forms of treatment, even prescription drugs sometimes, may yield only frustration and discouragement when the infection returns again and again.

To help prevent the return of thrush, give the newborn 100 to 300 mg of niacinamide daily and apply black walnut tincture locally. The newborn will get niacinamide (in the milk) through the mother's increased intake, but can also be given liquified dosages. All of the B vitamins are helpful (nursing mothers can significantly increase daily intake of B vitamins and vitamin C), and acidophilus is particularly important.[5]

Acidophilus (super strengths are available) should be taken by both mother and baby over a period of time to help eradicate the tenacious **Candida albicans** fungus which causes yeast infection. (Nursing mothers and their babies may wish to take the **L. bifidus** strain; if that doesn't help, they should switch to **L. acidophilus.**)

HEALING AND SECURITY BENEFITS OF BONDING

Much has been said about bonding and its long-range effects on all concerned. There are yet other benefits, healing benefits, derived from close personal contact. Mothers soon learn that any time an infant is not well, he wants to be held. What does one do when his arm has been injured? He holds the arm, cradles it, or simply holds a hand over the injured area. Why? Perhaps some unexplained things happen, but for sure healing comes from the warmth, the touch of healthy tissue giving positive feeling to the damaged tissue.

I recall a lovely lady, the national director of a behavioral science institute, who used to tell her students that elderly people, especially if they are infirm, should never sleep in the same beds or rooms with very young persons. The aged body draws heavily upon the fresh, positive, healthy energies of the young. She used to say also that when an infant is sick and the parents or others are well, the infant should be held to allow some parts of the baby's body to touch the flesh of a well person. This touching gives the baby an opportunity to draw on the positive energies of a system that is in better condition.[6]

I can see Moms everywhere nodding their heads in recognition of this truth, as they recall the days and nights when their sick infants had to be held. They will remember too that their infants always seemed to wake up when they were put into bed, especially when they were ill. A sick child feels much more comforted, both physically and emotionally, while being nourished by the touch of a healthy person. Most babies would rather sleep alone and in their beds IF THEY ARE WELL and if during their waking hours they feel secure in their relationships.

Security benefits come through good bonding with family members. Introduction to strangers is not usually a problem when bonding has established security. A person who stops long enough to spend some time watching and communicating with a baby or young child will be captured by his uninhibited responses. A baby who is well and comfortable accepts anyone who does not rush him or threaten his security. He doesn't care whether you are rich or poor, skinny or fat, short or tall, man or woman, bearded or bald.

Infants are very sensitive to another's spirit, and if your spirit is loving and kind, if you smile at him whether he comes to you or not, and if you give him time to feel your spirit, he will respond. If he cries or fears you, he may not be well, or perhaps you have hurried the relationship.

Seldom do children rebel against going to bed, not getting a bottle, etc., if they have been dealt with in a loving and patient manner and have had enough quality time spent to build a real sense of being cared about. This love and attention builds the security that allows them to make changes easily in young life.

Someone has suggested a formula for how often you should hug or physically respond to your child: if he's one year old, at least once an hour; six years, at least every six hours; and so on up to age 12, after which it is twice a day for everyone!

The intent is not to translate emotion into hard and fast rules, but it does demonstrate the fact that the younger the child is, the more frequently he needs this assurance of your love (he may resort to misbehaving if you ignore him "past his limit"). All of us need expressions of affection to thrive. Security through bonding promotes physical health and emotional healing in ANY individual.

POSTNATAL EXERCISES

Regaining a fun figure is important to new mothers. Wearing a snug girdle for about two weeks will help internal organs to slip back into place more quickly. Simple exercises (see Figure 67) done 15 minutes before an hour's rest or bedtime, on a regular basis, should not overtax a nursing mother who is trying to establish a milk supply.

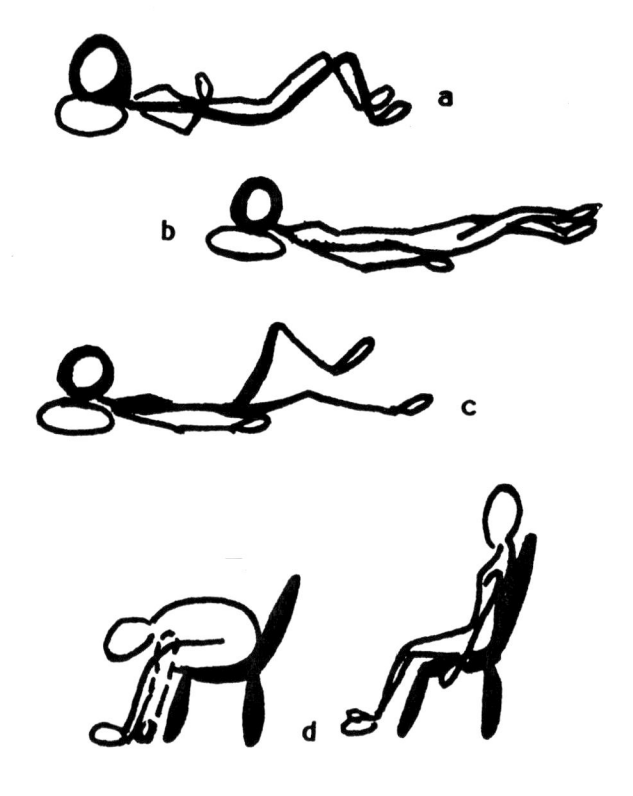

Figure 67. POSTNATAL EXERCISES. (a) Hands press on the abdomen while thoracic breathing is done, then while abdominal breathing is done. (b) Knees straight, legs crossed. Contract and relax buttocks and thighs. Anal and perineal muscles are drawn in tightly, as in kegel exercises. (c) One leg is straight, the other is lifted to a right angle and lowered slowly. Repeat with the other leg. (d) Sit straight in a chair, legs at right angles, feet on the floor. Bend forward to touch the floor, slowly sit up and straighten shoulders.

FEELING BEAUTIFUL BECAUSE YOU ARE

Exercise will help the mother feel good and look good, of course; however, after the baby is born mothers can expect many body changes, ways that the bearing of children has altered both personality and physique.

Some young girls work furiously to restore their figures to those of their teen years. (It may be that sight of something even better has not been imagined.) A healthy, beautiful, trim body is something to behold, yet the maturity brought on by motherhood adds special dimensions perhaps not contemplated by some women. It is no longer time to be, and perhaps to look, as she once was. A girl who has become a mother has an added beauty that draws immediate attention from others. She can still be trim and lovely, but developed curves and charm and depth of personality shine admirably through the changes that have taken place.

Just as everyone speaks of the glow that radiates from an expectant mother, there is something special in the countenance of the new mother. Many women display a new maturity that shows the dignity, wisdom, and warmth that come from having kept the commandment to bear offspring.

A woman is always more beautiful in body and spirit after she has given birth or adopted children and nurtured them. Giving unselfishly of love and time invariably brings glowing dividends. FEEL beautiful, because you REALLY are.

NOTES

[1] **Neuro-Vascular Dynamics** is an outgrowth of the research of Dr. Terrence Bennett, a chiropractor, who discovered in the 1930's that when specific areas on the body were contacted bimanually (one contact on the spinal area and the other usually near the organ), that the blood supply and activity of a particular organ would increase.

[2] Although mother's milk is best for almost all infants, the infant with **phenylketonuria (PKU)** will have to have a special phenylalanine-free formula, to prevent retardation due to his body's inability to metabolize this natural amino acid, a constituent of many proteins.

[3] Richard C. Hochberger, D.O., "A Complication of Circumcision," Osteopathic Annals 10 (April 1982) :54, 58.

[4] Bilirubin is a reddish yellow compound produced when red blood cells (**erythrocytes**) are destroyed. **Hyperbilirubinemia** is an EXCESS of bilirubin in the blood. This can be caused in the newborn by many things, including blood loss, blood group (ABO) or Rh incompatibility (maternal antibodies destroy the baby's erythrocytes), prematurity (the liver is especially immature), and many drugs (including aspirin). Even the routine vitamin K injections given the newborn to improve blood clotting ability can elevate the bilirubin level, perhaps seriously. (Many parents object to this injection, unless there is a bleeding problem.) Jaundice (yellowing of the skin, tissues, and body fluids) results from a high bilirubin count. Severe jaundice (large amounts of bilirubin) can damage brain and spinal cord cells, resulting in neurological impairment, such as spasticity, muscular incoordination, deafness, and mental retardation, or even death. (Hence, the exchange transfusion(s) for seriously affected infants.)

[5] See Adelle Davis, **Let's Have Healthy Children**, completely rev. and updated by Marshall Mandell, M.D. (Bergenfield, N.J.: New American Library, Inc., Signet Books, 1981), p. 257.

[6] A recent news article (**Salt Lake City** [Utah] **Deseret News**, 12 June 1984) reported the success a team of doctors in Columbia has had using a "kangaroo" treatment with premature babies: the babies are not placed in incubators and fed through tubes, but are wrapped against their mother's breasts, where they find food and warmth. Survival rates have been remarkable. (Babies weighing 1.1 to 2.2 pounds have been saved.) Perhaps the same principle applies here.

UNIT IV

Special Situations

CHAPTER 20

HIGHER RISK DELIVERIES

USING LANDMARKS

It may be wise to have already registered in mind a few helpful tips for managing any kind of higher risk birth, before these are dealt with on a separate basis.

A **dystocia** is something which makes labor or delivery more difficult, painful, or slow. **Fetal dystocias** are due to the size, shape, or position of the baby. When dystocias occur and there is need for internal management, look for **landmarks** (body parts that will tell you the positioning of the baby); they will help you to not do harm (such as trying to rotate in the wrong direction, etc.). Don't be afraid to feel gently for these landmarks—they will assist you in making safer decisions.

In a **face presentation,** for example, several bumpy parts, close together, can be felt. The mouth may feel like an anus, so go beyond to find the nasal bridge or saddle between the eyes, being careful not to push on an eyeball. Ears are identifiable, but check the root of the pinna (small prominence in front of the ear) to see if the face is to the right or to the left.

Fontanels (soft spots found at each end of the sagittal suture) and the direction of the **sagittal suture** clue you to rotational progress and flexion.

Knees do not have solid caps formed, and so are somewhat hollow, but elbows have a firm point.

Toes are almost the same length, fingers are not. Hands are often fisted; however, check further to distinguish between a fist and a heel: the foot extends in a firm mass before the toes are found and can be grasped at the ankle between the index and middle fingers easily.

If you confuse an extremity with the cord, remember that the cord will pulsate.

BREECH BIRTHS

Breech presentations at term occur only three to four percent of the time. It may be that a trend toward higher percentages of breeches has occurred in recent years. In a breech birth the baby is positioned with the head high in the uterus; consequently, the head will present last.

There are three types of breech presentations (see Figure 68):

1. **The complete breech.** The baby's arms are folded across its chest, the thighs are flexed on the abdomen, and the legs are crossed and flexed on the thighs. Buttocks present first.

2. **The frank breech.** The baby's arms may be folded across the front, or one or both arms may be behind the head or neck. The legs are straight up beside each ear or crossed in front of the face.

Higher Risk Deliveries 441

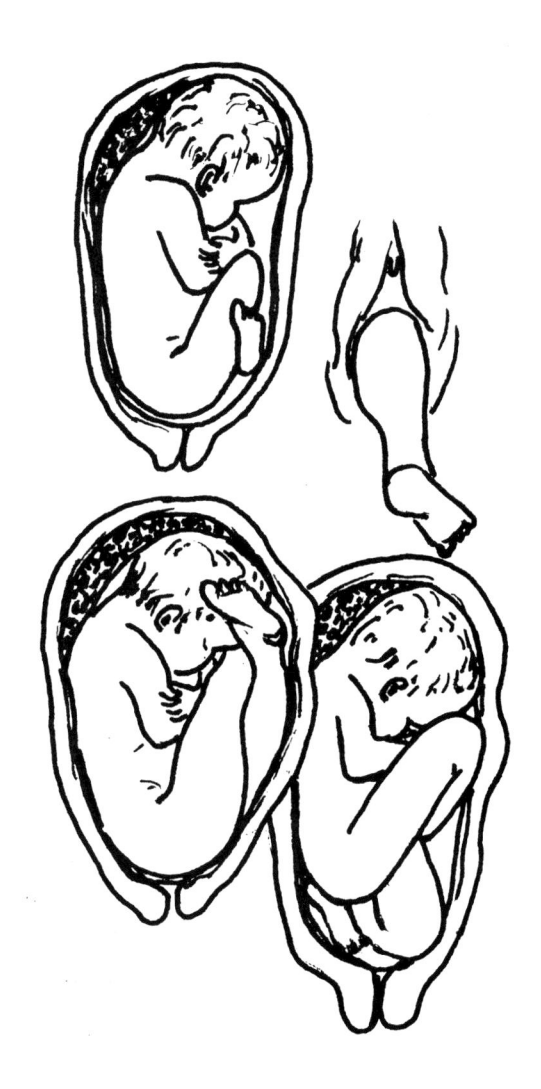

Figure 68. BREECH PRESENTATIONS. (**top left**) full or complete breech; (**top right**) footling breech (incomplete breech); (**bottom left**) frank breech; (**bottom right**) knee presentation (incomplete breech).

3. **The incomplete breech (foot/footling or knee presentations).** The baby's arms are usually in a fetal fold. One foot or both feet (**double footling**) or one or both knees are presenting.

It is believed that low-placed placentas are a major cause of breech presentations, and that about 14 percent of breech presentations follow breech births in previous pregnancies. This is referred to as **habitual breech.**

The loss of the fetus is usually due to: (1) excessive haste during second stage, (2) premature birth, (3) tears—due to forceps extraction--at the fetal cerebrum (brain) and in the spinal cord, followed by intracranial hemorrhage, and (4) prolapse of the cord.

If the gravida's abdominal muscles are very firm, you may not be able to diagnose a breech at first. About 10 to 15 percent are not diagnosed. Fetal heart tones will give you some indication, because of their location. These are heard at or above the mother's navel.

Breech babies often turn themselves to vertex (head-down position) prior to time for delivery. Breeches are about nine times more common at the 28th week than they are at term, and even after the 34th week **spontaneous version** occurs about one-third of the time in nulliparas (women who have not given birth) and two-thirds of the time in multiparas.

So, what if the baby is breech for delivery? If you have been taught and trained to deliver a breech, it is not any more difficult, IN MOST CASES, to deliver than a vertex posterior baby.

One reason physicians resort to cesarean delivery of breeches includes the fact that adequate training in natural delivery may not have been available in most instances. Today in medical schools the only breech procedure elaborated upon is the cesarean section. This is unfortunate.

Sometimes the parturient has not been psychologically prepared to assist all through the birth. Her help is vital. The result of a drugged mother is that fetal heart tones are lowered, perhaps too much to withstand what trauma or stress the baby may be called upon to go through for a few moments.

Many important factors enter into a well-managed breech birth. The first three-fourths of labor is very important. It is true that breeches can be precarious and difficult, but midwives who haven't been scared to death of them and who have been adequately trained to handle them do perform beautifully without compromising the baby.

Recently I held a beautiful nine-month-old boy in my arms who had been delivered breech by one of my advanced trainees. He was the son of a primipara, was six days overdue, weighed 9+ pounds, and was attended by two trainees and a therapist who administered several forms of therapy throughout labor. When they consulted with me prior to the birth, I advised them to not deliver the baby at home. The situation was high risk: the mother was a primigravida carrying her fetus breech, she was overdue, and indications were that the baby would be quite large. All else was perfect.

We know that due dates are approximate. The mother's weight gain was perfect. Prenatals were perfect. The whole program had been CAREFULLY followed, along with regular walks and exercise.

Father, mother, therapist, and midwives felt a definite, go-ahead peace of mind. What could I say? The back-up doctor refused to have anything to do with it.

The outcome? There was no bleeding, no tearing, no episiotomy, no panic—nine hours of labor from onset of contractions and a very beautiful, happy birth and baby. It was not "just luck." All parties were prepared, truly prepared, and had a confirmation that all was well and would go right. None of us ought to argue with that kind of feeling. Rather, we should always have the same qualifications and qualifying conditions whenever we step to the door of a birth.

Breech Version (Turning the Fetus)

I do not recommend manually turning the baby from a **podalic** (foot) to a **cephalic** (head) position. This maneuver is questionable, since: (1) spontaneous version to vertex often occurs, (2) the incidence of breech presentation at term is little different than when nothing is done, (3) the baby often returns to breech afterward, (4) it is difficult to turn a baby in those last weeks, and (5) THIS TYPE OF INTERFERENCE IS DANGEROUS.

A good midwife will keep watch over the mother, and if spontaneous version has not occurred by the 32nd week, it may help to put the mother on a slant board (12 inches high at the foot) for half an hour twice a day, or to raise the foot of her bed six inches at night. (This may help unless the placenta or cord prevents correction.) The midwife should then watch carefully for the change to vertex. When it occurs, the mother will lower the bed or discontinue use of the slant board in order to not encourage the baby's return to breech position.

Also, one therapist felt that holding the femoral pressure points for relaxation regularly during the last months of pregnancy may help breech babies to turn to vertex position at an appropriate time before delivery (see Chapter 15, Femoral Pressure Points).

MANUAL VERSION

To do a manual version, one must know the whereabouts of the placenta and cord, along with the length of the cord. Even ultrasonic equipment is not reliable enough, in most instances, to make this determination. The possibility of separating the placenta prematurely or of tightening a cord that may already be around the fetal neck makes version too risky. Sometimes a strong placental souffle or cord beat can be heard, but that is insufficient. NOTHING CAN GUARANTEE THAT MANUAL VERSION WILL BE SAFE.

The only time I would turn a fetus is when an arm or shoulder presentation is in the making (if there is a transverse lie), or if in a multiple birth the second fetus is in a transverse (horizontal) lie. To reach in, get the feet of the second baby, and thereby maneuver a footling into a sacrum anterior presentation is not too difficult. YOU are in control then; the cervix has been dilated by the first infant, the wet body can turn rather easily, and no problem is likely to present. IT MUST BE REMEMBERED THAT ONE NEVER "PULLS" OR FORCES the fetus anywhere! THE PULL-REST OR PUSH-REST MOVEMENTS accomplish a safer correction and lessen the possibility of injury to the mother or baby.

Some Important Points

Breeches are not all fatality prone.

Though higher risk, breeches can be handled safely if:

1. You are not afraid.
2. You have been trained well in the delivery of breeches.
3. You have an honest confirmation to go ahead.
4. You screen to eliminate cases of the incorrectable pathologies and higher risks of breeches, such as a history of precipitous deliveries, toxemia, hydramnios, maternal disorders, etc.

It seems certain that our Heavenly Father knew that once in a while certain little characters were going to be different and come down to earth topsy-turvy. He also knew that if they were meant to live, help would be provided to assist them in a safe journey. In true emergencies where no one else is available, divine help will intervene, even with breeches.

The latter was the case in my first delivery. Never would I have consented to help in the first place had I known the delivery was breech. However, it was an emergency, an unavoidable circumstance. The mother was doing all she could to get help by calling various services as well as a back-up trio of midwives, just in case no one made it in time. Only we, the trio, arrived in time. If all breeches were impossible, novices would not have been able to manage this one.

This was the very first baby I had ever delivered —and it was a complete breech. The husband had left for work and had to commute for over an hour, so was not available. The doctor's answering service was not answering, and the mother had heard that my partner and I were assisting her doctor, so she called us. She did not know that our training had only just begun, or that we had had no practical experience as yet. She needed help. We were available. She had planned a home birth, and though labor had set in rather quickly, she thought surely help would be coming. It did not get there in time, and I was elected to do the honors.

You can imagine my surprise when I palpated—for the first time in my life—and had to turn my head away from the mother to tell my assistant in subdued tones, "It isn't the head!"

She opened her mouth, then closed her mouth. And her eyes asked, "What?" I repeated nonchalantly and ever so quietly, "It isn't the head." With my free hand I made the illustrating finger-to-air drawing of buttocks, crack, buttocks.

Without apparent panic she swished around to the other side of the bed to whisper matter-of-factly to the other assistant. There was an instant of breath-holding, then matter-of-fact pursuance of our duties. I sensed each was glad they had volunteered MY services. However, at no moment did I sense the parturient suspected we were not old hands at this sort of thing. (Attendants, take note: This attitude is important in your work. Panic is forbidden. In an emergency, you do what has to be done.)

One assistant had experienced a home, doctor-attended, breech birth of her own, and while she made reference to the fact that we might have to put pressure on the fetal head through the abdomen, no other instructions were forthcoming. And I really cannot take any credit for that delivery. It was pure inspiration and guidance, because my hands did things they did not know to do (even to retrieving the limbs prior to the head), and the birth was extremely successful. Part of the success was due to the fact that the parturient had had three breeches before, and this was her twelfth baby. There was no uterine inertia, no cord prolapse, no laceration, and no more than very normal postpartum bleeding.

We "played it cool" to the end, for we did not want a frightened mother on our hands. We checked everything we knew to check and found everything just fine. Afterward, we went home and had heart attacks!

While this story is told in a light vein, and thank goodness we can smile about it years after its event, surely the reader can see what could have happened. Any birth, whether breech or anterior vertex (the most common and normal presentation), can have difficult and dangerous moments. Tragedy can be the outcome, even with proper training and the life-supporting equipment of the hospital. Therefore, to lessen these foreboding possibilities, be prepared to give competent help before you deliberately put yourself or anyone else in a compromising position.

I can't say enough about a midwife having to be in tune with a higher power, and having the integrity to abide by real promptings. She is no more infallible than any doctor is, and together they can do much to bring about miraculous outcomes in birth. However, both must be willing to be led not only by their expertise, but by inspiration.

Training, or the lack of it, and level of experience may find any practitioner in one of three positions:

1. To "know better" than to try a particular delivery on his or her own, and to discount a divine prompting to go ahead with the delivery.

2. To not know his or her level of competence, and to be misled by courage to think it is a divine prompting to go ahead on his/her own.

3. To be adequately trained or not, yet be superbly in tune with Providence and willing to follow these promptings.

We must do the best we can, but we must never deny that it is someone else who performs the miracles.

Let me remind us all of my old and familiar warning: If it is an emergency, the Lord will help and all will probably go well—no matter who helps, with whatever amount of training. But if you set out deliberately to have a home birth without plans and competent help, I do not know how many times the Lord will pull your chestnuts out of the fire.

Delivery Management of Breech Births

Along with a few fundamentals of procedure, one must use a lot of intuitiveness with regard to details in delivering breech presentations.

First of all, NEVER HURRY FIRST STAGE WITH ANY BREECH LABOR. The cervix needs plenty of time to dilate all that is possible. One advantage the home birth attendant has is that she knows how to rim and to encourage an even and full dilation prior to the bearing-down stage, and that is one of the major concerns with the breech birth (along with delivery of the head.)

BE ALERT TO THE POSSIBILITY OF A PROLAPSED UMBILICAL CORD (see Chapter 16, Prolapsed Cord), particularly if there is an INCOMPLETE or a COMPLETE breech. These do not cover (block) the cervical opening as completely as does the solid head or even the frank breech.

If one knee is presenting INITIALLY in the breech birth, the mother is put in a knee-chest position and the wayward knee is gently pushed back in and up against the baby's abdomen. Pelvic rocks will assist repositioning, and if the buttocks will present through the cervix, so much the better, as the buttocks are capable of dilating the cervix more adequately and more quickly.

If the buttocks are not dilating the cervix (**incomplete breech**), start both the feet down if you can (again, utilize the knee-chest position). When they reach the air, be sure to keep them very warm. COVER ALL EXPOSED PARTS UNTIL THE HEAD IS BORN. A warm towel will assist your handling of parts presenting.

NEVER ALLOW PREMATURE BEARING DOWN. Wait for the buttocks to open the vulva. The mother is encouraged to bear down enough to crown the perineum with the width of the buttocks, putting the fetal head nearer -0- station. The body is in position now for you to reach extremities more easily.

MANEUVERING THE EXTREMITIES

It is my belief that if the extremities can come down in a normal fashion before the birth of the head, there is less likelihood of injury to any part of the infant.

In the case of the **complete breech** (feet and arms folded in the fetal position)--and the **frank**

breech (feet up by the head), if possible--when the buttocks have not quite fully dilated the vulvar opening, the midwife reaches in with the palpating fingers to place them between the fetal abdomen and thigh--remember it is slippery and wet and is not impossible to work with--and then she follows the thigh down with a little presssure to urge the foot to slip through the center of the baby's crotch and out (see Figure 69).

At almost the same moment the other leg is urged in the same way, although one leg at a time. (When the feet are out, it is easier to carefully rotate the infant from a posterior position to an anterior one IF the toes are pointing up! You are in control and face-down positions are best in breeches.)

The mother pants at this point if there is an urge to push, while the midwife reaches for the hands. (Any time the midwife needs additional time to perform some duty, she tells the mother to pant. The mother cannot bear down with contractions if she is panting.)

Find each hand by reaching for the shoulder and sliding your palpating fingers to the inside of the fetal elbow, then working your fingers down the forearm (the baby's arm and hand will come downward as you "walk your fingers" from the elbow toward the hand). Many times one or both of the hands will be down momentarily as a reflex to the movement of the legs into another position.

Frank breeches can be more difficult, but not impossible. One difficulty comes if the arms are back of the head. This means that the circumference through which both the head and arms are to pass at the same time may present problems. Tearing of the cervix may result, and caution is

452 POLLY'S BIRTH BOOK

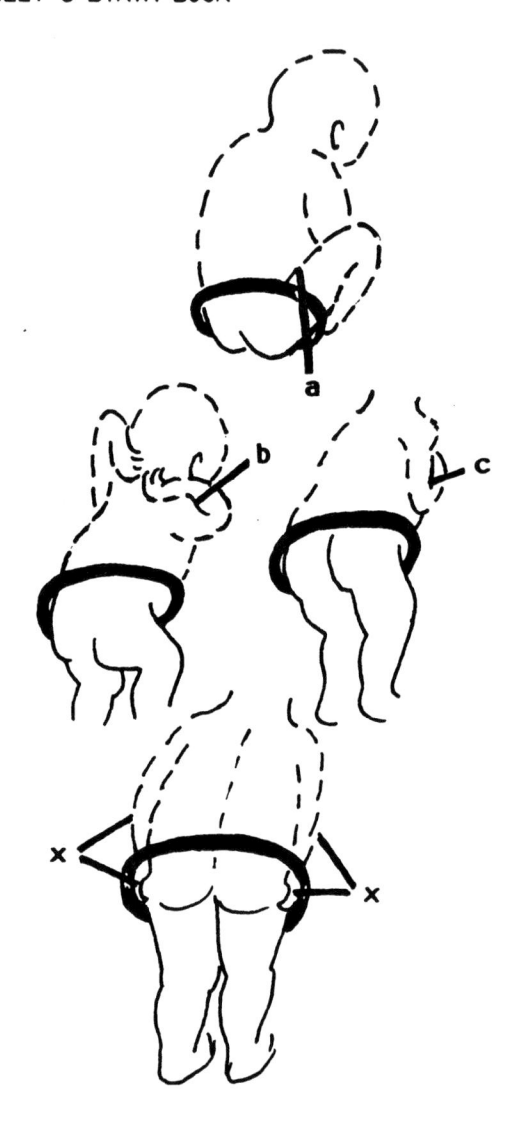

Figure 69. MANAGEMENT OF BREECH BIRTH. Work each foot through the vulva from the baby's thigh (**a**); follow the baby's arm down from the shoulder (**b**) and forearm (**c**) to get each hand out; hold the torso and arms here (**d**) to maneuver the shoulders and head out.

needed to keep the uterus from prolapsing and to prevent injury to the fetus.

ARMS BEHIND THE NECK IN A BREECH can usually be untwined by turning the torso, quite far, so that the face moves around in the direction of the arm which needs to be freed. Then slip your index finger around to the bend of the elbow and work your way down the arm to the hand. You can then turn the trunk back again and also do the same for the other arm if it needs to be freed.

If the LEFT arm is behind the neck, turn the torso CLOCKWISE to free it. To release the RIGHT arm from around the neck, turn the torso COUNTERCLOCKWISE. Remember to TURN THE BODY AND FACE TOWARD THE ARM THAT NEEDS TO BE FREED.

I want the hands to the sides of the fetal body so that I may hold them and the body together as the shoulders, one at a time, and the head are maneuvered. This position: (1) helps to prevent grasping the liver or kidney portion of the infant body too tightly, (2) gives better leverage, and (3) prevents the arms from being in the way.

IF YOU HAVE NOT BEEN ABLE TO GET THE LIMBS OUT, LET THE BIRTH CONTINUE NORMALLY.

COMPLETE THE DELIVERY WITHIN FOUR MINUTES AFTER THE UMBILICUS IS PRESENTED--TIME IS OF THE ESSENCE. The cord is particularly exposed to compression at the pelvic brim (the head is there now) and at the vulva. You have FOUR MINUTES to get the head out without causing possible brain damage; a maximum of EIGHT MINUTES to save life.

When the umbilical cord at the navel comes out, CAREFULLY PULL OUT A LITTLE ADDITIONAL CORD, being careful not to put stress on the fetal navel, but to give ample length for when the head comes through -0- station and out.

RATHER STRINGENT FUNDAL PRESSURE MAY HAVE TO BE APPLIED TO ASSIST THE BIRTH OF THE HEAD THROUGH -0- STATION AND TO MAINTAIN FLEXION (to lessen the chances of the chin or a wide diameter of the head becoming arrested at some point). This is where the assistants come into play. Palms of the hands are placed over the fetal head, and DURING BEARING-DOWN CONTRACTIONS it is pushed down and slightly out to encourage head flexion and passage THROUGH -0- STATION ONLY.

Care must be taken to apply this pressure ONLY as the head approaches -0- station. (Premature action could force the head between the arms or possibly deflex the head.) The mother must bear down with all these contractions, for her muscles will assist in the birth of the baby.

To ensure that secondary uterine inertia does not set in following birth of the legs and torso, SOMEONE MUST HOLD THE PITUITARY REFLEX on the mother's big toe until the head is born (see Chapter 15, Figure 38). This stimulates continued pituitary performance and contractions.

WAIT TO DELIVER THE SHOULDERS UNTIL AN ARMPIT BECOMES VISIBLE.

DELIVERING THE HEAD

The face must be down, and when the chin has passed the bony canal--if the head is not progressing rather rapidly through the floor--reach in, put your finger in the baby's mouth, and MOVE THE MANDIBLE (chin bone) enough for the chin to slip over the "perineal sweep" (inside surface of the perineum).

Higher Risk Deliveries   455

In delivering the head, an important maneuver must be understood to prevent spinal injury: HOLD THE INFANT BY THE BODY WITH ARMS AT THE SIDES. Holding the baby by the feet for the following maneuver puts tremendous stress upon a spine which has been curled in a fetal position for months. (Experts in the field of spinal health tell us that unforgiveable damage has been done by unthinking practitioners who have lifted infants by the feet and let the heaviest part of the body, the head, hang and stretch the previously uncurled spine--not to mention additional stress caused by using the legs to pull the head around and out of the birth canal. Don't you be guilty of this.)

TO DELIVER THE HEAD IN BREECH BIRTHS, swing the baby's body UP with slight tension, quite high, THEN DOWN, then BACK UP AGAIN, all in one smooth operation. Up, down, then back up. The mother's buttocks must be near the edge of the bed to carry out this maneuver successfully. The face, with this swinging action of the body, spans the internal perineum, then the downward sweep pulls the occiput forward, and as the infant is lifted the last time, the face appears outside.

Usually the whole head then slips out without popping out or projecting. If the maneuver has been carried out with just the slightest tautness put on the head, and with movements up and down as if they were all one movement, the outcome will be proper; otherwise, the face only will present, leaving the occiput retained.

When this happens, care and time can be taken to assist the birth carefully to prevent tearing or a traumatic emission of the head. Time is no longer too much of a problem if you keep the infant warm and do not allow the position of the body to threaten a retreat of the face. The weight of the buttocks and feet have helped thus far. Therefore, in this facial position, suctioning can be done. Baby Dear can get all the air he needs. He no longer needs the oxygen of the cord. The only problem now is to work with the vulva (especially the perineum) to free the back of the head. Go about this slowly, as you would if the baby were still inside and a cephalic presentation were about to crown normally.

MULTIPLE BIRTHS

Multiple pregnancy and delivery calls for close planning, screening, and weighing of risks and possibilities, plus superb prenatal preparations. Special precautions are taken. Competent attendants must be present and back-up personnel available. Delivery techniques differ, and more diverse (and perhaps quite complicated) situations could develop. Nevertheless, multiple births have been delivered safely at home, with all the advantages of home birthing.

I smile when people start panicking at the thoughts of delivering multiple births, especially in the home. I recall the news media carrying a story in the 1970's about a midwife who successfully delivered sextuplets under a bus on a hot, dusty road in Mexico. They were on the way to the hospital when the births occurred. The nurse suggested they get back in the bus and continue to the hospital, but the husband asked, "Why? Everything is all right. Let's turn around and go home!"

Some Important Points

Twins are found only about once in 80 pregnancies, and, of course, they come from a variety of physiological environments and circumstances.

Twins tend to birth prematurely (about 2 to 6 weeks), though this need not always happen.

There is usually greater demand on the mother for nutrition, folic acid, and rest (due to the increased weight, which brings on fatigue more quickly).

The Good Program is vital to discourage anemia, premature labor, toxemia (due to overload on the eliminative systems), and two potential problems due to the enlarged placental site(s): placenta previa and postpartum hemorrhage.

Twins (or each multiple fetus) come in their own sacs (with but rare exceptions), and each has its own umbilical cord, even though they may share a placenta. One placenta may be supplying the needs of two or more babies, or there may be a placenta for each fetus.

Binovular twins (from two ova) have separate placentas, and the incidence is influenced by the age and **parity** (how many previous births) of the mother, and also by heredity—from either mother or father. Binovular twins come from older mothers, as a rule, particularly those 35 to 40 years of age who have had several other children.

Monovular twins (from the same ovum) occur three to four times LESS frequently, and more often in mothers age 20 to 35 years, particularly in **primigravidas** and **secundigravidas** (mothers in their first or second pregnancies).

Fetal abnormalities occur twice as often as they do in single births. Variations in function or development or freak formations can occur, as they may in any pregnancy.

For instance, sometimes one twin will not develop and will decease, while the other one will live and carry until term. Sometimes, with monovular twins, one will take over the circulation and heart functions of the other, leaving a very abnormally small fetus. This happens when the umbilical cords enter one placenta too closely together and the **transfusion syndrome** occurs, starving one of the twins. It will sometimes be born in the membranes of the placenta, or it may deliver normally. (Do not become alarmed during delivery if you find the small, deceased one falling into your hands and collapsing there, or being born flattened or compressed by the further developed fetus. The deceased twin will still be at the stage of development from which it could no longer survive.)

Forty-five percent of the time both heads are vertex when labor begins. Forty percent of the time one fetus is breech and one fetus is vertex. Ten percent of the time both are breech.

Seventy-five percent of the time the FIRST presentation is vertex.

It seems that the left twin usually presents first.

Delivery Management of Multiple Births

The use of drugs during labor should be particularly avoided with all multiple births.

If labor is more than two weeks premature, pressure on the fetal head may cause bruising, since there will be less thickness to the scalp for padding.

If labor starts with premature rupture of the membranes, caution is the watchword for a prolapsing of the cord: until contractions set the first head or presenting part down far enough to occlude (block) the birth canal, frequent checks for the cord must be made.

Labor is usually shorter, but conducted normally--without undue haste or delay.

The cord of the first baby is cut immediately. It must be clamped twice and cut quickly to secure against the second fetus bleeding through a shared placenta, if this should be the case.

There may be two placentas, or one for each baby if there are more than twins.

Rarely is the first placenta born before the second baby, and bleeding is not usually heavy because the second baby is pressed against a contracting uterus anyway.

Only if the second baby is much larger than the first is there usually much of a delay (30 to 45 minutes) in the presenting of the second twin, and this time allows a little more dilation to take place. HOWEVER, a good midwife checks the position of the second infant to determine whether there is a **transverse** (horizontal) **lie.**

Should there be a transverse lie, **external version** (turning), if possible, should be done to promote either a vertex or podalic (foot) presentation. This should not be difficult; if it is, do a **podalic version** by reaching in and taking both feet in your hand between the thumb, index, and middle fingers, pointing the toes down, and carefully drawing the feet down while the mother is working WITH the contractions to NATURALLY bring about the birth. Arms are brought down beside the torso and the head is born; the cervix is already dilated, as is the vulva (see this chapter, Delivery Management of Breech Births).

Version of the second baby may cause **constriction ring closure** (see Chapter 17, Uterine Retraction Ring), so USE GENTLENESS (but not delay) in this maneuver.

If the FIRST baby is BREECH and the SECOND is VERTEX, caution is made to prevent the heads from locking as the first baby presents. THIS RARELY HAPPENS, but you should know of the possibility because early recognition is essential. (Auscultating fetal heart tones over the last two to three weeks is helpful in screening). A side position for the mother sometimes helps to maneuver the head of the second baby back up into the uterus a little to allow the head of the first to come down into the canal. THIS PRESENTATION CAN BE MOST DIFFICULT. It happens once in about 800 twin gestations. Back-up personnel should be present in or out of the hospital, since cesarean sections must sometimes be employed.

Rarely, though it happens, one twin will be born and another will remain in utero, alive and well, from several hours to several days or months. In this case, vital signs must be carefully monitored long enough to determine whether: (1) infection is building, (2) nursing promotes new labor, or (3) internal bleeding is a problem. The latter is less likely, inasmuch as the fundal/fetal pressure is adequate to preclude this happening.

Triplets (Or More!)

Though the birth of twins is more usual than the birth of triplets (or more), those on fertility pills or those from families with multiple birth histories should be aware of greater multiple birth possibilities. Similar difficulties are present in childbirth, and the same precautions, principles, and techniques of delivery--such as watching for a transverse lie of the succeeding fetus, etc.--will be employed with triplets (or more) as are with twins.

If the mother is "definitely" within eight days of term when labor begins, the maturity of each infant may be sufficient to try home birth IF a doctor is present AND all back-up measures have been taken. This would include special screening during all of the third trimester, and extra precautions planned for and executed.

Remember, warmth and bonding are essential. Enlisting the help of "the rest of the neighborhood" may be necessary to ensure warmth and care of the babies as they are born, especially if you were NOT expecting more than twins!

UNCOMMON PRESENTATIONS

Ninety-five percent of the time the fetus is positioned for a "normal," vertex birth. Only five percent of the time do uncommon presentations happen. At or near term the incidence of the various presentations is approximately as follows: **vertex,** 95 percent; **breech,** 3.5 percent; **face,** 0.5 percent; **shoulder,** 0.5 percent.

Since no one is immune from encountering an uncommon presentation, we will discuss them briefly.

Arm and Shoulder Presentations

Suppose you arrived on the birthing scene to find the amnion ruptured and an arm protruding into, or through, the vaginal cavity? Two assessments would dictate your actions: (1) the length of the extremity that is extending, and (2) the vigor with which labor is progressing.

An arm out to the elbow in an early labor with contractions up to about ten minutes apart could be handled with careful, deliberate moves.

One midwife, who was accompanied at a birth by her back-up doctor, encountered this kind of situation. During a normal, six-hour labor the midwife checked for dilation and found a fetal hand and arm in the vagina. She didn't bother to awaken the doctor, who was asleep on the couch in the TV room downstairs, but instead she felt carefully to find the elbow and correct bend of the arm in relationship to the infant's body.

She bent the arm, pointed the hand in the right position to slide across the chest, and gently worked the arm back into the "fetal position." Then the shoulder and body had to be moved slightly (by using the left hand on the mother's abdomen and the full right hand internally) to help the fetal head slip more securely into the pelvic inlet. Placed thusly, it would remain there and not allow the hand to slip through again.

Had there been hard, fast contractions forcing a shoulder, or an arm and shoulder, through the cervix and vagina she may never have chosen the technique she used above. And had she been unable to handle the situation herself, she undoubtedly would have summoned the back-up doctor immediately.

A parturient knee-chest position may or may not have been effective. It would certainly be worth a try to put a mother in this situation into that position while transporting, to see if some distress could be lessened until a C-section could be effected. (A normal, live baby in a transverse position cannot be delivered vaginally.)

Face Presentations

It is easy to understand why it is important to maintain some of the flexion of the head as the occiput crowns at the vulva if the woman is delivering on her back. The face must not rise too soon and cause a wider angle of the head to crown and to lacerate tissue.

A woman in a squatting position for delivery during the perineal crowning does not seem to have this problem. The position of her own body in the squat supports the natural evacuation of the fetal head and body. See Chapter 14, Figure 29 (Curve of Carus), then see it again when turned appropriately to correspond with the squatting position, in which gravity and the curve direct the occiput more effectively.

If in a vertex presentation sufficient **flexion** does not occur prior to deep engagement, either on its own or with the attendant's help, the result will be a transverse head arrest or a malpresentation (face/brow presentation) (see Figure 70).

Poor flexion is revealed by the easily-detected presence of the **sagittal suture** and both fontanels--especially if there is sufficient dilation--showing the full top of the fetal head presenting through the pelvic brim. By pressing on the forehead with contractions prior to full engagement, adequate flexion can be encouraged. Sometimes a few pelvic rocks will do the same thing in early second stage, or as soon as the lack of flexion is discovered to be persistent.

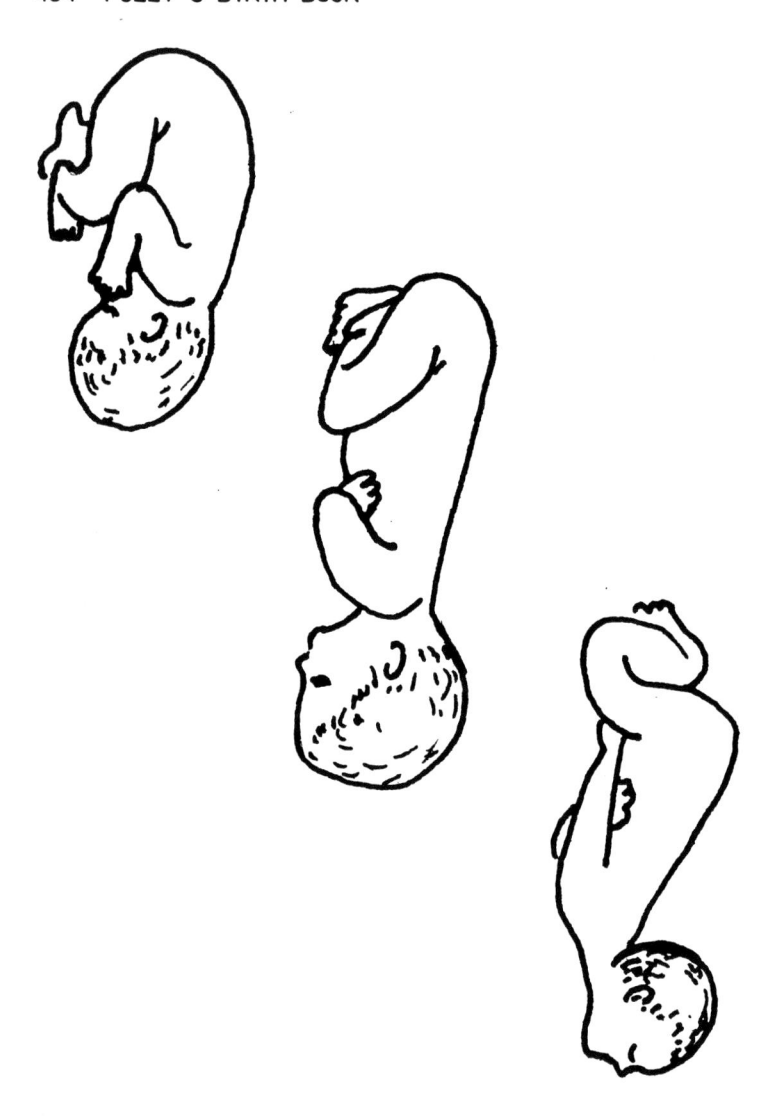

Figure 70. FACE PRESENTATION. A normal, vertex presentation requires good flexion (**top**). Insufficient flexion (**middle**), uncorrected, results in a transverse head arrest or, with full extension (**bottom**), a malpresentation (face, brow, or chin presentation).

Higher Risk Deliveries 465

On occasion, you will discover that somehow flexion did not take place, but instead, **extension** of the head came through and you are palpating numerous little bumps or peaks and valleys in a confined area. These represent nose, chin, brow, cheek bones, and puffy eyelids. Yes, a **face, brow,** or **chin presentation** is in the making. At this point, if the labor is progressing right along, the safest thing to do is to allow the birth to proceed. As a rule, this will happen without too many complications: most deliver spontaneously, thank goodness!

A chin that is directly posterior (down) when it passes the sacral promontory MUST rotate for birth to proceed. Spontaneous rotation (chin to the symphysis pubis) and easy delivery can be expected in about two-thirds of these less-frequent cases. The head flexes and comes out with the face up; the next contraction lifts the occiput out. There MAY be perineal tears with face presentations.

In cases of face presentations, about one-third will show that pelvic inlets are too small, or **contracted.** The doctor usually wants an x-ray before deciding on vaginal delivery, especially when there is a large baby. And sometimes--when the gravida's abdomen is pendulous at term--you can anticipate a face presentation.

Although delivery may proceed without complication, the birth itself is hard on the baby and his neck. Do expect rather heavy edema of the nose, mouth, and brow, and possible breathing or feeding problems until the edema lessens.

The last time I encountered a face presentation was when I was consulted with by another midwife, who was on the scene and had watched the delivery from the onset of labor. She wanted a confirmation of her findings. She was correct in her diagnosis (of the face presenting), and we told the parents what was happening and gave them the choice of either continuing delivery at home or transporting.[1]

Home birth parents are informed in detail about these many potentials and can make logical decisions when they are called for. This mother had had dystocias with her last birth and needed to be assured that we were not going to press her to remain at home if she felt the need for hospitalization. Risks are incurred with any malpresentation, and in this case the parents chose to transport because of the possibility of neck injury and certainly of edema, which is to be expected at the brow and particularly at the nose and lip areas. (Such swelling can cause immediate postpartum problems, since babies are nose-breathers.)

Obstructions, and some malpresentations, bring stress upon the fetus and the mother. But as long as birth is imminent and the obstruction has been taken care of, even if a malpresentation is unavoidable, the safest and healthiest thing to do for all concerned is to allow the infant to be born.

NOTES

[1] In this case, where transporting was carried out, the back-up doctor called for immediate x-rays to determine whether the head was small enough to safely pass through -0- station and whether the head was in rotation. However, the fetus was continuing to move right along and the parturient was rushed into the delivery room, where the baby was born within the next few minutes. Ten minutes later, the x-ray technician came running down the hallway toward the delivery room, waving the x-ray in the air and calling out to the physician, "The head is too large! It can't be born vaginally! It'll never make it!" It was apparent that transporting had assisted with rotation and tilting, and the head passed through the pelvis very nicely--which goes to show that maternal repositioning often assists nature in the correction of dystocias.

CHAPTER 21

MALFORMATIONS, INJURIES, AND ABNORMALITIES

BIRTH DEFECTS

It is rare that a midwife will encounter many severe birth defects in her work. This may be due to the stepped-up preventive program home birth parents undertake. However, because so many drugs are used now and adverse environmental factors affect all of our lives, it is not impossible that you will need a few tips to guide your actions if you attend the birth of a malformed or defected infant.

As a midwife, you need to develop the skills for handling delicate moments, such as telling parents that their infant has an injury or might have a defect. I have had a few cases of irregularities at birth, and with the few I have had, it has been my nature to talk to the infant in a matter-of-fact way that will not evoke feelings of maternal guilt. "You little stinker, what have you here? Why, I believe you've got an extra opening! You surely have. Look, Mom...."

Cleft Palate and Cleft Lip

A **cleft palate** is usually a genetic defect; however, Cortisone can also cause this defect. It occurs when the **nasal palate** (roof of the mouth) does not join during growth of the fetus. It is important to check each newborn for this obscure defect. Using a good light and a gloved finger, feel the roof of the baby's mouth. There may be a **cleft** (opening) on one side or both sides, and the **soft palate** may be cleft slightly or severely. When the baby nurses, the milk will come back through its nose, causing the infant to choke and become cyanotic (turn blue because of lack of oxygen).

When both the **cleft lip** and the **cleft palate** are present, a more severe disunion has occurred, and prompt medical attention must be given. Surgery is usually not performed until the infant has built some circulatory defenses. (Remember, the newborn's liver does not function well for about six months.) The infant is watched until his hemoglobin level is good and the baby is better able to handle surgery. This may mean waiting as long as 18 months. Several operations may be necessary to repair the cleft palate.

The cleft lip can be dealt with sooner--anywhere from the 10th day to the eighth week. The mother should be shown how to feed the baby in an upright position and how to handle other feeding problems so she can feel secure at home with the infant feedings (the hospital is helpful in giving these instructions).

Cosmetic surgery to correct these cleft problems is very effective. In severe cases, dental plates may be applied the first week after birth.

Such infants can be fed with reasonable care. If the infant has trouble breast-feeding, a large, soft nipple can be contrived, with mother's milk, to give plenty of suckling experience.

Retardation

Mongolism (Down's Syndrome) is a form of retardation that is indicated by slanting eyes, broad hands and short fingers, and a broad, short skull. The degree of retardation varies considerably from child to child. If you KNOW that the newborn has this defect but the parents do not immediately notice the symptoms, it may be better to let them gradually come to sense the condition. If you feel prompted to tell them, use tact and sensitivity. BE SURE your diagnosis is correct. If you are not sure, have a physician confirm your findings and handle informing the parents.

Anencephaly is a severe form of physical retardation in which an infant's development was arrested. An anencephalic baby will have a deformed head that ends just above the eyebrows. The top part of the head isn't there, and there is no brain. Do not expect this infant to live. About seventy percent are females.

Spinal Defects

If you ever deliver a child that has any kind of opening, abnormal growth, or protrusion from the spine (it will usually be at the bottom of the spine, or at the back of the neck), it should be wrapped with a nonadhering dressing: a warm, moist cloth that does not press the part, but does support it. Carry the infant without touching or pressing the area spoken of. Take note of whether there are any leg movements in the child (which may give cause to believe there is extensive spinal damage), and transport to the hospital.

BIRTH INJURIES

Swelling

Two kinds of swelling can occur on the head of the newborn. First, if the part of the baby's head that fits into the cervix has the venous blood supply shut off for very long as dilation proceeds, that area, starved of blood, may become edematous (swollen) and congested. This swelling, the **caput succedaneum,** will appear immediately after birth. Swelling can also be caused when the fetal head rotates, or it can even develop when the head is fitted for any length of time against the vaginal outlet.

The caput succedaneum is present at birth and may cross the sagittal suture (the place where the two top skull bones meet). It usually is gone within two or three days. When you touch it, it feels soft and does not have specific edges. If there should be two caputs, they will be **unilateral** (found only on one side).

Second, the **cephalhematoma** is a swelling on the fetal head where blood has gathered between the skull and the scalp; this swelling is caused by friction and subsequent injury to the membrane covering the skull bone. If the head has to pass through any difficult bony place, especially a **contracted** (irregular) **pelvis,** and it collapses enough to finally go through, the cephalhematoma will develop.

This condition usually develops 12 to 14 hours after birth, not immediately afterward. It generally needs no treatment. The swelling eventually

Malformations, Injuries, and Abnormalities   471

lessens and disappears as the blood is absorbed into surrounding tissue. Once it is gone, you may feel a ridge around where it had been.

Unlike the caput succedaneum (which usually disappears within a few days), the cephalhematoma tends to grow larger and will persist for weeks. This swelling does not cross over the sagittal suture, and it does have a definite outline-- again, unlike the caput. **Double cephalhematomas** are usually **bilateral** (one on each side of the sagittal suture).

Both of these conditions can be successfully treated by placing a gauze saturated with arnica tincture over the affected area and capping it with plastic to keep it moist (see Appendix D, For Hematomas).

Laceration of the Liver

Laceration of the liver may occur in a breech delivery that is not managed well. The newborn's liver is very large, and as you grasp the infant's body to deliver the head, you must be careful not to grasp too vigorously. A frank breech MAY give this kind of outcome when the upright legs press against the rib cage in delivery. If the liver has been torn or ruptured, the baby will become gray and will go into shock. With IMMEDIATE surgery, doctors are able to save some babies with this injury.

Breech delivery is a lost art, except among midwives who are trained well. You can learn to manage a breech effectively. Be sure that you learn well so that serious injuries such as this one do not occur.

Erb's Paralysis (Erb's Palsy)

Under the clavicle at the side of the neck is a complex of nerves that can be injured when the baby's neck is twisted or stretched. Injury to this **brachial plexus** results in **Erb's paralysis.** It usually occurs as the birth attendant tries to deliver the baby's shoulder. (This injury can also happen in breech deliveries when trying to deliver the head.) While you rarely see such injuries in a home birth, no matter where the birth takes place, someone who is not sufficiently trained may panic because of inexperience with a large infant whose broad shoulders are stubborn (whether in the vertex or breech position), and may unwittingly injure the infant.

If you are not sure whether there has been an injury, you can usually tell by closely observing how the infant moves his arms. If there is an injury, the upper arm will hang limply and close to the body, the forearm will be extended and rotated inward, and the palm of the hand will face away from the body. The elbow also points out. The baby may be able to move his fingers and perhaps his hand, but not his arm.

WHAT TO DO:

> Treatment for Erb's Paralysis calls for immobilizing the affected arm in the manner shown in Figure 71. This outward rotation and position of the arm is to be maintained carefully, even during feedings and baths. You can work the injured arm with very gentle massage and very slow movement. A slight injury usually heals in a few weeks, though it can take months if the injury is severe. If there has been extremely severe damage, the arm may atrophy and stay short.

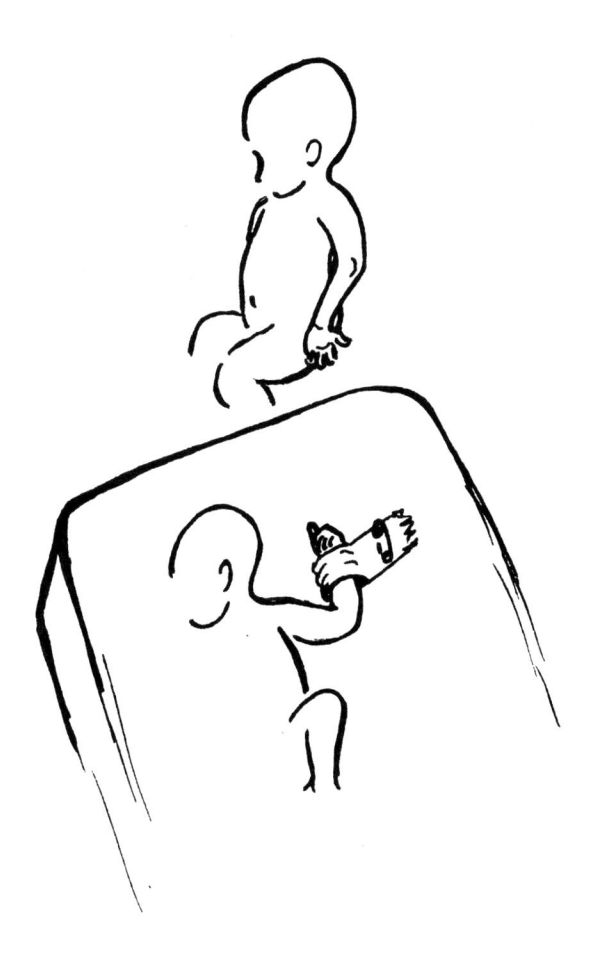

Malformations, Injuries, and Abnormalities 473

Figure 71. ERB'S PARALYSIS AND TREATMENT. Tape a padded bandage around the baby's wrist, rotate his hand toward his body and move it up beside his head (fingers up, palm facing the side of the head). Pin the bandage to the sheet or crib to keep the arm at right angles to the body. If the baby is not in bed, the arm should be held in this position.

UTERINE ABNORMALITIES

Anteflected Uterus

If putrefaction of lochia occurs, it may mean the mother's uterus has tipped forward, or **anteflected**, and the upper two-thirds of the uterus has trapped the drainage. (The uterus can also tip in a backward direction, or **retroflect**.) When normal drainage is impaired, bacteria breed rapidly and cause inflammation, itching, pain, odor, and eventually fever.

Most women can feel the small, firm ball of the fundus at the top of the symphysis pubis (overweight people may find it more difficult to find) when they palpate abdominally. A midwife will be able to examine internally and determine if the uterus is anteflected. She may assist the mother to help the uterus drain properly as follows:

> Have the mother do knee-chest positions for a day or two to "relax" the uterus into normal position. She should quickly get as comfortable as possible in this position, then, almost immediately afterward, reach back with one or both hands and gently part the buttock cheeks and the vulva. Air will quickly be drawn into the vagina, where there has been somewhat of a vacuum. She will hear this introduction of air. She should then release the cheeks immediately. She should feel the uterus slip into place.
>
> It may take going through this exercise a time or two to accomplish the desired results. Ten minutes after doing the above, the mother should slide down onto her abdomen and rest for a few minutes, then turn over and get up. Drainage should occur within a short time.

Malformations, Injuries, and Abnormalities

This knee-chest exercise may be done several times a day for a day or two. It may take as long as several weeks of doing the exercise several times a day before the uterus will remain in proper position.

If the knee-chest position exercise does not alleviate the drainage problem, manual drainage may have to be done by the midwife. It is done with the use of a speculum to hold the vagina open:

1. Use a sterile DeLee suction hose or boil a clear plastic enema hose for ten minutes. Cool on a sterile cloth.

2. Douche with calendula tincture diluted in warmed, sterile water, or with a strong calendula or yellow dock tea.

3. Wash the perineum and the labia (major and minor) with soap and warm water and rinse well with clear water, then rinse with calendula tea or tincture. This external cleansing is important, since this area is frequently the source of bacteria that can be carried inside the body. Insert the closed speculum, then open and secure it.

4. Now introduce the sterile plastic tube through the vaginal canal and into the uterus. Remember that the INTERNAL os must be passed before reaching the trapped lochia, so carefully and gently guide the tube through the isthmus. When the lochia is tapped, drainage will occur. Lochia will pass more freely if the end of the tube outside the body is held below the level of the uterus. The mother may sit on the edge of the bed in a reclining

position. GENTLENESS IS IMPORTANT to prevent perforating the uterus.

5. If the mother has developed a temperature, time is of the essence in combatting infection. Act accordingly.

Prolapsed Uterus

A **prolapsed** (low-hanging) **uterus** is one that has come down into the birth canal. If someone kneads the fundus improperly, it can cause the uterus to prolapse or even **invert** (come out).

The following remedies will produce tone, comfort, and healing for the woman with a prolapsed uterus. This program will usually prepare the uterus for more pregnancies, but must be continued between pregnancies until the uterus remains secure.

WHAT TO DO:

1. Lift no children, nothing heavier than a spatula for six months.

2. No intercourse for 45 to 60 days, depending on the degree of prolapse and the amount of progress made.

3. Sitz baths a.m. and p.m. Add 3 T. ginger and 3 quarts strong white oak bark tea. (Simmer 2 cups bark to 3 quarts water for 40 minutes, then strain and add to the bath. This will make 3 gallons all together.)

4. Douche daily before or after sitz baths, alternating some of the following formulas:

    MINERAL WATER (1 cup in 1 quart water); twice weekly.

Malformations, Injuries, and Abnormalities 477

> BAYBERRY-GLYCERINE TINCTURE (1/2 cup in 1 quart water) or BAYBERRY TEA (1 quart); each a.m.
>
> WHITE OAK BARK-GLYCERINE TINCTURE (1/2 cup to 1 quart water) or COMFREY TEA (1 quart); as an alternate treatment.
>
> COMFREY-GLYCERINE TINCTURE (1/2 cup to 1 quart water) or COMFREY TEA (1 quart); as an alternate treatment.
>
> MYRRH AND SKULLCAP TEA or LOBELIA TEA (1 cup herb to 1 quart warm water, steeped and strained); at any time for tenderness.

5. Trampoline (use the small one):

> 10 bounces 5 times a day for 2 weeks, with legs together, FEET REMAINING ON THE TRAMPOLINE (not bouncing above it). (If the uterus protrudes through the vagina, use a snug sanitary napkin for support.)
>
> 20 bounces 5 times a day for 2 weeks, LIFTING THE HEELS ONLY OFF THE TRAMPOLINE (not the toes).
>
> 50 jumps 3 times a day for 2 weeks, LIFTING THE FEET 2 INCHES off the trampoline (and thereafter each day of the year). Adjust this therapy to the individual.

6. Knee-chest position:

> Daily, after 1 p.m. and again upon retiring—for 10 minutes each time.

> IMPORTANT: Immediately after getting into knee-chest position, reach back and part the buttocks enough to allow air to draw into the vagina, then let go of the cheeks so they will close again. You will feel the uterus relax into position. After 10 minutes, slide down onto your stomach for a while to rest.

7. If constipated, 2 LB capsules before breakfast and 2 upon retiring. Use enemas to evacuate the bowels instead of bearing down.

8. Increase parsley intake with meals and in teas (2 cups daily) or in capsules. (Do not drink parsley tea if nursing. It dries up the milk flow.)

9. Increase dandelion intake; use in salads, green drinks. Dandelion tablets may be taken out of season.

10. Drink 1 cup ginseng tea in the morning (if not nursing, add parsley).

11. Drink red raspberry, St. Johnswort, and comfrey teas, 3 times during the day.

12. Take 2 tablespoons mineral water twice a day in juice. Adjust this to your own needs. Do not take a mineral water that flushes the bowels.

13. Eat no white flour or refined sugar products. Eat two steamed vegetables per meal, all others raw. Eat plenty of raw fruit.

Inverted Uterus

An **inverted uterus** is one that has been "turned inside out!" You may have stages of **incomplete inversion** (inversion of the top of the uterus, or fundus), **complete inversion** (the inverted fundus reaches or extends through the external os), or **prolapse of the inverted uterus** (the entire organ is outside the vulva). Sometimes the placenta remains attached to the inverted uterus. (This certainly would be true in the case of the **adhered placenta**.)

In many cases there is severe pain, and almost always there is profuse bleeding with inversion. Severe shock for no apparent reason following birth calls for looking quickly to see if there is a craterlike hollow just above ("behind") the symphysis pubis, or palpating internally for a protrusion into the cervix (the uterus may be obscured inside the vagina as an incomplete inversion).

An inverted uterus results from several things, ranging from improper pressure on the fundus and lack of uterine integrity to a prolapsed uterus involved in a traumatic or precipitous birth, etc. It is most apt to invert if undue effort is made to bring about the presentation of the placenta (such as pulling on the cord): in other words, POOR MANAGEMENT OF THIRD STAGE. (Inversion may occasionally recur with subsequent births.)

Brave fathers or attendants who sometimes feel they are ready to deliver a baby alone because they have witnessed a birth or two or have read a lot about birth are apt to make the mistake of hurrying a birth or of pulling out the placenta. Those who have "pulled them out" and brag about it because nothing adverse did happen probably didn't realize that the placenta had already separated and was "sitting there" ready to be lifted out of the vaginal nest into which it had slipped. Others, even physicians, who have prematurely separated placentas (pulled them out) have much more bleeding than is necessary. Hemorrhage and, on occasion, inversion takes place.

One mother delivered her first child in the hospital and after seventy-two hours of trauma was left with a partially prolapsed uterus. There were so many adverse experiences and outcomes from the birth that she lacked trust in anyone to make repairs, afraid they would take her uterus out, and she refused to go back to the hospital way of handling things. She conceived easily, and had four more children, but all were precipitous births. The cervix in late months literally hung out past the vulva and there was constant concern about infection and premature labor. Her home birth doctor and attendants worked carefully and constantly with her to prevent these things, and her outcomes were good. She did, however, have increased difficulty with intercourse following the birth of the first child.

WHAT TO DO:

>This can be a cause of very serious postpartum shock, and has to be corrected immediately. Treatment for shock should accompany any attempt to correct or to transport (see Appendix B, Shock: Symptoms and Treatment.)

>TO REVERSE THE INVERSION, not enough can be said about STERILE CONDITIONS. Prognosis is good if this can be executed promptly. It is painful. If the placenta is still attached, it will cause too much extra bleeding to

separate it at this point. If possible, leave it attached.

Put the entire hand under the uterus and go inside the vagina. The palm will hold the uterus, but DO NOT stuff it back into place. Begin at the junction of the cervix and corpus, and use the thumb and finger tips--gradually and with gentleness--to "gather" and reinsert the uterus FROM THE EDGES, a little at a time. The top, or fundus, of the uterus is replaced LAST.

"Stuffing" adds to the trauma and will probably end in another immediate prolapse or inversion. Instead, do as directed for two to five minutes, then carefully remove the hand. If the placenta should still be attached, healthy contractions brought on by herbs will help it to separate. Be sure NOT to put any pressure on the fundus, but allow the placenta to separate on its own volition if it will.

A careful check of the placement of the uterus should be made following the presentation of the placenta. It goes without saying that first aid for bleeding will have been employed from the beginning (see Chapter 17, Hemorrhage).

"HYALINE MEMBRANE DISEASE" (RESPIRATORY DISTRESS SYNDROME)

"Hyaline membrane disease" (respiratory distress syndrome, RDS) is due primarily to immature lung development, resulting in the lack of good blood oxygenation in the pulmonary (lung) circulation. (The lungs of affected infants have hyalinelike membranes; hence, the common name.) Even at term, that which allows the lungs to inflate properly following birth (**surfactant**) can be deficient, leaving the lungs (or a portion of them) small and stiff (underinflated, and also hard to inflate) until they mature enough to produce the needed surfactant. In the meantime, the blood is not getting all the oxygen it needs, and other difficulties arise as the newborn's system responds to and tries to compensate for this respiratory inadequacy—calling for the support systems of the hospital. Treatment depends upon the severity of the "disease"/distress. (If death does occur, it is almost always within 72 hours of birth.)

There is a tremendous rate of hyaline membrane disease in newborns today. One might not go to the texts necessarily, but to those who observe these cases and make inquiry into the results of postmortem research:

1. Hyaline membrane disease occurs most frequently in babies born at 32 to 33 weeks of gestation (about 35% have it).

2. Nearly all babies born at six months have it.

3. It occurs in babies for whose mothers the **Betamethasone** level was not high enough. (Betamethasone is a drug used to assist the baby's lung development; it is given to women threatening to deliver prematurely.)

4. The **lecithin** level must be twice that of **sphingomyelin** (a natural component of the secretory system) to insure the maturity of the lungs and to prevent RDS.

5. Infants weighing 1,000 to 2,500 grams (about 2 to 5 1/2 pounds) have the highest incidence of hyaline membrane disease.

Malformations, Injuries, and Abnormalities   483

6. Infants of diabetic mothers are predisposed to it.

7. Babies from mothers whose amniotic membrane had been ruptured more than 48 hours (labor induced or cesarean delivery effected) are more likely to have it.

8. Babies born cesarean are more likely to have it.

9. When the calcium level is low, the baby often has it.

We in the home birth movement in Utah have a good record of not having to deal with this problem, except in two cases that have come to my attention over the years. There could have been more; however, we feel that the rate is so very low. This doubtless is due to the prenatal precautions taken by the gravidas we deliver. In prenatal visits we recommend that rather heavy dosages of certain supplements, especially vitamin E, and alfalfa herbal drinks be taken (see Chapter 9, Preventive Supplementation). Enough vitamin E (encapsulated with lecithin) taken by the mother insures that the proper **L/S ratio (lecithin** to **sphingomyelin)** is maintained. In MOST instances, we are able to avoid all of the above circumstances in home birth planning.

CHAPTER 22

CESAREAN SECTIONS

There are numerous disadvantages to **cesarean section,** a procedure of taking the fetus (usually with forceps) through incisions in the abdominal and uterine walls. This operation, if repeatedly used, usually limits the number of births to a family. It prevents the first half-hour bonding so essential to the emotional welfare of both mother and child. It also eliminates the immediate postnatal nursing of the newborn, with its attendant benefits. (Delay in feeding the newborn of the mother who prefers nursing her offspring may predispose it to hypoglycemia.) There can be serious depression of the newborn and postpartum depression of the mother brought on by the use of anesthesia. And, importantly, the struggle of birth is pre-empted.

Prematurity of the newborn is often found in this delivery because the due date used to schedule delivery was either incorrect or it did not reflect the maturation needs of that particular fetus. Also, the "hyaline membrane disease" is frequently found in the newborn delivered by cesarean section.

One foreign-born woman was sensitive to the need for the physical and psychological struggles built into natural childbirth. When she witnessed a cesarean section in the United States, she hurried to apply firm pressure to the baby's head and body, in squeezing motions, to simulate a natural birth. It might be said that the baby is denied the feeling of being born when it is delivered by cesarean section.

The mother that delivers by cesarean section is denied necessary psychological and maternal feelings of having given birth. A mother in **A Superior Alternative** said she was alienated to the point of subconsciously feeling her baby belonged to someone else, questioning in her mind "their" approval of her undressing the baby to check it over.

Often cesarean sections are scheduled to accomodate office hours—so the physician will not be called in the night to deliver a baby—or to dovetail appointments, meetings, trips, conventions, and the like.

C-sections have been on the rise for many years. This is an intervention that medical professionals use too often in childbirth. Because it is major surgery, it calls for anesthesia and its risks are higher than for vaginal delivery. The use of fetal heart monitors is believed to be a major cause for this intervention. Natural childbirth is certainly the preferred method, and there is much less chance of having a cesarean section when deliveries are made at home.

If you are reluctant to consider cesarean delivery, you are among a sharply increasing number of parents, physicians, and researchers who are reporting that repeated C-sections are almost always unnecessary. In fact, they are so convinced that most first-time C-sections done today are totally unnecessary, that several in-depth studies are underway. **The Clarion Cesarean Prevention,** published by the Cesarean Prevention Movement in Syracuse, N. Y., expresses belief that when a cesarean is NECESSARY, it can be a lifesaving technique for both mother and infant; however, vaginal birth after cesarean (VBAC) is safer for both, in most cases, than is routine repeat-cesarean.

Those in the movement know that given adequate emotional support and education, 90 to 95% of women can deliver their babies as nature intended. They also believe that poor nutrition, smoking, alcohol, and medications taken during pregnancy and labor contribute to unnecessary cesareans. Published quarterly, **The Clarion** reports from numerous ongoing studies, conferences, published medical reports, and personal parental experiences of successful vaginal births after C-sections. Triplets, VBAC, total weight over 11 pounds, were delivered successfully at the Brigham and Women's Hospital in Boston in October of 1983.

A long overdue resistance to unnecessary cesareans is now being brought about through knowledge and experience in this area of childbirth.

Those assisting in the prenatal care of a woman who plans on natural childbirth can help the gravida prevent many of the problems that seem to call for C-sections. Still, a C-section may be considered necessary in the following cases:

1. THE MOTHER'S PELVIS IS TOO NARROW. This is rare, but women who have had rickets usually need a C-section. True cephalopelvic disproportionment is very rare and cannot often be used as an excuse for C-sectioning.

2. UTERINE INERTIA PERSISTS and vital signs begin to fail. This problem is usually preventable by maintaining good muscle tone through exercise, proper nutrition, sitz baths throughout pregnancy, and conceiving babies at least two years apart.

3. THE FETUS WILL NOT MOVE DOWN INTO POSITION to allow the head or presenting part to press against the cervix, preventing cervical dilation. (In most cases this can be dealt with by using the techniques discussed in Chapter 15, Obstructed Labor.) When the baby is in an abnormal position (transverse lie), normal delivery is prevented. (This sometimes happens in primigravidas and very young parturients.) BREECHES, for the most part, do not fall into the category of malpositioning, although many practitioners consider anything but anterior vertex as a malpresentation; therefore, many breeches are now unnecessarily taken by C-section.

4. PLACENTA PREVIA HAS OCCURRED (see Chapter 11, Placenta Previa).

5. THERE IS A LIFE-THREATENING ABRUPTIO PLACENTA (see Chapter 11, Abruptio Placenta).

6. INDUCTION OF LABOR BECAUSE OF TOXEMIA OR ECLAMPSIA FAILS, necessitating immediate delivery in order to save the mother's life (see Chapter 16, Eclampsia).

7. THE UTERUS HAS RUPTURED in the rare case of hydramnios (excessive amniotic fluid), or ruptured due to excessive amounts of Pitocin given during labor.

8. AN INOPERABLE PELVIC TUMOR OBSTRUCTS THE BIRTH CANAL.

9. THE BABY IS IN STRESS and cannot be treated by any natural method. Stress in this instance could be a true knot in the cord, exceptionally high emotional stress on the mother's part (which in turn may cause a response of meconium staining prior to the onset of labor), an accident which injures mother and/or fetus, or a noncorrectable prolapsed cord.

When C-sections must be done, the **"bikini"** incision over the lower abdominal and uterine segments is preferred over the **classical,** or vertical, incision. Fewer "window" stretches are found in the tissues and better healing experiences occur with "bikini" section. And, it is less likely to rupture with future pregnancies. The classical incision is used appropriately in special circumstances.

Fetal deaths in utero sometimes NATURALLY cause early termination of pregnancy. This is usually no cause for C-section, and is rarely cause for induction of labor. (Nature sets in motion the process of elimination in a very normal way. It can be handled at home very easily by preparing for an eventuality of overbleeding.)

APPENDICES

APPENDIX A

ASEPTIC TECHNIQUE

Aseptic technique involves taking measures to prevent contamination of clean or sterile areas, so as to not introduce bacteria into the body. Hands introduced internally to palpate and deliver should be scrubbed prior to each time they touch the parturient, then washed afterward.

As a result of numerous studies over the years, practices of scrubbing with strong agents to insure cleanliness in surgery and obstetrics are ever changing. It appears that successive scrubs at a time with antiseptic preparations cause at least three problems: (1) destruction or impairment of natural body defenses, therefore (2) an increase in bacterial counts on the skin, and (3) dermatological abrasions and infections.

Probably most hospitals in the United States have made studies to help deal with these problems. Typical tests have included taking a bacterial count on the surgeon's hands prior to scrubbing, then five minute scrubbings and bacterial counts are alternated several times to determine the effectiveness of such scrubs, as well as the surface damage to the extremities. Bacterial counts actually increased with repeated scrubs, because bacteria introduced following scrubs lived for successively longer periods of time and multiplied more rapidly, due to the fact that natural body defenses were impaired and could no longer protect the environment as well. When anything but WATER was used, body defenses were made much less effective in preventing contamination or in giving protection to the individual's own blood stream.

Probably pHisoHex or a mild soap (Dial or Safeguard) that contains nothing stronger than small amounts of hexachlorophene would suffice for initial scrubbing. This should be followed by clipping fingernails, cleaning underneath them thoroughly, scrubbing again with a soft brush and warm soapy water for 3 to 5 minutes, and thorough rinsing under warm, RUNNING water.

Williams Obstetrics warns that the use of gloves ". . . even in conjunction with other precautions, does not entirely eliminate the possibility of introducing bacteria into the genital tract, since organisms may be carried up from the vaginal outlet by the sterile, gloved finger."[1] Also, on occasion the glove tears, so hand cleanliness is of paramount importance.

After thorough washing and rinsing past the elbows, the gloves are put on by picking up the first sterilized glove (right, if right-handed) with the left hand. It is touched only where the cuff has been turned back before packaging. Never touch the outside of the glove with a bare hand. The right hand is now gloved and it picks up the remaining glove in the same manner and slips it on the left hand. A lubricating jelly (the container is handled by someone else) or olive oil helps ease the discomfort of vaginal exams. It is applied to the glove, not the vulva. Discard gloves following each use and scrub each time

Aseptic Technique

prior to a vaginal examination. Do not touch doorknobs, clothing, the gravida, bedding, or ANYTHING between scrubs and examining.

If your storage of gloves is depleted, and for some reason others are unobtainable, or if you find yourself at the scene of an accident, disaster, or precipitous birth, don't choke if you have to work without them. Do everything possible to clean the hands (with at least running water) and try not to touch the mother any more than is absolutely necessary. (Hence, the importance of having a first aid kit containing moist, sterile wipes in the car.)

I have also known a few practitioners who did not use gloves, but who were meticulous in striving for asepsis. I asked one if he had ever had a case of infection (childbed fever) with his patients. He smiled and said emphatically, "No! You go to the hospital to get those!" I also saw the same doctor reprimand a couple who kept examining between his visits in a prolonged labor. He wanted them to know the dangers they were imposing upon the wife and baby by frequent palpations, whether they were being cautious or not.

Common sense and a healthy sense of responsibility are the most important criteria in aseptic measures.

Instruments, especially the teeth on hemostats and forceps, must also be scrubbed with a brush in hot, soapy water, then rinsed thoroughly. Soak instruments in a good germicidal solution, dry, and store in a sterile towel. At the scene where they are to be used, they must again be placed in a sterile solution unless they have not been opened following sterilization (autoclaving or oven preparation). (Clean instruments may be wrapped carefully in a sturdy cloth, folded in foil, and baked at 125° F for 2 hours, or pressure cooked at 10 pounds for 10 minutes. Do not unwrap them until you are ready for their use.)

Apparently some doctors are not careful in observing standard hand-washing procedures. A study reported in the **New England Journal of Medicine** found that in one intensive care unit, doctors and nurses washed only 41 percent of the time, in moving from patient to patient, while handling urine bags, intravenous dressings, respiratory equipment, and patients in general. "Physicians were among the worst offenders." All this in spite of the fact that "Hand washing is considered the single most important procedure in preventing [hospital-caused] infections, and it has been recommended after contact with every patient by both the Centers for Disease Control and the American Hospital Association."[2]

Parents usually want to know what they can do to prepare the home for delivery. You can perform a valuable service for them when you visit the home, prior to term, if you will teach them what to do. The bathroom floor and all fixtures should be washed with a germicidal solution at the time the midwife is called. Wastebaskets are emptied and washed. Perhaps newspapers could be used on table tops where clean, sterile towels will be used to lay out instruments. The floor (or carpet) that the parturient will use between the bathroom and her bedroom should be freshly cleaned. Even then, she may want to use clean socks on her feet when she walks in these areas, then remove them when she gets in bed. Bed linens should have been properly cleaned and stored as has been suggested (see Chapter 13, Home Birth Supplies). The bed will be changed by the midwives at the appropriate time. The birthing room should be dusted; bare

floors, windowsills, and door frames should be
wiped with a damp cloth.

In spite of the assumption that Americans with
indoor plumbing bathe frequently, the value of
cleanliness should be stressed. It is especially
important that the mother bathes prior to her
delivery, even though she may possibly be in and
out of the tub a few times during labor. Clean
clothing is always used following baths. And, of
course, all infant wear should have been
unpackaged and prewashed to remove any fabric
fillers or handling contaminants.

NOTES

[1]Williams Obstetrics, 14th ed., p. 410.

[2]Richard K. Albert, M.D., and Frances Condie, M.S., "Hand-Washing Patterns in Medical Intensive-Care Units," **New England Journal of Medicine** 304 (June 11, 1981) :1465-66.

APPENDIX B

VITAL SIGNS

We speak of vital signs as being important information in the health care of people. What are they? What part do they play in pregnancy and childbirth?

Vital signs are those physical indicators that tell us whether or not the body is functioning properly. The disruption of one or more vital organs or systems alerts us to serious problems in the making or problems that already exist, which, uncorrected, will bring about serious consequences, including death.

In order that vital organs may do their part in sustaining life, they must each adequately perform certain duties. We are able to measure the performance of these duties quite well.

RESPIRATION

A person must breathe to sustain life, so **respiration** must occur on a regular basis to accomodate the pace and demands of the rest of the body under the stress of different activities. If the lungs are denied **oxygen** or clean air in any degree, this causes a negative chain reaction in other systems which rely upon the lungs' (and skin's) performance to supply oxygen to every part of the body. (The skin is the largest organ of the body and it works right along with the lungs in the performance of "breathing"; thus, clean skin is important.)

Respiration in the adult usually runs between 16 and 20 breaths per minute to provide adequate amounts of oxygen to the body. More or less activity will alter this figure. Lack of oxygen to the brain cells, for instance, will cause damage (mental retardation) and even death in those cells.

A blueness (**cyanosis**) appears in the part of the body that does not receive sufficient oxygen. The body can usually cope with such stresses if the oxygen insufficiency is not too great and if it is not prolonged for more than a few minutes--usually 3 to 7 minutes--at a time. (Smokers and industrial workers who labor with asbestos and other high risk materials impose recurring respiratory stresses that ultimately reach crisis proportions.)

Normally, the level of **carbon dioxide** runs slightly higher than the level of oxygen in the body, but too much carbon dioxide would contribute to the adverse chain reaction spoken of earlier. In that case, the body would become **acidotic** (pH becomes too acid, upsetting the chemical balance of the body) and die.

VASCULAR AND CIRCULATORY SYSTEMS

Heart and Pulse Rates

The **vascular system** (system of vessels, particularly blood vessels) and **circulatory system** (vessels and organs that circulate blood and lymph fluids) are vital systems in the work of sustaining life.

A process of **osmosis** transfers oxygen from the lungs to the blood stream. That great pump in the body, the heart, pushes the oxygenated blood through vessels of varying sizes (large arteries down to minute capillaries) to the outermost layers of the skin. The vascular system also returns wastes to be disposed of through the lungs and through other organs and body parts.

The heart's rate of pumping and the strength with which it pushes the blood through the vascular system is measured to determine if the frequency and vigor of the pumps (or beats) is adequate to meet the demands of whatever activity the body is presently engaged in.

We count the **pulses** (pulsations) of blood, and gauge the intensity with which they course through the blood vessels, with the finger tips. **Pulses** (pulse locations) can be seen and lightly palpated all over our bodies: on the side of the neck, at the wrists, in the groin, on the ankle--any place where a large enough vessel comes close to the surface of the skin. By counting the **pulse rate,** we can determine if that system is intact and performing on a regular, uninterrupted basis. (Stepped-up activity, or rest, will also alter the pulse rate.)

THERE IS A WAY TO TELL IF A WOMAN IS BLEEDING INTERNALLY! There is little excuse for not detecting a hidden hemorrhage. It can be done, especially if the volume of loss is very much. Several signals are given us.

When there is a SIGNIFICANT LOSS OF BLOOD from the normal blood stream, what happens? The heart says, "Woops! I'm not getting enough return to work with, so I'd better push harder to get the blood I DO HAVE to everywhere it must go!" And so, the pulse rate rapidly increases to try to compensate for the loss. What does this tell you? It says that WHENEVER THE PULSE RATE, which is normally between 60 to 70 counts per minute, RISES SHARPLY TO 20 BEATS OR MORE ABOVE NORMAL, you have, according to the circumstances (amount and swiftness of the loss of blood), a certain length of time in which to apply measures that will alter the situation--before that chain reaction (shock) sets in over the body and causes death.

In short, the loss of very much blood is accompanied with an increase in the pulse rate. Then, if immediate alterations are not made, there will not be enough blood for the heart to pump and the beats will slow down and stop! A POUNDING pulse (an early sign of trouble), the RAPID BUT FAINT pulse, and the IRREGULAR pulse (late signs of trouble) all reveal information that is vital. (Other disorders, such as emotional shock, infection, fever, heart disease, heart attacks, etc. can cause these same reactions.)

Blood Pressure

Blood pressure can be measured and the disturbance of normal rates can be detected when the **blood pressure cuff** and the **stethoscope** are properly used (see Chapter 8, Blood Pressure). In the normal, well adult, individual pressure will run between about 113 mm Hg (millimeters of mercury, the standard of measurement) systolic pressure over about 75 mm Hg diastolic pressure to about 125 mm Hg systolic over 80 to 82 mm Hg diastolic pressure (about 113/75 to about 125/82). (**Systolic pressure** is the pressure of the blood during the **systole,** the CONTRACTING phase of the heart's pumping action, in which blood is driven from the heart. **Diastolic pressure** is the blood pressure during the **diastole,** the RELAXING and DILATING phase of the heart's pumping action, in which the heart cavities are filled with blood.)

Various circumstances of emotional or physical stress can change these scores rapidly to outside acceptable levels. They return to normal, though, with recovery from the stress. However, in pregnancy, especially, ANY CHANGE IN AN INDIVIDUAL'S NORM that REMAINS higher than 30 MM SYSTOLIC OR 15 MM DIASTOLIC indicates an abnormal or serious condition, one that endangers the heart and blood vessels, and the fetus and gravida. A blood pressure that continues high (about 100 mm diastolic and 160 mm systolic, or more), is very dangerous and must have IMMEDIATE attention. **Hypertension** (high blood pressure) must be treated and monitored regularly, since there are rarely any symptoms apparent to the individual.

TEMPERATURE

A careful, periodic check of vital signs in pregnancy and childbirth includes taking the body temperature. Body temperature normally runs about 98.6° F. However, each person has his own norm that runs withing a few tenths of a degree over or under this figure. Temperature up to 102° F is not dangerous unless it remains high over a period of several days. It may even be the body's way of taking care of minor disturbances. Higher temperatures are more significant, and the cause must be determined and dealt with promptly.

* * *

Important, then, is KEEPING RECORDS of each client's normal vital ranges, in order to distinguish what FOR HER is normal and what is not, and how significant the difference may be. Any time there is internal or external interference with any of the vital systems, signs of the interference will be made manifest. These should be picked up and appropriate first aid administered.

The midwife owes the safety and successful management of births a careful study of vital organs and their direct communications to her. She should hear what they are saying to her when all is well, and she should hear the warnings in the event of malfunctions. The wise use of herbs, physical therapy, or supplements as first aids can only be safely administered when one knows what is going on and which, if any, first aid is called for.

SHOCK: SYMPTOMS AND TREATMENT

Serious disturbance to any vital system (respiration, heart, blood pressure, pulse, temperature) will bring on shock in an individual. Some degree of shock accompanies, or follows, any serious accident or injury. Shock is caused by bodily reactions that slow down or stop circulation: the consequent blood (and therefore, oxygen) insufficiency to vital organs is serious. If shock becomes irreversible—and it can reach this point rather quickly—it will be fatal.

As soon as lifesaving first aid is administered in any given situation--clearing air passageways, restoring breathing, stopping bleeding, restoring normal body temperatures (hypothermia or heat stroke)--take necessary measures immediately to prevent shock. Always think of shock as being inevitable.

(The shaking legs of the mother following delivery are a mild form of shock and must be dealt with right away. The mother chills when labor is concluded, and she must not be allowed to lose too much body heat. Warm blankets and jars filled with hot water can be placed on top of the blanket, alongside her legs.)

Signs of shock in any situation are:

1. Weakness.

2. Rapid but weak pulse.

3. Pale face.

4. Cold, clammy skin (though the person may be perspiring at the forehead and palms); chills.

5. Thirst.

6. Nausea.

7. Shallow, irregular breathing.

8. Very low blood pressure (this is a LATE SIGN).

WHAT TO DO:

1. DEAL IMMEDIATELY WITH THE LIFE-THREATENING INJURY, ETC., FIRST.

2. The head of the person should be at or below body level. This may be accomplished by elevating the legs and hips. DO NOT LOWER THE HEAD IF IT HAS BEEN INJURED, OR IF THE NECK COULD BE BROKEN!

3. Cover the person to protect from loss of body heat. Do not allow the person to chill.

4. Seeing the injury (an inverted uterus, for instance) usually increases shock, even in the "brave ones," so do not let them look! Pain also increases shock. Handle injuries or the victim gently. REASSURE THE PERSON IN SHOCK.

5. If the person IS CONSCIOUS, and is NOT VOMITING, and does not have abdominal injury, give a **shock solution:** HVC (1 T. vinegar, 1 T. honey, and 1/2 tsp. capsicum) in 8 ounces of water. If this is not available, but salt and soda are, measure carefully: 1 tsp. table salt and 1/2 tsp. baking soda into 1 quart of water. Give all the person can or will drink. (These can be premixed, and should be included with both car and home first aid supplies.)

6. Transport. If you have given the above-mentioned first aid, the person will probably be in pretty good shape by the time you have reached help. In pregnancy or parturition, if you have been able to resolve the crises, and prevent shock, continue with the matters at hand.

APPENDIX C

SAMPLE RECIPES FOR THE GOOD PROGRAM

TRANSITION DIET

Following are some recipes that make introduction to the Good Program diet a pleasurable experience. Nearly all of your favorite recipes may be adapted to good food menus. Use carob instead of chocolate, and honey or pure maple syrup instead of sugar (which takes out your B vitamins and calcium, etc.). Even yellow D sugar (dark brown cane sugar) is not as highly processed as other refined sugars. (ANY sweetener is used in moderation.) Go to your health food store and get two or three good recipe books, and learn to really come alive with good, clean, live food again.

After a few weeks of experimenting and of expanding ideas, preparation time for food will lessen and a general freedom from kitchen chores will give you at least two new horizons. The obvious benefit is a feeling of well-being, with more strength and energy and less feeling of "heaviness" or "fullness" following meals, and more cheerful countenances found on all those who are participating in "the new life." A second horizon opens up when you discover that preparing food and eating are not all there is to life!

There will now be time to develop and expand and enjoy your other talents and gifts. There will be more time for your family, for learning, for giving of self--a new self that will now feel more like giving!

BREAKFASTS WILL NEVER BE THE SAME AGAIN!

Petra's Auflauf

- 2 cups cooked rice
- 1 apple, chopped
- 1/2 cup chopped dates
- 1/2 cup raisins
- 1/2 cup nut cream (cashews blended in blender with 1/4 cup peanut oil or other oil)

Mix well. Bake or steam for 1/2 hour. Sesame nut cream is great, also. Serve with strawberries, orange slices, and bananas.

Whole Grain Cereals

Especially in the winter, whole grains are a delight for breakfast. Cook whole wheat or other grains like you do rice. Millet, instead of rice, makes a different and tasty breakfast or pudding. (Millet is also great in soups, and is used for a binder.)

There are a number of delightful cereals made from whole, rolled, cracked, mixed, and ground grains: wheat, barley, rye, triticale, oats, millet, amaranth, rice, corn, etc. The protein in grain cereals may be supplemented with nuts, sesame, sunflower, flaxseed, etc.

Soak all grains to release needed enzymes before cooking for cereal. You can conserve time and energy by bringing the cereal to a boil the night before, covering, and turning the unit off. Reheat or finish cooking briefly in the morning.

Grapenut Crunch

Sprout wheat to the length of the kernel only (about 2 to 3 days), grind in a food grinder. Spread and dry on a tray, crumble, and you have your own grapenuts. (To make a tasty cracker, use chunks or broken squares of the dried grapenuts—before crumbling—and sprinkle with Spike or vegetable seasoning.)

Apple Topping

Use Apple Topping on your oatmeal and you will never use milk again!

Per serving:

    1/2 apple, unpeeled
    8 almonds
    3 pitted dates
    1/3 cup water

Blend just until nuts are chopped into less than pea-sized bits. Pour over hot oatmeal.

Pancake Toppings

Try the following toppings on pancakes and waffles:

    apricot puree (from fresh or bottled apricots)
    apricot-pineapple puree
    pear puree with coconut shreds
    berries in their juice
    applesauce with dates or raisins
    peaches (fresh or bottled)

Maple Syrup

    1/4 cup hot water
    1 cup honey
    a few drops (1/2 tsp.) maple flavoring

FRUITS ARE FUN!

Extravaganza

Picture in your mind what a dreamolicious plate this must be with all its rich colors:

    2 Satsuma plums (dark purple plums)
    pear wedges
    orange wedges or rings (wash, but do not peel)
    grapes (green or red or purple)
    bananas (cut in oblong, 1/2-inch slices)
    apple rings or wedges
    fresh or bottled cherries
    apricots or peaches (bottled or fresh) or nectarines
    pineapple rings or chunks draped with a spearmint twig
    fresh coconut chips (or unsweetened coconut)

Serve with a nut cup and/or raisin, date, nut, banana, or zucchini bread.

Nuts used should be unheated (raw) and clean.

Soy beans, roasted and slightly salted, are also delicious with this plate.

Pineapple Gondola

Slice a fresh pineapple in half; leave top leaves on the halves. The pineapple can easily be cut into four long gondolas. Spray-wash the leaves, nooks, and crevices of the pineapple exterior carefully before slicing. Remove all the pineapple from the "boat" shell. Prepare and mix the following fruits:

> banana circles
> cantaloupe balls or wedgelike chips
> seedless grapes
> pineapple pieces (from the "boat")

Use pineapple juice or the juice of 1 cup blended red raspberries to make a sauce. The sauce is blended in the blender with a banana to make it gravy-thick. Add honey to taste. Mix with the fruits, pour back into gondolas, and sprinkle with coconut. (Strain raspberry seeds if they are objectionable.)

Watermelon Basket

Wash a small or large (depending on size of family or number of guests) watermelon. Cut carefully in half lengthwise to near the center. Stop cutting to leave 1 1/2-inch space for the handle on each side. The handle is cut up and across the top of the melon. (Instead of cutting lengthwise through the center of the melon, I lift the knife HIGHER ON THE MELON to make a little deeper basket to hold more fruit.) Scoop out the watermelon and seeds. Save the melon to return to the basket with other fruit. You will want to scoop out all the pink meat so only the white of the rind will be left. Be careful not to break the handle, but turn the melon on its side to drain, or fill it with paper towels to dry. Combine other fruits with watermelon squares or balls and fill the basket. Melons with yellow (orange), white, and green meats are good combinations. Bananas and grapes also are good. For variety, use whipped cream, nuts, and shredded coconut to stir into the fruit meats before returning the mixture to the watermelon basket.

Fruit Malts

MALT #1

    5 fresh or frozen apricots
    1 cup pineapple or pineapple juice
    10 almonds
    2 T. honey
    1 banana

Blend—on liquefy.

Serve chilled. Good anytime, especially for breakfast.

MALT #2

    1 cup berries
    1 cup pineapple
    1 cup papaya juice or coconut milk
    2 heaping T. protein powder
    1 cup water if a more bland taste is desired
    honey (optional)

Blend (liquefy).

MALT #3

    1 large banana
    10 almonds
    5 apricots (or any fruit or berries, canned or frozen)
    1 cup water or apple juice

Blend (liquefy).

As you can see, any fruit or juice combination is great, and the nuts add a complete protein.

MAIN DISHES

Lentil Loaf

>   2 cups cooked lentils
>   1 cup soy milk
>   1/2 cup oil
>   1 1/2 cup crumbs
>   1 egg
>   1 cup nuts (any kind)
>   1 tsp. salt
>   1/2 cup grated carrots
>   1/2 cup celery, chopped
>   1 cup cooked oatmeal or garbanzo beans for binder
>   3/4 tsp. sage
>   1 T. onion

Mix well; bake at 350° F in an oiled loaf pan for 1/2 hour.

Cooking With Soybeans

I highly recommend the **Soybean Cookbook** by Dorothea Van Gundy Jones (New York: Arco Publishing, Inc., 1979), an excellent little paperback. It tells the story of the soybean, explains the nutritional value of soybeans, and gives dozens of recipes for everything from salads to desserts.

Soybeans come in about 160 varieties. This economical protein food is called "the meat that grows on vines," and it is versatile in that it provides flour as well as milk:

Soybeans not only contain high-quality protein, but their protein content is much higher than that of other foods. Compared with other protein foods, soybeans contain

- 1 1/2 times as much protein as cheese, peas, or navy beans
- 2 times as much protein as meat, fish, or lima beans
- 3 times as much protein as eggs or whole wheat flour
- 11 times as much protein as milk

Two pounds of low-fat soy flour are equal in protein content to

- 5 lbs. of boneless meat.
- 6 doz. eggs.
- 15 qts. of milk.
- 4 lbs. of cheese.[1]

Soybeans should not be eaten raw. Petra Sukau has a trick for making boiled soybeans taste soft and delicious, for those who have a slightly difficult time cooking them enough to soften them, or for those who have a hard time digesting so much protein at once. She says, "Soak them overnight in three times as much water as beans, put them on a towel to dry, then freeze them on a cookie sheet. To cook: add 1 part water to 1 part beans, boil slowly for 1 1/2 to 2 hours."

Baked Soybeans

2 1/2 cups cooked soybeans
3 1/2 cups tomatoes (drain juice into sauteed onions)

Add:

1 cup sauteed onions
1/4 cup oil
1/4 cup brown sugar
2 tsp. salt

Cook until thick. Then add:

    1/4 cup lemon juice
    1 tsp. sweet basil
    1/2 cup tomato paste

Bake 1 1/2 hours at 350° F.

Tomato Cups

Wedge around the tops of large tomatoes, scoop out the insides, and fill with Summer Fair Salad (alone, or mixed with cottage cheese).

Green Pepper Cups (Raw)

Fill with Summer Fair Salad, cooked bean salad, or baked beans.

Green Pepper Cups (Cooked)

Try any of the following variations:

1. Scoop out seed section, fill with lentil loaf mixture. Cook at 350° F for 1/2 hour.

2. Fill with cubes of zucchini squash, onion, and tomato. Add a pinch of garlic powder, celery salt; top with bread crumbs. Cover. Bake at 350° F for 40 minutes.

3. Fill with celery chips, tomatoes, and cheese. Cover and bake for 1/2 hour. Uncover and bake for another 10 minutes. Cover with crumbs or potato chips (optional).

4. Fill with chili and bake.

Many similar combinations will please the whole family.

Vegetable Plate Pinwheel

Any huge plate you prepare with a colorful arrangement of vegetables or fruits will disappear FIRST in any meal. A complete meal of such can be served with whole wheat crackers or nuts to the satisfaction of good health. (Don't say you cannot affort to use fruits and vegetables because they are too expensive! You cannot affort NOT to use them! I can go to the grocery store and buy five sacks of fresh produce and pay less for them all than I can when I buy just one sack full of meat, cheese, canned goods, etc.)

Cut in interesting wedges, flowers, strips, and slices, and arrange the following vegetables (washed, but unpeeled) in a complementary color arrangement on a large platter or tray:

    turnip wedges
    celery
    tomato wedges or little salad (cherry) tomatoes
    cucumbers (scrape lengthwise with fork, then slice round)
    zucchini slices, sprinkled with Jensen's Broth or Seasoning powder
    yellow crookneck squash slices
    radishes
    carrots
    beet shreds
    red onions or little green onions
    olives
    green pepper rings
    broccoli sprigs
    cauliflower silhouettes
    any other vegetable you like raw

Serve with a dip, or add a center dish of cheese cubes on toothpicks.

Summer Fair Salad

    1 6-inch zucchini
    4- to 6-inch yellow crookneck squash
    8 red radishes
    1 medium green pepper
    1 cucumber
    2 tomatoes
    2 stalks of celery with leaves
    1 medium carrot, shredded

Chop above vegetables into 1/4-inch bits and serve with Golden Harvest Salad Dressing. (They may be tossed with the dressing.) If used for a main dish, add 1 cup kidney beans or garbanzo beans.

Ruby Delight Salad

    2 medium, fresh, washed, raw beets (unpeeled)

Shread with tiniest salad shredder. Serve as a side dish with NOTHING added or with honey (3 T.) and apple cider vinegar (2 T.). It will do wonders for your liver!

Tossed Salad Supreme

    any three lettuces (endive, red, iceberg, etc.)
    thinly sliced cauliflower flowerets
    chopped broccoli
    cucumber
    tomatoes
    celery
    carrot shreds
    green onions
    shredded radishes
    zucchini slices
    red cabbage
    sharp cheddar cheese
    imitation bacon bits

DRESSINGS

Basic Recipe for Soy Mayonnaise

    1 cup cold water
    3/4 cup soy milk powder
    1 tsp. salt
    1 cup oil
    1/3 cup lemon juice

Put water, soy powder, salt, and lemon juice in blender, add oil VERY SLOWLY in a tiny stream as blender liquefies on high speed. You will know you have enough oil when the hole in the center joins together in the first blurp! Turn blender off and serve.

To this basic recipe can be added:

    onion (fresh, dried, or powdered)
    garlic
    pimento, olives, and onions (tartar sauce)
    parsley

Golden Harvest Salad Dressing

    3/4 cup Basic Soy Mayonnaise or Miracle Whip
    1 T. Jensen's Broth or Seasoning powder
    3 T. lemon juice

Thousand Island Dressing

Add to basic mayonnaise recipe these options:

    1 stalk celery
    olives
    tomato paste
    a little honey
    more lemon juice
    water
    onion and pickle

Mustard Variation

Add to basic mayonnaise recipe:

    1/2 tsp. cumin
    3/4 tsp. turmeric

Avocado Dip

    1 peeled and mashed avocado
    1 tsp. Jensen's Broth or Seasoning powder
    1/3 to 1/2 cup salad dressing
    2 T. fresh lemon juice

Oil and Vinegar Dressing

We always like this particular dressing tossed into the salad because of the evenness of the taste and distribution when done in this manner. Use equal amounts of each. FIRST pour the oil over the salad and toss gently, but well. THEN add any seasoning you like, such as Spike. THEN add the vinegar. For a large salad use 5 T. (or more) oil and 5 T. (or more) of vinegar. If you like a more bland taste of vinegar, add 2 T. water with the vinegar.

TREATS

Carob Nut Log

    1/2 cup carob powder
    1/2 cup toasted soy flour
    1/2 cup ground mixed nuts (raw or dry roasted)
    1/2 cup chopped pecans
    1/2 cup sunflower seeds
    1/2 cup sesame seeds
    3/4 cup honey
    2 tsp. sesame oil

Combine and mix well. Shape into balls or logs and store in the refrigerator in plastic or foil.

Carob Bread Pudding

    2 eggs
    2 cups whole wheat bread crumbs
    2 cups milk
    1 cup raw sugar or honey
    4 to 6 squares unsweetened carob bar
    1/8 tsp. salt

(Carob sweetened only with licorice will taste sweet, but will cut down on sugar intake. You may eliminate the raw sugar if you use a sweetened carob bar.)

Blend eggs, diced carob, raw sugar, and milk in blender. Pour mixture over bread crumbs and let stand until the bread is softened. Bake in moderate oven (350° F) until set--about 30 minutes.

Candy Bars

    graham crackers
    1 cup freshly ground peanut butter
    1/2 cup honey
    sweetened carob bar(s), melted

Mix honey and peanut butter. Break each graham cracker half into 2 pieces. Spread honey and peanut butter mixture between crackers. Roll in melted carob. Place on waxed paper and refrigerate until set. Peel from paper and serve. To keep and ration, wrap each separately and freeze.

Trail Mix

>   date nuggets
>   almonds
>   raisins
>   pumpkin seeds
>   dried banana slices
>   peanuts
>   cashews
>   (any other nuts you like)

Shortcake

Drip fruit jams over homemade bread and add whipped cream.

GREEN DRINKS

Basic Green Drink

>   2 sprigs of peppermint or spearmint
>   1 handful tender dandelion leaves
>   1 handful celery leaves

Add pineapple juice and honey to taste. Blend (liquefy), strain, and chill.

To the above ingredients may be added any favorite herb or combination of herbs for a variety of tastes.

Jeanne's Blend Green Drink

Use only the freshly picked, young, tender leaves in season. The following amounts will serve about 16 to 20 people (3 to 4 quarts). (It can also be stored in the refrigerator two to three days for a cleansing fast.)

Sample Recipes for the Good Program

If you cannot find all the herbs, use whatever you can find. (For fewer servings, use smaller amounts of everything.)

- 1 handful of tender dandelion leaves (not in blossom)
- 3 handfuls wheat grass
- 3 handfuls marsh mallow leaves (rich source of zinc)
- 3 handfuls redroot (wild amaranth) leaves
- 3 handfuls purslane (rich source vitamin A)
- 3 handfuls parsley
- 3 handfuls pineapple mint (makes good tea)
- 3 handfuls spearmint
- 3 handfuls shepherd's-purse
- 3 handfuls nettle ("stinging," excellent source of iron)
- 2 medium sprigs of filaree (especially good for nerves)
- 4 medium comfrey leaves
- 1 handful lemongrass
- 1 handful hound's-tongue (great for cough syrup)
- 1 handful brooklime (great kidney herb)
- 3 handfuls alfalfa tops
- 3 sprigs catnip
- 3 handfuls Johnson grass
- 3 handfuls yellow dock (both wide and narrow leaf)
- 3 handfuls couch grass (quack grass)
- 3 handfuls wild millet (foxtail grass)
- 3 handfuls plantain
- 3 handfuls lamb's-quarters

Wash the herbs in deep, cold water baths briefly; tear into pieces. Add 2 cups of the combined herbs you have gathered to 1 quart of water; blend at high speed. Let the juice sit for a few minutes, covered, then strain thoroughly. DO THIS FOR EACH BATCH UNTIL ALL YOUR HERBS ARE USED.

SAVE the herbs from each batch until all batches are blended, then return the herbs to the blender, cover with water, blend again, and strain again. Add this also to the first juices.

Add 1 quart pineapple juice to the combined juices. (Pineapple and papaya contain superior digestive enzymes and are good fruit juices to combine with herbs or vegetables satisfactorily.) Some tender herbs are already delicately sweet, but you can add a bit of honey if the pineapple or papaya do not make it sweet enough.

Store any fresh herbs you do not use in a plastic bag in the refrigerator. They last three to four days, as do other greens, but are at their best fresh from the field or yard.

Jeanne's Blend is one of the most delicious, delectable tastes I have ever experienced. It is packed with nutrition and energy pickup. In pioneer days when "bitters" were known to be good for health, people would have thought anything that tastes as good as Jeanne's Blend could not possibly be good for you. But believe me, it is. It is an excellent drink for picnics, long drives, juice fasts, breakfast, or whenever.

CANNING RECIPES

Freezer Jams and Jellies

    1 pkg. MCP pectin
    2 cups berries (or unsweetened Concord grape juice)
    1 to 2 cups mild-flavored honey
    1 tsp. instant vitamin C powder

Stir pectin and vitamin C into the crushed fruit or juice. Set aside for 1/2 hour. Stir honey in, bottle, and freeze. (For a thicker consistency, add more honey.)

Iris's Home Canning Method

DO NOT USE THIS METHOD FOR TOMATOES OR VEGETABLES --ONLY FRUIT:

> PEEL RIPE FRUIT. Scald fruit in boiling water 20 to 40 seconds, depending upon ripeness, then plunge in cold water. Cut fruit in half --pears squeeze right out of their skins! Place in a bowl of water with lemon juice or vitamin C added (to prevent darkening) until ready to pack into bottles.
>
> PACK FRUIT IN BOTTLES. Add 100 to 250 units vitamin C (ascorbic acid--the heat would spoil the natural kind) and one rounded tablespoon of honey per quart. You may want a little more honey if the fruit is really tart. Fill bottles up to fill line with water. Wipe tops well and put preboiled lids on.
>
> TIGHTEN LIDS AND PLACE IN A COLD PACK CANNER KETTLE, with hot water over the top of the jars. Bring canner to a full, rolling boil.
>
> REMOVE FROM HEAT. Leave lid on and let sit for thirty minutes. Then remove bottles from canner kettle to cool.

This timing works well at 4,500 feet; adjust for altitude, if needed. Cooled bottles that have not sealed (lids bulge slightly and will "pop" when pushed in) can be refrigerated and used first.

NOTES

[1] *Soybean Cookbook*, p. 9.

APPENDIX D

HERBAL PREPARATIONS

HERBS FOR FEMALE PROBLEMS

Problems connected with female systems can be helped immensely by taking a good combination of herbs designed for that purpose. Such things as amenorrhea, irregularity of menses, excessive flows, and too frequent menses or prolonged menses are particularly helped with a good **female corrective**. Cramping, swelling, and other discomforts can be eliminated with prolonged use of the female corrective. Add such supplements as vitamins E, B complex, and C to round out the needs created by individual problems, such as the inability to conceive and carry a fetus to term. Although it is said that FREQUENTLY amenorrhea (no menses) or irregular menses are due to the system's carrying parasites, menstrual regularity can be assisted by using the female corrective following the riddance of parasites.

Female Corrective Formula

A formula widely used in the Intermountain West is an excellent female corrective. Use 1 part each of the following herbs: cramp bark, blessed thistle, cayenne, false unicorn root, ginger, red raspberry leaves, squawvine, and uva ursi, and 3 parts goldenseal root. Powder the herbs, encapsulate them in "00" gelatin capsules, and take 2 twice a day or, if needed, three times a day.

To Rebuild an Unhealthy Vaginal Floor

HERBAL BOLUSES

Vaginal tissue can be strengthened and healed between births with the use of herbal boluses. Herbs are mixed, shaped like tampons, and put into the vaginal cavity overnight or during the day. They can be made and stored in the refrigerator in a tight container. Three at a time are brought to room temperature before use. Following are two of many combinations suitable for rebuilding vaginal tissue.

Always use finely powdered herbs in boluses. Mix the powders, add just enough mineral water (or oil) to form a doughlike consistency, and mold into tampons the shape and size of your thumb. Insert three boluses into the vaginal cavity. Follow with a natural sponge with a six inch string sewn through it for easy removal. The sponge prevents the boluses from slipping out during evacuations of the bowel or bladder.

1. Olive oil, wheat germ oil, white oak bark, comfrey root and leaves, marsh mallow root, mullein, black walnut leaves, gravel root, wormwood, lobelia, skullcap, and ginger. (A similar commercial salve, B F & C Ointment, can be applied to a tampon and inserted overnight.) Use equal parts of the powdered herbs and blend with the liquids.

2. Comfrey roots and leaves, slippery elm, white oak bark, flaxseed (powdered), yellow dock. Mix with mineral water.

I would suggest that you alternate types of boluses from time to time.

After an initial three-week period of relatively steady use, follow a different schedule. Try using boluses only at nights three times a week for about six weeks. Use yellow dock tea douches following their use to cleanse the vagina.

For Varicosities of the Vulva

WHITE OAK BARK TINCTURE

White oak bark is an astringent. Varicosities shrink when the tincture is applied locally (wear a snug-fitting sanitary napkin). Make a gallon of tincture at a time, if you like. Glycerine will preserve it without refrigeration. Use the following proportions and multiply for desired amount of tincture. The basic recipe is:

   2 T. white oak bark to 1 cup of water.

To make ONE GALLON of the tincture:

   Use 1/2 of the amount of water (1/2 gallon) over 2 cups white oak bark. Simmer 45 minutes. Strain off the tea. Pour the other half of the water (1/2 gallon) over the dregs and simmer for another 45 minutes. Strain and combine the teas now prepared. Add 1/4 cup pure vegetable glycerine (a healing and preserving agent) to each cup of tea. Mix well.

HERBS FOR ILLNESS, INFECTION

Herbal Composition Powder

This multiuse formula is said to have been used by the families of Brigham Young. It works advantageously on the pituitary gland and would be good in childbirth. Grind, or powder, the following:

- 4 oz. ground bayberry
- 4 oz. poplar bark
- 4 oz. pine bark
- 2 oz. ginger
- 2 oz. cloves
- 2 oz. cinnamon
- 1 oz. cayenne pepper (capsicum)

Black Walnut Tincture

Simmer the hulls of black walnuts in water (2 cups hulls to 1 quart water) for 45 minutes. Add 1/4 cup pure vegetable glycerine to each cup of strained tea. This tincture can also be preserved by substituting vinegar (1/2 cup to the quart) for glycerine. Apply locally to fungal, viral, and bacterial infections.

For vaginal douches, add 1/3 cup of the above tincture to 1 quart of warm water. A saturated tampon (undiluted tincture) is inserted overnight.

Garlic Powder Douche

1 tsp. garlic powder is added to 1 to 2 quarts warm water.

Garlic and Cayenne Enema

Add 1 tsp. garlic powder, 1 tsp. cayenne to a full enema bag of tepid water. Warm water tends to nauseate. Cayenne does not sting internally or very much when evacuated. It stimulates the peristaltic nerves to accomodate good bowel cleansing. These need not be high enemas, but three bagfuls of this solution should be used during one trip to the bathroom.

LB Formula

Herbs found in the **LB** (liver and bowel) **Formula** are the following:

- 1 part barberry bark
- 1 part goldenseal
- 1 part cayenne
- 2 parts cascara sagrada bark
- 1 part ginger
- 1 part lobelia herb or seeds
- 1 part red raspberry leaves
- 1 part turkey rhubarb root

Powder and encapsulate. This combination not only softens stools for complete evacuation, but it heals and nourishes bowel tissue. It is not a laxative, as such.

For Bladder and Kidney Ailments, Toxemia

Soak the following herbs for 6 hours (or overnight), then barely heat (do not even simmer), for 30 to 45 minutes:

- 1 oz. licorice root
- 1 oz. yarrow
- 1 oz. marsh mallow root
- 2 oz. hydrangea
- 1 oz. couch grass (quack grass)
- 1 oz. corn silk
- 1 oz. cleavers
- 1 oz. sanicle

A strong syrup is made by straining the herbs and adding 1/4 part pure vegetable glycerine and 5 to 6 ounces of rice bran syrup. To this, add 1/5 part brandy.

This is taken orally. If you use the mixed powdered herbs, take 2 capsules three or four times a day. If you use the syrup formula: for 7 to 12 year olds, 1/2 tsp. three times a day between meals; 12 to 17 year olds, 3/4 tsp. three times a day; adults, 1 dessert spoon to 1 T. three times a day.

For Mastitis

Apply mullein oil mixed with lobelia powder to the afflicted breast between feedings; cover and add warm heat. I am told that Canary Island women rub castor oil on packed breasts and that it also helps increase the secretion.

HERBS FOR HYDROTHERAPY

1. During pregnancy and parturition a tub bath containing 3 T. ginger soothes and relieves tension and soreness.

2. Peripacs dipped in very warm ginger water (1 T. to 2 quarts water) not only relieve tension, but promote healing.

3. Sit on a "donut" in a warm sitz bath of ginger water for relief of a broken coccyx.

4. Mineral water applied to 4-inch square pads and placed at the vulva with each change of sanitary napkin also relieves soreness and promotes healing of all small lesions, lacerations, and sutured areas at the perineum.

5. White oak bark tea, an astringent, is very helpful in sitz baths for the person who suffers from varicosities at the vulva. Mineral water would also work well.

6. Lobelia tea in sitz tubs and in enemas is especially helpful to relieve pain.

7. Black walnut tea is excellent for the treatment of warts, lesions, or for yeast-caused tenderness near the vaginal opening. Black walnut tincture (or strong tea douches) has already been suggested for yeast-infected vaginal cavities.

HERBS FOR CHILDBIRTH

For with the Five-Week Antenatal Formula

It is difficult to suggest certain amounts of oral aids due to the physiological make-up of individuals. While the majority may do very well with the five-week antenatal formula, an individual person may need extra amounts of one or more of the ingredients therein. In this case, she may have realized this early in pregnancy and will have taken, say, squawvine all along, or wild yam, or whatever. Then again, as term approaches, an individual may feel the need for an additional something to calm persistent Braxton Hicks contractions and to give a sense of preparedness. The following combination seems to prepare the gravida both physically and spiritually for delivery. It is taken daily during the two weeks before labor, and is prepared as a tincture and preserved in glycerine, mineral water, or vinegar. Refrigerate after preparing.

VIBURNALGIA TINCTURE (a homeopathic preparation)

    1 part blue cohosh
    1 part cramp bark
    1 part cloves
    1 part pulsatilla (windflower herb)

Use 1 tsp. in warm water, morning and night, or 1/2 tsp. after each meal.

Sometimes a person seems to subconsciously "hold back" in labor. If labor is beginning to drag on, take 1/2 tsp. of the tincture. It will do wonders. Then, if the placenta is stubbornly retaining, take 1 tsp. every half hour. (Twice is usually sufficient.)

For Use with Pressure Points

Dip finger tips into a small dish of one of the following preparations before holding pressure points:

TINCTURE OF WORMWOOD. (Patted on only, NOT RUBBED in.) The camphor ingredients of wormwood will enhance the use of pressure (acupressure) points.

LINAMENT. The following linament is excellent for acupressure or when applied to sore, aching muscles, etc.

    3 qts. wormwood tincture
    3 oz. wintergreen
    1 pt. witch hazel
    1 oz. tincture of cayenne (optional)

Antispasmodics

At least two tinctures are frequently referred to as antispasmodics. The one used in childbirth at the beginning of labor (to relieve pain) is the LOBELIA/CAYENNE tincture (Tincture #1).

ANTISPASMODIC TINCTURE #1

Combine 2 parts lobelia to 1/4 part cayenne, cover with vinegar for 10 days. Shake each day. Strain and store the tincture. (Antispasmodics are a must for family home storage. They last indefinitely.)

Dosage: 5 drops tincture in 1 cup of water. (More than this given at one time will tend to nauseate the mother; however, greater amounts of lobelia tincture can be taken in enemas (3 T. to the quart of water). This preparation is excellent when used as an emetic (to promote vomiting), or for the person with asthma or a heavy catarrh buildup.

ANTISPASMODIC TINCTURE #2

This tincture is used to relieve pain, cramps and spasms, persistent coughs, and lockjaw. It contains the following powdered herbs:

   1 part crushed lobelia seeds
   1 part skullcap
   1 part skunk cabbage
   1 part gum myrrh
   1/2 part black cohosh
   1/2 part cayenne

Mix these well in a (quart) bottle, then stir into the mixture enough apple cider vinegar to cover it generously. Shake well each day for 10 to 14 days. Strain and bottle in smaller containers if you wish. Use 3 to 5 drops orally, or use more when poured over wounds, applied in pacs, or rubbed over cramping areas.

This is excellent for coughs. Add 1 tsp. tincture to 2 ounces (only) of water, drink twenty minutes apart, for three times. Also, three drops inside the cheek of a lockjaw victim will release that condition.

Herbal Preparations 531

HERBS FOR THE NEWBORN

Mucus-Cutting Formula, Stools

Heavy mucus in the stools of the newborn is uncommon, but when the baby is experiencing heavy mucus in the nose and throat, there is bound to be some in the stools. Sometimes meconium does not expel as it should. Give an enema (with an infant syringe) of the following to cut the mucus safely:

    2 tsp. olive oil
    2 tsp. mineral water
    1 to 2 tsp. chlorophyll

Do not worry that this will harm the newborn. If you put petroleum jelly on the tip of the syringe, expel any air in it, and VERY carefully insert the 2-ounce ear syringe, this formula will cut mucus immediately, and in a healing way.

Mucus-Cutting Formula, Nose and Throat

Heavy mucus in the nose and throat is often found in the newborn whose mother has consumed a lot of milk during pregnancy. Choking and cyanosis is alarming and dangerous. If this seems to be a problem, the following formula can be used, even in the first hours after birth:

    2 drops of chlorophyll
    1 tsp. sterile (distilled or boiled) water

Mix and use an eyedropper to put ONE DROP in each nostril. Remember that babies are nose breathers, so more than that at a time might pose a problem.

For Hematomas

Hematomas are reported to disappear within a few hours if a four-inch gauze is saturated with arnica tincture and placed over the swelling. A plastic cap (be very cautious with its use) can be improvised and tied under the chin to keep the tincture moist and effective.

For Feeding Problems

For infants who can't nurse and for small children with feeding problems, liquefy the following:

- 1 cup sunflower seeds that have been soaked overnight in 1 quart water
- 1 heaping T. carob powder
- 1 rounded tsp. bone meal (calcium source)
- 1 T. brewer's yeast
- 1 T. molasses (when the child is constipated) or 1 T. heated honey
- 1 T. oil (soy or sesame)
- 1 T. lecithin

Supplement this formula with vitamins E and C and garlic oil, in the bottle. Add 1 tsp. acidophilus[1] for each ounce of formula.

Sore Baby Bottoms

Apply the salve of calendula, mullein, comfrey, plantain, and marsh mallow to clear rashes and scalded diaper areas. (CMM Ointment is essentially the same salve.)

NOTES

[1] The **Lactobacillus** organism supplement generally best suited for infants and young children is **L. bifidus**, which comes from mother's milk. (This is especially good for infants who haven't been able to nurse, or who have been weaned very early.) **L. acidophilus** is also beneficial for growing "friendly" intestinal bacteria, and in times of illness it may even be preferred. (These strains are not taken together, as they compete with each other. You may have to alternate according to the infant's needs.)

INDEX

A

Abdomen
  alcohol intoxication through, 425
  incision of
    abortion, 27
    C-section, 92, 484, 488
  muscles, 242, 287, 326
  newborn, distended bladder, 409
  pain
    abruptio placenta and, 186
    anterior lip and, 369
    with bleeding, 186
    eclampsia and, 302
    ectopic pregnancy and, 190
    mistaken for threatened abortion, 194
    pendulous, face presentations and, 465
    placing newborn on mother's, 351
Abdominal aorta, 379
Abdominal band (binder), 380, 389, 430
Abdominal breathing
  during labor, 280-81
  prenatal, postnatal exercise, 159, 161-62, 434
Abortion
  "The Case Against Easier Abortion Laws," 29n
  definitions, 26-27
  induced, 25-29
    boy vs. girl fetuses, 115
    complications, 27-28
    contemplating, anecdote, 25-26
    mental/emotional problems and, 29n, 355
    methods used, 27
    screening, 85, 95

Abortion (cont.)
    statistics, 28
    uterine damage from, 95
  spontaneous (miscarriage)
    accidental, 191
    causes, 88-90, 186, 191
      abruptio placenta, 186
      amniocentesis, 115
      ballottement, 76, 80
      contraceptives, 40
      diabetes, 208
      early palpation, 77
      ectopic pregnancy, 189
      intercourse, 37-38, 89,, 186
      placenta previa, 186, 191
    in second, third trimesters, 88, 192
    threatened, 158, 192-94
      conditions mistaken for, 194-95
  therapeutic, 27, 28, 29
Abuse, of body, 33, 34, 134
Accident(s)
  C-section and, 488
  gloves unavailable, 493
  miscarriage and, 191
  premature labor and, 191
Acid neutralizers, 150, 175
Acidophilus, 183, 195, 431, 532
Acidosis, 368, 497
  diabetes and, 209, 210, 211
  silent, fetal deaths due to, 211
Acupressure. See Femoral pressure points, Foot therapy, Sacral pressure points.
Adhered placenta. See Placenta, adhered.
Adrenalin, 154
Affection
  birth of natural, 355
  needed to thrive, 433

Afterbirth, 71, 383. See also Placenta, Amnion.
  evaluating the, 382-86
Afterpains, 415-16
Age,
  of fetus, 107n
  screening, 83, 87
Agrimony, 177
Air embolism, 182, 317, 340n
Airola, Paavo, 14, 44n
Albert, Richard K., M.D., 495n
Albumin, 128, 197
Alcohol (Alcoholic drinks)
  C-sections and, 486
  depressant, 146
  Humphrey's Law of Conservation and, 292n
  screening, 86, 96, 97
Alcohol (Isopropyl or rubbing)
  in birth supplies, 220
  sterilizing agent, 220, 386n
Alfalfa, 150, 152, 198, 200, 219, 287, 483. See also LaVay's Pregnancy Tea.
  properties of, 150, 152, 198
Allergies, 86, 99, 423
Aloe vera, 169
Alternatives, arguments for birthing, 23
Aluminum pans, 149
Amaranth, 203, 505
Ambu bag, 227
American Hospital Association, 494
American Medical Association, 21
Amino acid metabolism, 430, 436
Amniocentesis, 114-15
Amnion (Amniotic membrane, Amniotic sac, "Bag of waters"), 68, 69, 70, 71-72, 73
  advantages of intact, 242, 253, 327
  over baby's face, 72, 327
  embryo outside, anecdote, 117
  examining after birth, 383, 384
  fluid within. See Amniotic fluid.
  mucous plug protects, 251
  protects against infection, 199, 253
  retained fragments, 361-63, 370

Amnion (cont.)
  retained fragments (cont.)
    false unicorn, 158, 362, 363
    ring forceps, 255
    turning placenta to prevent, 358
  rupture, 72, **242**, 251, 253, 319
    artificial, 52, 72, **225**, 327-29
      arguments against, 327
      hospital routine, 52
      indications for, 72, 327
      procedure, 327-29
      hand flushed out, 328
      place of rupture (high, low), 72, 199, 314, 315
    premature, 199-200
      amniocentesis and, 115
      healing of, 199-200
      with multiple births, 458-59
    prolonged, 52, 199, 253
    hyaline membrane disease and, 483
    umbilical cord flushed out, 200, 253, 314-15, 316, 319, 328. See also Umbilical cord, prolapsed.
Amniotic fluid, 68, 71-72, 169, 239, 253
  assists dilation, 239, **242**
  discoloration of, 300-301, 302. See also Meconium staining.
  excessive, 231. See Hydramnios.
  flow after membrane rupture (flush vs. dribble), 72, 199, 200, 253, 255, 314-15, 319-20, 328, 329
  pH, 72
  protects baby, 72, 199, **242**, 253, 327
  replaces itself, 71, 200
  sphingomyelin in, 346
  withdrawal of, 27, 114
Anaphylactic shock, 100
Anatomy, obstetrical, 59-75. See individual entries.
Anderson, Dr. Anne, 51
Anemia, 100, 175-77
  blood loss and, 118, 176
  borderline, 155

Anemia (cont.)
  checking for, 86, 109, 117, 118, 176
  cow's milk and, 423
  iron-deficiency, 100, 351
  nutritional deficiencies and, 118, 176, 197
  replenishing iron, 177. See also Iron, sources.
  sickle cell, 110
  stripping cord and, 351
Anencephaly, 469
Anesthesia, C-section, 484, 485
Anesthetics, 46, 332, 392-93
Angelica, 208
Animal flesh, amativeness and, 44n
Animal protein, 136, 428
Anteflected uterus, 66, 415, 474-76
Anterior (cervical) lip, 277, 298-99, 369
  Pitocin and, 291
  recurrence, 291, 298
  management, 298-99
Anterior positions. See Occiput, positions.
Anterior rotation, ROP position, 245. See also Rotation.
Antibodies
  Rh, 204-5, 436n
  screening, 109-10, 205-6
  ultrasound and, 112
Anti-D gamma globulin, 205
Antiseptic herbs. See Calendula, Goldenseal, Myrrh, White oak bark.
Antispasmodic tincture(s), 366-67, 386n, 529-30
Anus, 63
  imperforate, 402
  sphincter laceration, 330, 332, 390
Apgar score, 84, 305, 341, 342, 343, 344, 401
  determining, 342, 343
Appendicitis, 194
Appetites of the flesh, 34, 44
Apple pie, 145
Apple cider vinegar. See Vinegar.
Arching exercises, 159, 163
Arizona mother, twins anecdote, 112

Arm(s)
  Erb's paralysis, 472, 473
  maneuvering, breech presentation, 451, 452, 453, 455
  presentation, 19, 229, 461-63
    doctor asleep, anecdote, 462
    turning fetus, 445
Arnica tincture, 471, 531-32
Arrest, head. See Transverse head arrest.
Asbestos, respiratory stress and, 497
Aseptic technique, 288, 397, 491-95
Asparagus, 419
Aspiration
  meconium, 300
  olive oil, 333
  vacuum, abortion method, 27
  vitamin E, 346
Aspirin, 48-49, 436n
Association of Maternal Child Health, 112
Asthma, 99-100, 530
Astringent herbs. See Bayberry, Black walnut, Calendula, Comfrey, Juniper berry, Mullein, Nettle, Red raspberry, Sanicle, Shepherd's-purse, Squawvine, St. Johns-wort, Uva ursi, White oak bark, Yellow dock.
Asynclitism
  anterior, 235
  posterior, 235
Attendants, birth, 4, 9, 237-38, 250, 255, 265, 287, 290, 479
Auscultation
  in labor, 257-58, 320
  multiple pregnancy and, 126, 460
  with naked ear, 123
Authority
  harass, berate, intimidate, 6
Autoclave, 223, 493
Autonomic nervous system, 146, 387n

B

Baby. See Fetus, Newborn.
Back. See also Spinal defects, injuries.

Back (cont.)
 ache, 98, 174, 254
  in labor, 254, 266-68, 296
 adjustments, 268-71, 416
 exercises, 159, 162-63
 therapies
  inferior sacral acupressure, 295-96
  for respiration (thorax rub), 342, 344
  sacral pressure points, 266-68
  uterine reflex points (Neuro-Vascular Dynamics), 416, 417
Bacteria
 intestinal, 195, 429, 532
 introduced into vagina, 228, 253, 475, 492
 multiplication of, 121, 134, 491-92
 in urine, 121
Bag of waters. See Amnion.
Baking soda, shock solution, 503
Ballet dancer, inertia in, 287
Ballottement, 76, 77, 80
Baptist, John the, 146
Barberry, 171, 177, 526
Barley, 203, 505
Baths
 after membrane rupture, 253
 breech, vertex deliveries in, 272-73
 daily, 182
 for distressed infants, 348, 349
 effect on labor, 254-55, 272, 285
 hot, fainting and, 173
 sitz. See Sitz baths.
Bayberry, 156, 477, 525
 for bleeding, 151, 362, 376
 properties of, 158
Beach, Dr., 11, 16n
Bearing down
 in breech birth, 449, 450, 451, 454
 coaching, 325-26
 cord prolapse and, 319-20
 to deliver placenta, 357, 358
 hemorrhoids and, 100, 179, 340n
 mother cannot, if panting, 451. See also Panting.

Bearing down (cont.)
 pelvic build and, 90-91, 294, 325, 326
 premature, 262-63, 369, 450, 454
 therapies assist, 294
Beauty, from motherhood, 435
Bedrest
 premature membrane rupture, 200
 threatened miscarriage, 192, 193
Beef extracts, 287
Bendectin, 49
Bennett, Dr. Terrence, 436n
Betamethasone, 482
BF & C Ointment, 169, 422, 523
Bicarbonate of soda, 182
Bilirubin, 425, 426, 436n
Bimanual compression, 374, 379
Binding powers of heaven, 34
Binovular twins, 457
Biofeedback, 377, 387n
Biparietal diameter, 230, 239, 319-20
"Birth" (poem), xx
Birth(s)
 extraction. See Extraction delivery.
 precipitous. See Precipitous birth.
 premature. See Premature birth.
 previous, screening, 83, 90-94
 process of. See Labor.
  overview, 238-47
 struggle important, 484-85
Birth canal. See Cervix, Pelvis, Vagina, Vulva.
 anatomy, 59-64, 246
Birth certificate, 412
Birth control, 38-42
 anecdote, need a rest, 39
 contraceptives, 40, 85, 95-96
 methods using restraint, 39-42
 nursing and, 42
Birth defects, 467-70. See also specific abnormalities.
 diabetes and, 209
 drugs and, 48, 49, 50, 96, 100, 467, 468
 encountering, 467
 feeling of guilt and, 467
 newborn evaluation and, 409

Birth defects (cont.)
  screening, 87, 101
  testing for (amniocentesis),
    114, 115
  umbilical vessels and, 354
Birth injuries, 470-73. See
  also specific injuries.
Birthing bed, 216, 217, 256, 399
Birthing chair, 321
Birthing room, preparation of,
  256, 350, 494-95
Birthing supplies, 216-21
  midwife's kit, 221-27
  portable maternity kit, 214-16
Blackberry leaves, 202
Black cohosh, 154, 155, 530
Black walnut, 183, 431, 523
  tincture recipe, 525
Bladder, 62, 102, 104, 526-27
  anatomy, 37-38, 63, 64, 65
  catheterization, 65, 409
  control, exercise for, 161
  distended, newborn, 409
  infections. See Urinary
    tract, bladder infections.
  rupture, 64-65
Blanching of perineum, 331, 333
Blechschmidt, 25
Bleeding. See Hemorrhage.
Blessed (holy) thistle, 156,
  208, 219, 420, 522
Blessings, 7, 33, 346, 377, 387n
Blindness, 213, 408-9, 413
Block, Polly, xx, xxi, 15, 24n,
  29n, 55n
Blood
  anemia. See Anemia.
  building, 181, 207, 208, 382
  circulation. See Circulatory
    system.
  clots, 95, 112, 181, 193
    following birth, 371-72,
      373, 374, 377, 393
  loss. See Hemorrhage.
  pressure, 118-20, 499-500
    dangerous levels, 129, 368,
      500, 502
    high. See Hypertension.
    low, 154, 502
    monitoring
      in labor, 255, 257
      prenatal visits, 116, 117,
        118-20

Blood (cont.)
  norms, 119-20, 368, 411n,
    499
  toxemia and, 128, 129, 130,
    302, 305
  Rh, ABO incompatibility. See
    Hemolytic disease, Rh-
    negative factor.
  sugar, 120, 209, 210, 211,
    411n. See also Diabetes,
    Hypoglycemia.
  tests, 109-10. See also
    related topics.
  transfusions, 205, 206, 381,
    436n
  type (group), 84, 109, 381.
    See also Rh-negative
    factor.
Bloodroot, 208
"Blowout" lacerations, 92, 330,
  389
Blue cohosh, 156, 208, 226, 528
  for inertia, 285, 286
  properties of, 154, 157
Bonding, 30, 341, 355, 431-33,
  461, 484
Bony cage, Bony canal. See
  Pelvis.
Borage, 208
Bowel(s), 87, 100-01, 128, 134,
  135, 148, 158, 332. See
  also Constipation, Diarrhea.
Brachial plexus, 472
Bradycardia, 311
Braxton Hicks contractions,
  253-54, 266, 528
Breakfast plate menugraph, 139
Breasts. See also Breast-
  feeding.
  changes in pregnancy, 80, 168,
    169
  newborn, 71, 400
  stimulation, for hemorrhage
    control, 362, 376
Breast-feeding (lactation), 94,
  407, 417-23
  advantages of, 38, 94, 423
  afterpains and, 415, 416
  anecdote, roommate, 417-18
  as a contraceptive, 42
  cleft palate and, 468, 469
  diabetes and, 209, 210

Breast-feeding (cont.)
frequency, first few days, 407, 418
herbs for, 157, 419-20
hypoglycemia and, 407, 418, 484
increased appetite, 175
inverted nipples, 94
let-down reflex, 154, 421
lochia and, 415
mastitis, 421-22, 527
milk coming in, 168, 418, 427
milk drinking and, 145, 420
precluded, 422, 436n, 532
sexuality during, 35
sore nipples, 157, 168, 422
stimulates uterine contractions, 362, 376, 407, 415
substances to avoid, 418-19, 478
supplements during, 176, 178
supply problems, 419-20, 420-21
weaning, 423
Breathing. See also Respiration.
abdominal. See Abdominal breathing.
fetus, in utero, 340n
following birth. See Respiration, newborn.
in powders, infant, 425
Breech presentation, 229, 440-56, 461, 471
anecdotes
fasting father, 38
my first delivery, 446-48
not just luck, 443-44
C-section and, 443, 487
delivery management, 449-56, 471
designating position in, 232
diagnosing, 126, 231, 442
fetal loss and, 442
foot therapy and, 275, 276, 454
frequency, 440, 461
important points, 445-56, 448-49, 450, 453, 454, 455, 471
midwives can handle, 19, 443, 446, 471
types of, 229, 440, 441, 442
version. See Version, breech.

Brigham and Women's Hospital, 486
Brigham tea, 154
Bulb syringe
for suctioning the newborn, 215, 226, 342, 386n, 413
warnings, 182, 183, 226, 386n
Burdock, 177
Buttbones, 61, 62, 103. See Ischial tuberosities.
Byrd's Method of Resuscitation, 347, 348

C

Caffeine, 145
Calcium, 146, 174, 172, 483, 504
sources of, 150, 151, 152, 157, 203n
Calcium ascorbate, 152, 167n, 178, 189, 203n
Calef, Dr. Victor, 29n
Calendula, 213, 226, 475, 532
for bleeding, 371, 374, 375, 378
Callander, R., 16
Canada snakeroot. See Wild ginger.
Cancer, 96, 99, 107, 110, 146, 147, 423
Candida albicans, 431
Cankers, 157, 430-31
Canning recipes, 140, 520-21
Cannon, Walter B., 292n
Capsicum. See Cayenne.
Caput succedaneum, 470-71
Car, maternity kit for, 214
Carbonated drinks, 145
Carbon dioxide, 327, 497
Cardiac failure, 97, 98, 369
Cardiopulmonary resuscitation (CPR), 23, 346-47
Cardiovascular disease, 95-96
Carling, Ann, 55n
Carob, 504, 516-17, 532
properties of, 146
Cascara sagrada, 171, 419, 526
Cassette recordings, 256, 427
Castor oil, 329
Catheters, 222, 288, 318-19, 409
Catheterization
bladder, 65, 288, 409
of lochia, 474-76

Catnip, 151, 198, 202, 219
  with fennel, for colic, 419,
    427
  for threatened miscarriage,
    192, 193, 200
Cat's reflex, 408-9
Cayenne (Capsicum), 171, 172,
    180-81, 195, 201, 208, 226,
    278, 286, 312, 379, 522,
    525, 526, 529, 530
  for bleeding, 151, 187, 189,
    193, 305, 362, 371
  for hemorrhoids, 180, 340n
  in HVC, 291n, 503. See also
    HVC.
  properties of, 151
Celery leaves, 202
Cell salts, homeopathic, 303,
    382
Century, 177
Cephalhematomas, 470-71
Cephalic presentation, 229. See
    also Vertex presentation.
Cephalopelvic disproportionment,
    235-36, 486
Certified Nurse Midwives, 54
Cervix (also External os), 63,
    66-67, 365
  anterior lip. See Anterior
    lip.
  bleeding from, in early labor,
    186, 306-7
  cancer, 99
    Pap smear, 107
  damage to, from abortion,
    27-28
  dilation, 66-67, 252, 258, 259
    anecdote, not hurting, 261
    with breech birth, 449, 450
    foot therapy and, 291n
    full, 260-61, 284, 293
      bear down prior to, 262-
        63, 369
    lack of progress in, 264,
      284-85. See also
      Uterus, inertia.
    measuring, 259, 260, 263
    Polly-Jean formula and, 155
    precipitous birth and, 330
    prevented, 289, 290-91, 298-
      99, 311, 487
  effacement, 66, 258, 259, 260
    foot therapy and, 274

Cervix (cont.)
  erosion, incompetence, 89
  purse-string suture, 90
  external os, 66-67, 68, 365
    position in early labor,
      258, 260
  internal os, 67, 187, 188, 365
  laceration of, 263, 298-99,
    306, 307, 369, 371
  previous, foot therapy and,
    276
  lower uterine segment and,
    action in labor, 67, 365
  mucous plug, 251, 252
  pain at, ectopic pregnancy
    and, 190
  palpation in early pregnancy,
    77, 104
  prolapsed, anecdote, 480
  "reach to China," 258, 261
  rimming. See Rimming,
    cervical.
  softening, 79, 258, 261
  superficial rings, 260
Cesarean section, 92-93, 484-88
  anecdote, foreigner and, 484-
    85
  breech presentation and, 443,
    487
  diabetes and, 209, 211-12
  disadvantages, 484-85
  fetal heart monitors and, 113,
    114, 485
  hospital routine and, 52, 53,
    286, 291
  hyaline membrane disease and,
    483, 484
  incision, 84, 92, 484, 488
  indications for, 131, 187,
    188, 199, 209, 235, 286,
    306, 311, 460, 486-88
  vaginal birth after, 92-93,
    485-86
Chamomile, 201
Charcoal, 175
Chemotherapy, 99
Chestnuts from the fire, 61, 449
Chia seed, 202
Childbed fever, 361-62
  anecdote, 493
Childbirth. See Labor,
  Crowning, controlled and
  delivery.
Childbirth Without Fear, 16

540 POLLY'S BIRTH BOOK

Chills, 200-203, 502
Chinese saying, 184
Chiropractors, 416, 436n
Chocolate, 145-46, 504
Chorion, 69, 70, 327
Cinnamon, 525
Circulatory (Vascular) system, 70, 148, 160, 346, 481, 497-500. See also Blood.
  fetal, newborn, 46, 70, 311, 350, 352, 353
  transfusion syndrome, 458
  varicosities. See Hemorrhoids, Varicosities.
Circumcision, 423-24
The Clarion Cesarean Prevention, 486
Cleavers, 526
Clitoris, 64, 65, 371, 400
Cleft palate, lip, 402, 468-69
Cloves, 525, 528
Clubfooted infants, 313-14, 402
CMM Ointment, 532
Coaching, 280-82, 293
  eclampsic mother, 303
  pushing, bearing down, 325-26
Coccyx, 60, 61, 97, 106, 245, 309-10, 527
Cohen, Nancy Wainer, 15, 92, 131n, 132n
Coitus. See Intercourse.
Colby, Benjamin, 16
Colds, 202-3
Colic, 427-28
Colostrum, 168, 418, 427
Coma, 128, 197, 210, 211, 302
Comfrey, 150, 152, 200, 201, 203, 219, 287, 299, 398, 421, 477, 478, 523, 532
  properties of, 150, 177, 194
Common Sense Childbirth, 15
Complications, 5, 7, 24. See also specific conditions.
Composition powder, 286, 524-25
Conception
  age, of fetus, 107n
  estrogen and, 154
  Pill doesn't prevent, 40
  postpartum. See Birth control.
  sexuality changes after, 34-35
Conceptus, 68, 69, 70, 76-77, 89-90, 95, 117, 169, 193, See also Amnion, Amniotic

Conceptus (cont.)
  fluid, Chorion, Fetus, Placenta, Umbilical cord.
  implantation, 107n, 187, 189-90, 339n
Condie, Frances, M.S., 495n
Confessions of a Medical Heretic, 15, 55n, 107n
Congressman, anecdote, 21, 22
Constipation, 100-101, 135, 171-72, 195-96
  infant, 428-29, 532
  preventing, treating, 100-101, 171-72, 180, 195, 330, 478
Constriction ring. See Uterus, retraction ring.
Contaminants, food, 136, 207
Contraception. See Birth control.
Contractions. See Labor.
Controlled crowning. See Crowning, controlled.
Controlled substances, 18, 391
Convulsions, 100, 128, 301, 302, 303, 304-5, 386
Cord. See Umbilical cord.
Coriander, 208
Corn silk, 526
Corpus, 66, 67. See also Uterus.
Cortin, 154
Cortisol, 51
Cortisone, 468
Couch grass, 519, 526
Cough, 202, 203, 530
  to separate placenta, 360
CPR. See Cardiopulmonary Resuscitation.
Cradle cap, 404
Cramp bark, 522, 528
Cramps, 66
  herbs to relieve, 150-51, 158, 522-23, 530
Crowning, 238, 244, 246, 309, 332-34
  controlled, and delivery, 332-39
  episiotomies and, 46, 331-32
  techniques
    anal push, 334, 336
    perineal press, 334, 337
    preventing premature extension, 334, 336

Crowning (cont.)
 therapies to assist stretching, 325, 377
 antenatal, 228-29, 329. See also Exercises, prenatal, Sitz baths.
 peripacs, 273, 297, 299
 rimming, 297, 333
C-section. See Cesarean section.
Curve of Carus, 246
Cyanosis, 212, 302, 312, 335, 468, 497, 531
 preventive supplementation, 151-53
 vitamin E for, 346
Cysts, vaginal exam, 106

D

D & C. See Dilation and curettage.
Dairy products, 145
Dandelion, 478
 properties of, 150, 177
Danger signals, 185
Davis, Adelle, 15, 436n
Decidua, 68, 69, 117
Deer tallow, 174
Deficiencies, nutritional, 175-78
Deformities. See Birth defects.
Dehydration, 171, 196, 429
DeLee suctioning device, 342, 475
Delivery. See Labor, Crowning, controlled and delivery.
 of placenta. See Placenta, separation.
Demerol, 47, 53
Dentist, 13
Depressants, 146. See also Drugs.
Depression, 47, 96, 350, 484
DES (diethylstilbestrol), 49, 112
Descent, 238, 239, 245
Deseret News, 436n
Diabetes, gestational, 211
Diabetes mellitus, 208-11
 hyaline membrane disease and, 483

Diabetes mellitus (cont.)
 mortality, 88, 89, 209, 210, 211
 screening for, 86, 93, 98, 211
Diaper rash, 430-31, 532
Diarrhea, 157, 172, 180, 429
Diastolic pressure, 118, 119, 500
Diethylstilbestrol, 49, 112
Digestion, 149, 151, 157, 171, 198
Dilation and curettage, 27-28, 85, 95, 361
Dilation
 cervical. See Cervix, dilation.
 perineal. See Crowning.
Dill, 420
Dinner plate menugraph, 139
"Dipsticks," 120
"Dirty" Duncan placental separation, 385, 386
Disaster, 5, 23, 493
Disease, 70, 135
 screening for, 86, 97-101
Disinfectant, 216, 221, 399. See also Germicidal solution.
Diuretic, 157, 195
Dizziness, 382
Doppler equipment, 79, 113, 114, 123
Douches, 182, 183, 475, 476
Down's syndrome, 114, 409, 469
Dreams, 42, 387n
Drive angle in labor, 262, 263
Drugs, Medication, 45-55. See also Aspirin, Bendectin, Betamethasone, Cortisone, Demerol, DES (diethylstilbestrol), Ergonovine, Morphine, the Pill, Pitocin, Thalidomide, Thiouracil, Xylocaine.
 alternatives to, 45-46, 54-55, 55n
 average use, in pregnancy, 48
 breast-feeding and, 418-19
 C-section and, 46, 53, 484, 485, 486
 effects on fetus, 46-47, 48, 49, 436n, 443, 484. See also Birth defects.
 anecdote, 50

Drugs (cont.)
  home birth mothers don't ask for, 55n
  inducing labor, hospital routine, 52-54. See also Labor, inducing.
  laws about, 18, 391
  local anesthetics, 46, 332, 392-93
  marijuana, 147-48
  miscarriage and, 89
  multiple births and, 458
  parents want birth without, 4
  reference books, 16, 50
  screening, 14, 83, 84, 85, 86, 90, 91, 95-96, 98, 99, 100, 121
  stimulants, depressants, 146
Due date, 52, 81-82, 87, 443
  Naegele's rule, 81
Dystocia, 288, 439

E

Echinacea, 201, 363
Eclampsia (severe toxemia), 121, 127-31, 301-5. See also Pre-eclampsia.
  C-section and, 487
  management of, 303-5
  signs, stages, 302
  whether to transport, 301
Ectopic pregnancy, 114, 189-90
Edema, 41, 185, 195-96, 288, 470-71
  toxemia and, 122, 128, 129, 130, 185, 195
Effacement. See Cervix, effacement.
Electrolytes, 72, 382, 429
Eliminative systems, 133-34
Eloesser, Leo, 15
Els, Jan, 48
Embryo, 74-75
Emergency
  birthing kit, for car, 214-16
  divine help with, 6, 449
  equipment, 7, 192
  preparedness, 12, 23, 225, 391
  rooms, notorious for delays, 381
Emergency medical teams, 6
Endocrine system, 134, 209, 210

Endocrine test, 78, 80, 126
Enema(s), 194, 208, 261, 288
  herbs for, 157, 176, 195, 198, 287, 525-26
Engagement, 238, 239, 261
  determining, 233-36
Ensign, 29n, 44n
Epilepsy, 86, 100
Episiotomy, 64, 224, 330-32, 391
  first baby without, 12
  local anesthetic, 46, 332
  scars, 92, 276
  stitched too tightly, 30
Epsom salts, 419
Erb's Paralysis, Erb's Palsy, 472-73
Ergonovine, 366
Ergot, 364, 377, 386n-87n
The Essential Guide to Prescription Drugs, 16
Estner, Lois J., 15, 92, 131n, 132n
Estrogen, 41, 70-71, 154, 155
Eternal perspective, 34, 42-44
Everywoman's Book, 14, 44n
Examinations
  prenatal, 116-32
  vaginal, 76-77, 102, 103, 104-7, 125
Exercises
  postnatal, 433-34
  prenatal, 158-64
Ex-lax, 419
Expulsion, 238, 247, 335, 338-39
Extension, 238, 244, 245, 246, 464, 465
  preventing premature, 334, 336
External os. See Cervix.
External rotation. See Rotation, external.
Extraction delivery, 53, 84, 92, 286, 442
Eyes
  newborn
    examining, 408-9
    mother's milk in, for inflammation, 410n
    silver nitrate, Argyrol in, 213, 226, 406, 410n-11n, 413
  tubal pregnancy symptom, 190
  visual disturbances, 185, 195-96, 302

F

Face presentation, 239, 461, 463-66
  anecdote, 465-66
  chin designates position, 232
  edema with, 407, 465, 466
  palpating, 439, 465
Fads, 8, 153
Fainting, 173
Faith, 5, 6, 304
Fallopian tubes, 66, 67, 190
False labor. See Labor, false.
False unicorn, 156, 226, 522
  properties of, 158
  for retained placenta, fragments, 158, 359, 362, 363
  for threatened miscarriage, 192, 193
Family planning. See Birth control.
Fatigue, 80, 173, 457. See also Tiredness.
  in labor. See Labor, conserving energy in.
  persistent, 153
Feeling beautiful because you are, 435
Female reproductive organs. See Reproductive organs, female.
Femoral pressure points, 265-66, 445
Fennel, 219, 419
  properties of, 151, 427-28
Fenugreek, 177
Fertility pills, 87, 101, 460-61
Fetal heart monitors, 53, 113, 114, 132n, 485
Fetalscope, 79, 221
Fetus
  abnormalities, malformations, 96, 114, 115, 117, 178, 192, 212, 457. See also Birth defects, specific conditions.
    ultrasound anecdote, 111-12
  circulatory system. See Circulatory system, fetal.
  death in utero, 117, 126-27, 488. See also Abortion, Stillbirth, specific conditions (Diabetes, Ectopic pregnancy, Venereal disease, etc.).

Fetus (cont.)
  development of, 73-74, 78, 123, **124**
  drugs and. See Drugs, effect on fetus.
  head, 230
    arrest, in labor. See Transverse head arrest.
    delivery. See Crowning, controlled.
    descent. See Descent.
    disproportionment. See Cephalopelvic disproportionment.
    engagement. See Engagement.
    extension. See Extension.
    external rotation. See Restitution.
    flexion. See Flexion.
    internal rotation. See Rotation, internal.
    molding, 59-60, 299, 308, 330, 339n
  heart rate, heart tones (FHR, FHT), 79, 123, 125, 257-58
    bearing down and, 325-26
    death in utero and, 127
    location, **124**, 231, 232, 442
    multiple pregnancy and, 126, 460
    stress and, 297-98, 311-13
    knows when to be born, 51
  lightening, 82, 123, 175, 239
  nutrition. See Nutrition, fetal.
  position, presentation, 229, 231-33. See also specific presentations.
  quickening, 80, 81-82
Fever, 100, 134, 194, 202, 203n, 361-62, 476
Fillmore, Utah, 55
First aid, 23, 201, 225, 331, 391, 501
Five-week formula. See Polly-Jean Five-Week Antenatal Formula.
Flaxseed, 171-72, 330, 505, 523
Flexion, 229, 238, 239, **464**
  assisting, 294, 308-9, 334, 337, 463
  in breech delivery, 454
  face presentation and, 463, **464, 465**

Flexion (cont.)
  transverse head arrest and, 307-9, 464
Folic acid, 152, 175, 176, 178, 457
Fontanels, 230, 252
  newborn evaluation, 408
  palpating, 294, 308, 440, 463
Food
  additives, 136, 207
  in Good Program, 133-49, 504-21
  testing, for digestive stress, 144
Footling presentation, 229, 441, 442. See also Breech presentation.
Foot therapy, 202, 288
  in breech birth, 275, 454
  with eclampsic convulsion, 304
  uterine reflex, 273-77, 291n
Forceps
  abortion technique and, 27
  midwife's instruments, 224, 352, 393, 493
    Allis, 225
    Kelly hemostatic, 223, 224
    Keyhole (ring), 224, 225, 366-67, 391
    Rochester-Pean hemostats, 223
    suturing (needle holder), 225, 391, 393
    thumb (tissue), 226
  obstetric
    extraction delivery. See Extraction delivery.
    fetal loss due to, 442
Foreskin, 423-24
Forewaters, assist dilation, 252
Formaldehyde, 144
Fourth stage of parturition, 388-411
Freezer jams, jellies, 520-21
Fruit
  Good Program, 136, 139, 140, 143, 145
  recipes, 140, 507-10, 521
Fundal height, 66, 82, 123, 124
  multiple pregnancy and, 125
Fundal lift, 356, 357

Fundus, 66, 67, 123, 124. See also Uterus.
  apply pressure to, in breech delivery, 454
  height. See Fundal height.
  kneading, 388-89
  hemorrhage control and, 372, 373, 377, 378, 380, 388-89
  improper, 357, 366, 370
  placenta delivery and. See Placenta, separation.
  prolapse, inversion. See Uterus, prolapsed, inverted.
Funis. See Umbilical cord.

G

Gag response, 408
Galt, Edith J., 15
Garrey, Matthew M., 16
Garlic, 172, 183, 195, 525-26
  properties of, 194, 201
Genitalia, 64, 65, 400, 402
Germicidal solution, 213, 215, 223, 493, 494
Gestation, 176
  length of, 81-82, 107n, 123, 124
  stewardship, 43
Gestational diabetes, 98, 120
Ginger, 158, 171, 183, 202, 226, 522, 523, 525, 526. See also Wild Ginger.
  in baths, 228-29, 329, 476, 527
Ginseng, 154, 415, 478
Girdle, 433
Gloves, 213, 221, 492, 493
Glucose, 72, 120, 211, 411n
Glucosuria, 120
Glycogen, 209
Goldenseal, 171, 183, 425, 523
  properties of, 194, 201, 208, 363
Gonorrhea, 212
  blindness and, 213, 409, 413
Good Program, 90, 133-67, 457
  recipe ideas for, 504-21
Gordon, Dr. Hymie, 25

Govan, A. D. T., 16
Grains, 141, 505-6
Grand multipara, 19
 inertia and, 287
 no longer felt pregnant,
  anecdote, 116-17
Gravel root, 523
Great American diet, 87
Green drink, 518-20

H

Haire, Doris, 112
Hand scrubs, 104, 213, 228, 258,
 429, 491-92, 494
 scrub supplies, 221
"Happiness in me," 184
Harmful substances, 96-97. See
 also Drugs.
Hawthorn berries, 202, 208
Hazell, Lester D., 15
Headaches, 96, 100, 134, 302
 severe, continuous, 185, 195-96
Head arrest. See Transverse
 head arrest.
Heartburn, 175
Heart disease, disorders, 86,
 96, 97-98, 369
Heart rate
 fetal. See Fetus, heart rate.
 maternal. See Pulse rate.
Heat loss, 350, 502
Heavenly Father, 75, 446
Hellman, Louis M., 16, 213n
Hematocrit, 109, 338
Hematoma, 470-71, 531-32
Hemingway, Isabel, 15
Hemoglobin, 468
Hemoglobinometers, 118
Hemolytic disease, 114, 205-6,
 426, 436n
Hemorrhage, 367-82
 anemia and, 100, 176. See
  also Anemia.
 avoiding, 375-76
  points to memorize, 369-70
  Polly-Jean formula and, 155-56
 causes, kinds of postpartum
  bleeding, 370-73

Hemorrhage (cont.)
 from lacerations, 306, 371-72, 373-74, 390. See
  also specific types,
  Lacerations, Suturing.
 placenta/uterine related,
  372-73, 374, 480. See
  also Fundus, kneading,
  Placenta, abruptio, adhered, previa, retained,
  second, separation,
  trapped.
 controlling. See also
  specific complications.
  points to memorize, 375-80
 from hemorrhoids, varicosities, 100, 179
 herbs for, 154, 158, 371, 374,
  376, 378-79, 415. See
  also specific situations.
 in first, second stage, 186,
  305-7
 individual tolerance levels,
  367-68, 369, 382
 internal (obscured), 118, 190,
  372, 386n, 498-99
 miscarriage and, 127, 186,
  191, 488. See also
  Abortion, spontaneous.
 postpartum, 413-14
 shock, 367-69. See also
  Shock.
 transporting, 368, 381. See
  also specific conditions.
 treatment following, 381-82
 umbilical clamping and, 352,
  459
Hemorrhoids, 178-81, 340n
 bearing down and, 100, 179,
  340n
 bleeding from, 100, 176, 179
Hemostats, 179, 223, 224, 352,
 393, 493
Hepatitis, 90, 110, 422
Herbal preparations (Appendix
 D), 522-32
Herbally Yours, 16
Herbs, 54, 149, 501. See also
 specific herbs, conditions.
 act slower, but sustain
  longer, 376
 anecdote, Ann Carling, Joseph
  Smith, 55n

Herbs (cont.)
  Certified Nurse Midwives not trained to use, 54
  harassment laws about, 18
  parents desire, in home birth, 4, 19
  with penicillinlike properties, 150, 194
  preparation of, 149
  in emergencies, 362, 363
Heredity, 400
  multiple birth and, 87, 457, 460-61
Hernia, umbilical, 430
Hesperidin complex, 88, 191, 203n
Hexachlorophene, 492
Hip dislocation, 409-10
Hochberger, Dr. Richard C., 423, 436n
Hodge, C., 16
Holy thistle. See Blessed thistle.
Home birth
  advantages, 6, 8, 12, 20-21, 45, 54-55, 55n, 151, 236-38, 255, 261, 418, 483
  here to stay, 23
  hyaline membrane disease and, 151, 483
  legislation, 17-24
  parents entitled to competent help, 4
  preparation necessary, 4, 5, 6, 216-21, 494
  reference books, 14-16
  safety, 3-4, 5-6, 20-21
  supplies, 214-27
Home nursing file, 8, 201
Homeopathic cell salts, 303, 382
Honey, 140, 145, 504
  in HVC, 291n, 503. See also HVC.
Hops, 154
Horizontal lie. See Transverse lie.
Hormone(s), 70-71, 88, 142-43, 153-55, 170, 171, 210. See also Estrogen, Oxytocin, Progesterone.
  endocrine tests for pregnancy, 78, 80
  herbs for, 154
  triggering labor, 51, 91, 236

Hospital, 5, 20, 448
  childbirth "routine," 46, 47, 52-54, 285-86
  delays, 3, 381
  hand-washing, infections, 491-92, 494
  anecdote, 493
  home birth safer than, for low risk mothers, 6
  support systems needed. See Transporting, specific conditions.
Hound's-tongue, 203
How to Raise a Healthy Child... In Spite of Your Doctor, 15, 203n
Huckleberry, 177
Hugging, "formula," 433
Humphrey's Law of Conservation, 292n
Husbands
  approach wife on mental level, 31
  as coach, 280
  a word to, 34-37
  should be with wife during childbirth, 10-11
  tell this to, 39
HVC, 215, 226, 291n, 503
  for bleeding, shock, 189, 190, 286, 291n, 375, 382, 503
  for energy, 291n
Hyaline membrane disease (Respiratory distress syndrome, RDS), 151, 481-83, 484
Hydramnios, 209, 211, 235, 487
Hydrangea, 526
Hydrocephalus, 235
Hydrogen peroxide, 425
Hydrotherapy, 8, 54, 272-73, 297, 367, 527-28. See also Baths, Peripacs, Sitz baths.
Hyperbilirubinemia, 205, 386n, 436n. See also Jaundice.
Hypertension (high blood pressure), 95, 129, 157, 196, 500. See also Blood pressure.
  screening, 86, 94, 98, 120
Hypoglycemia, 139, 154, 175, 207, 210
  delay in feeding newborn and, 407, 411n, 418, 484
Hypothyroidism, 89, 419

Hysterectomy, 187
Hysterotomy, 27

I

Ice
  for hemorrhage, 193, 203n, 219, 375-76
  suturing and, 393
Idaho Midwifery Council, 21, 22
Idaho State University, 48
Ilium, 60, 61, 275. See also Pelvis.
Implantation. See Conceptus, implantation.
Imperforate anus, 402
Induction of labor. See Labor, inducing.
Infection. See specific types.
Inferior sacral acupressure, 295-96, 299
Inferior symphysis pubis touch, 295, 299
Inferior vena cava, 173
Ingals, A. Joy, 15, 410n
Injuries, birth. See Birth injuries.
Innominate bones, 60, 61. See also Pelvis.
Instituto Indigenista Interamericano, 15, 23
Instruments, midwife's, 221-26, 227. See also Forceps, Sterilization.
Insulin, 154, 209
Intercourse. See also Marriage
  act.
  abstention, 33
  anecdotes, 34, 38, 39
  birth control, 39-42
  can be binding experience, 40
  postpartum, 414
  cause of miscarriage, 37-38, 89, 186
  men fulfilled more quickly, 43
  painful, with ectopic pregnancy, 190
  during pregnancy, 37-38
  taboo in some cultures, 37
  premature membrane rupture and, 199

Intercourse (cont.)
  prolapsed uterus and, 476, 480
  routine, 32
Intermountain area, 17
Internal os. See Cervix, internal os.
Internal rotation. See Rotation, internal.
Interracial marriage, 110, 235
Intuition (Intuitiveness)
  midwife's, 17-18, 129, 449
  woman's, mother's, 78, 116, 323, 428-29
  anecdote, 116-17
Inverted uterus. See Uterus, inverted.
Involution, 414
Irish moss, 177
Iron
  in cord blood, 351
  deficiency, 170, 175-77. See also Anemia.
  excesses of, 177
  fetal needs, 100, 176, 351
  maternal needs, 100, 109, 170, 176
  supplements, 153, 176
  sources, 146, 150, 153, 157, 177
  vitamin C needed with, 176, 178
Iron orotate, 153
Ischium, 60, 61. See also Pelvis.
  ischial spines, 60, 61, 62, 105
  zero station and, 62, 239, 243. See also Stations of progress, Zero station.
  ischial tuberosities, 60, 61, 62, 102, 103, 246-47
Isthmus, 66, 67, 364, 365. See also Uterus.
Itching, 169, 182, 397, 474
IUD, 40, 85, 95

J

Japan, women in labor, 281
Jaundice, 206, 425-26, 436n
  treatment, 419, 425-26
  vomiting and, 197, 199

548 POLLY'S BIRTH BOOK

Jewelweed, 398
Johnson, Jeanne, 155
Johnson, Deloy, 321, 340n
Juniper berries, 131, 194-95

K

KAL, 153
Kegels, 161, 434
Kidneys, 70, 134, 177
  disease, 86, 89, 98
  edema and, 122, 195
  herbs for, 131, 194-95, 526-27
  toxemia and, 98, 122, 128, 197
Kimball, President Spencer W., 30, 44n
Kit
  midwife's, 221-27
  portable maternity, 214-16
Kneading fundus. See Fundus, kneading.
Knee bends, 159, 323
Kneecap test, 130
Knee-chest position
  anteflected uterus and, 474-75
  arm presentation and, 462-63
  knee presentation and, 450
  prolapsed cord and, 253, 315-16, 317, 320, 340n
  prolapsed uterus and, 477-78
Kneeling, delivery position, 322
Knee presentation, 441, 442, 450. See also Breech birth.
Knots
  umbilical. See Umbilical cord, knots.
  suture, 394, 396
Kochia, 177

L

Labor
  anticipating, preventing, correcting problems in, 297-320, 360-67
  coaching. See Coaching.
  conserving energy in, 278-79, 280-82, 285, 286-87, 292n, 300
  contractions, 239, 253-54, 257, 262, 278-79, 280-82,

Labor (cont.)
  283-84, 321. See also Bearing down, Cervix, dilation.
  Braxton Hicks, 253-54, 266, 528
  directional force of, 242
  effect of position on, 262, 263, 321
  relieving discomfort of. See Labor, therapies to assist.
  resting between, 278-79
  timing, 257
  dilation, effacement. See Cervix, dilation, effacement.
  duration of, 90-91, 236, 261, 262, 263, 299, 325
  every birth different, unique, 283
  excessive bleeding. See Hemorrhage.
  expulsion of baby, placenta. See Crowning, controlled, Placenta, separation.
  false, true, 251, 253-55, 256
  first stage, 251-92
  "fourth" stage, 388-411
  inducing, 51-54. See also Pitocin.
  maternal position in, 262, 263, 321-24
  mechanism of, 238-47. See also Descent, Flexion, Engagement, Rotation, internal, external, Expulsion.
  membrane rupture and. See Amnion, rupture.
  preliminaries (first stage), 255-64
  progression of, 283-84
    lack of progress, 264, 284-85
    obstructions, 11, 91, 184, 261, 266, 282, 288-91, 298-300, 307-10, 311, 387n, 487
    stations of progress, 239, 243
  pushing, 324-26. See also Bearing down.

Labor (cont.)
  second stage, 293-340
  signs of, 251, 253-55
  slow, "poky," 250, 264, 284, 285
  therapies to assist, 264-82, 294-97
  third stage, 341-87
  transition, 284, 293-94
  when to call the midwife, 251
Labor log, 256-57, 411n
Lacerations, 389-90
  awareness of, 321, 329-30, 333
  bearing down cautions, 262-63, 326, 339n, 369
  bleeding from. See Hemorrhage, Suturing.
  "blowout," 92, 330, 389
  cervical, uterine, vaginal. See Cervix, Uterus, Vagina, laceration of.
  episiotomy and, 330-32
  pericare, 397-98
  precipitous birth and, 330, 371
  preventing. See Crowning, controlled, therapies to assist stretching.
  previous
    foot therapy and, 276
    screening, 84, 92
  unhealthy vaginal floors and, 62, 329
Lactation. See Breast-feeding.
La Leche League, 420
Landmarks, 258, 439-40
LaVay's Pregnancy Tea, 150, 152, 174, 192, 193
Laws, 17, 29n, 110, 391, 412-13. See also Legislation.
Laxatives, breast-feeding and, 419. See also LB formula.
LB formula, 171, 180, 195, 208, 478, 526
L.D.S. Church, 387n
L.D.S. Hospital, Rupert, Idaho, 321
Lecithin, 72, 152, 346, 482, 483
Lecithin-sphingomyelin ratio, 152, 346, 482, 483
Left occipital positions. See Occiput, positions.
Legal awareness, 9, 95, 192, 257

Leg cramps, 152, 174
Legislation, regarding midwifery, 17-24. See also Laws.
Legumes, 137, 141
Lemongrass, 202
Lemon juice, 130, 141, 202, 419, 426
Let-down reflex. See Breast-feeding.
Let's Have Healthy Children, 15, 436n
Leukorrhea, 106, 157, 182
Licorice, 154, 526
Lightening, 82, 123, 175, 239
Lilly, Eli, 48
Liver, 99, 112, 177, 178, 179
  herbs for, 150, 156. See also LB formula.
  infant, 47, 176, 425, 436n, 453. See also Jaundice.
  laceration of, 347, 471
LOA. See Occiput, positions.
Lobelia, 127, 156, 171, 183, 226, 477, 523, 526, 527, 528, 530
  properties of, 151, 157
  tincture, 174, 193, 198, 278
Lochia, 66, 387n, 389, 414-15
  drainage, anteflected uterus, 474-76
Lockjaw, 386n, 530
Longitudinal lie, 229
Long, James, W., M.D., 16
Lullaby of the Womb, 427
Lumbar roll. See Back, adjustments.
Lungs, 134, 179, 496-97, 498. See also Respiration.
  disease, screening, 86, 99, 100
  newborn, 352, 404, 481-82. See also Hyaline membrane disease.
  nicotine and, 146
Lymphatic system, 134, 179, 201

M

Magnesia phosphorica, 303
Magnesium, 146, 151, 157
Male Practice, 15, 50, 107n, 132n

Malpresentation, 19, 93, 289, 463, 464, 466, 487. See also specific presentations.
Manual for Suturing Knots, 391
Maple syrup, 144, 504, 507
Marijuana, 85, 147-48
Marriage act, 30-44. See also Intercourse.
  "anything not offensive," 32-34
  begetting major reason for, 32
  counsel by religious leaders, 30, 37, 38, 39
  frequency, 32
  instituted by God, 33
  levels of, 30, 32, 33, 44
  perversion of, 34
  restraint. See also Intercourse, abstention.
    during gestation, lactation, 37-38
    have you considered, anecdote, 39
  family planning, 33, 39-42
  from routine intercourse, 32
  sexual drives good, necessary, 30
  woman's sexual desires, 31, 32, 34-36
Marriage counseling, 33-34
Marriage vows, not license to use wives, 32
Marsh mallow, 183, 219, 422, 527
  properties of, 420
Mastitis, 421-22, 527
Maternal & Child Health Nursing, 15, 411n
Maternity kits. See Birthing supplies.
Mayo Clinic, 25
Meadowsweet, 177
Measles, 90. See also Rubella.
Mechanism of labor. See Labor, mechanism of.
Meconium, 168, 300
Meconium staining, 218, 300-301, 302, 363
Medication. See Drugs.
Medicine
  merry heart doeth good like a, 184
  practice of, 17, 331, 391
Melchizedek Priesthood, 387n

Membrane(s). See Amnion, Chorion.
Mendelsohn, Robert S., M.D., 15, 48, 49, 50, 55n, 95, 107n, 115, 132n, 203n
Menopause, 210
Menstruation, 66, 87, 102, 176, 210
  amenorrhea, 76, 80, 522
  due date and, 81, 107n
  herbs for, 522-23
Mexico
  midwivery training, 23
  sextuplets, anecdote, 456
Midring constriction. See Uterus, retraction ring.
"The Midwife," xxi
Midwife(ves), 3, 4-5, 6-11. See also specific situations.
  assistance of, with first baby, 12
  capable of screening, 19, 20
  Certified Nurse, 54
  definition, 3
  doctors should utilize, 23
  do preventive care not practiced by others, 21
  dreams, 387n
  go in pairs, 9
  help shape attitudes toward birth, 12
  how to choose, 13-14
  important role during labor, 255
  instills confidence in labor, 3, 8
  kit, 221-27
  knows limitations, 213
  life-saving resource, 23
  motto for, 7-8
  performs valuable service, 12, 213
  primary duty, 3
  reasons for becoming, 12-13
  successfully handle difficult situations, 19
  training, 4-5, 6-7, 17-18, 23-24
  uses natural methods, 45, 54
  a word to, 8-11
Midwifery
  compassionate service, 7-8

Midwifery (cont.)
 conference, Idaho State
 University, 48
 Council, Idaho, 21, 22
 legislation regarding, 17-24
 not used to perform abortions,
 28
 women and, 11-13, 17-18
Milk
 congestion from, 145, 420
 cow's, infants and, 423
 mother's. See Breast-feeding.
Milk of magnesia, 419
Millet, 141, 505
Mind over matter, 377, 387n
Minerals, 121, 170, 175, 179,
 379
Mineral water, 213, 398, 422,
 425, 478
Mint herbs, 151
Miscarriage. See Abortion,
 spontaneous.
Mistletoe, 226
 for bleeding, 338, 372, 375,
 376
 properties of, 151, 154, 208,
 366
 retained placenta and, 359,
 362-63
Molding, 59-60, 308, 330, 339n
Mongolism. See Down's syndrome.
Morning sickness, 49. See also
 Nausea, Vomiting.
Mortenson, Elda P., 55n
Motherwort, 156, 287
Motto for midwives, 7-8
Mt. Sinai Clinic, 29
Mucous plug, 251, 252
Mucus, suctioning. See
 Suctioning.
Mullein, 523, 527, 532
 properties of, 151, 177
Multiple birth, 101, 456-61
 delivery management, 458-60
 diagnosis of, 125-26
 screening, 87, 101, 456,
 460-61
 transverse lie in, 229, 461
 cord prolapse, 315, 458-59
 correcting, 289-90, 445,
 459-60
 triplets or more, 460-61
 anecdote, sextuplets, 456

Myles, Margaret F., 16
Myrrh, 183, 201, 425, 477, 530

N

Naegele's rule, 81, 87
Narrow birth canal. See Pelvis,
 build (narrow).
Nature, 115, 143, 195, 285, 308,
 335, 418
 corrects problems, 7, 250, 311
 expels nonviable fetus, 127,
 191, 488. See also
 Abortion, spontaneous.
 midwife assists, 7, 45, 199,
 311
 slow labors and, 250, 285
Nausea, 27, 100, 201, 278, 375,
 530. See also Vomiting.
 herbs for, 150, 157, 158, 198,
 291n
 pregnancy and, 49, 80, 171
 sign of shock, 502
Navel. See Umbilicus, Umbilical
 stump.
Neonatal deaths, 88, 94, 210
Nerves, 266, 342, 344, 397. See
 also Tension.
 herbs, supplements for, 148,
 152, 158, 197. See also
 Nervine herbs, Sitz baths.
 injury to (birth), 409, 472
 peristaltic, 195, 429
Nervine herbs, 151, 156, 157,
 158, 398, 427
Nettle, 151, 177
Neuro-Vascular Dynamics, reflex
 points, 416, 436n
Newborn
 birth defects. See Birth
 defects.
 birth injuries. See Birth
 injuries.
 bonding, 355, 431-33
 circumcision, 423-24
 cleaning, dressing following
 birth, 401-6
 establishing respiration, 342,
 344-47. See also Respiration, establishing,
 Suctioning.

Newborn (cont.)
  examining, evaluating, 401-2, 407, 408-10
    Apgar evaluation, 341, 342, 343, 344
    eye care following birth, 406, 413. See also Eyes, newborn.
  feeding, 407, 418, 419, 428, 532. See also Breast-feeding.
  heat loss, 350
  jaundice, 206, 419, 425-26, 436n
  measuring the, 401
  postpartum instructions, 408, 412-13
  sex organs, 71, 400, 402
  signs of prematurity, post-maturity
  suggestions for care and comfort of, 423-33. See also specific topics.
    colic, 427-28
    constipation, 428-29
    crying, 426
    diarrhea, 429
    mucus-cutting formulas, 531
    scalp care, 404, 405, 406
    sore bottom, 532
    swaddling, 402-3, 404
    swelling, head, 470-71, 531-32
    umbilical hernia, 430
    unusual odors, 429-30
    yeast infection, thrush, 430-31, 532
  umbilical stump, 352, 424-25
  vital signs, 408, 411n
  weighing the, 400
New England Journal of Medicine, 494, 495n
Newly-weds, anecdotes, 25-26, 34
Niacinamide, 183, 431
Nicotine, 146
Nipples, 168
  inverted, 94
  sore, 157, 422
Nose breathers, babies are, 407
Nourishment, during parturition, 285, 300, 369, 376
Nursing. See Breast-feeding.
Nutmeg, 372

Nutrition, 4, 8, 54, 78, 87, 133-49, 150-53, 179
  C-sections and, 486, 487
  fetal, 70, 72, 100, 176, 178, 313-14, 327, 386n
  multiple pregnancy and, 101, 457
Nuts, Good Program and, 139, 141, 143

O

Obstetrical texts, selected references, 16
Obstetrics Illustrated, 16
Obstruction of labor. See Labor, obstructions.
Occiput, 230, 232
  crowning, 334, 336, 337
  positions, 232, 233
  rotation, 244, 245. See also Rotation.
Odors, 240-41
  baby, unusual, 429-30
  lochia, 415, 474
  urine, 121-22
Olive oil, 157, 169, 221, 274, 349, 422, 492
  antenatal preparation with, 228, 329, 330
  for cleaning the baby, 218, 219, 401-2, 424
  for nourishment, 198
Ophthalmologist, 409
Ophthalmoscope, 227
Orange blossoms, 202
Organ transplants, 75
Osmosis, 70, 498
Otoscope, 227
Ovaries, 66, 67, 190
Overdue. See Due date, Post-maturity.
Overweight. See Weight, excessive.
Ovulation, 40-42, 67
Oxygenation, 157, 324
  vitamin E assists, 150, 152, 346
Oxygen unit, portable, 227
Oxytocin
  natural, 154, 376, 387n
  synthetic. See Pitocin.

Index 553

P

Palpation
  abdominal
    ballottement, 77
    cephalopelvic disproportion-
      ment, 235-36
    engagement, 234
    fetal position, 231-32, 258
    uterine, determining preg-
      nancy, 76-77
  vaginal. See Examinations,
    vaginal.
  warning against, with placenta
    previa, 188
Pancreas, 177
Panic, forbidden, 366, 447
Panting, 237, 325, 333, 334-35, 451
Papaya, 202
Pap smear, 107
Paralysis
  Erb's, 472-73
  facial, 409
Paramedics, 6, 305, 379, 381
Parsley, 177, 183, 423, 478
  properties of, 151, 177
Parturition. See Labor,
  Crowning, controlled and
  delivery, Placenta, separa-
  tion.
Passion flowers, 202
Passwater, Richard, Ph.D., 152, 167n
Pediatrician, 342, 343, 408, 413
Pelvic rocks, 159, 163, 164
  for labor dystocias, 308-9, 318, 320, 450, 463
Pelvic veins, 173
Pelvimetry, 97, 99, 103, 105
Pelvis
  anatomy, 59-62 (60, 61), 63, 243. See also individual parts.
  build
    assessment, 90-91, 97, 99, 102-6
    cephalopelvic disproportion-
      ment, 235-36, 486
    contracted, 235
    narrow, 90-91, 106, 266, 294, 299-300, 486
  cavity, 59, 60, 61, 63

Pelvis (cont.)
  engagement. See Engagement.
  expansion
    exercises, 159-61, 163-64
    labor therapies, 294-96, 322-23
    sitz baths. See Sitz baths.
  floor, 161, 244, 246, 308
  inlet, outlet, 59, 60, 61, 63, 243
Penis, 409, 423-24
Pennyroyal, 154, 155
Peppermint, 151, 175, 208
Pericare, 397-98
Perineal Press Technique, 334, 337
Peripacs, 180, 273, 297, 299
Perineum, 62, 63, 64
  blanching of, 331, 333
  compress, for hemorrhage control, 372, 376-77
  crowning. See Crowning.
  incision of. See Episiotomy.
  laceration of, 329-30, 371-72, 394, 395
  prevention, 325, 326. See also Crowning, controlled.
  "sweep," 64, 246, 297, 454
  therapies for stretching. See Crowning, therapies to assist stretching.
Periwinkle, 208
Petra Sukau, 511
Petroleum jelly, 113, 182, 429
Pharmacology in Nursing, 16
Phenylketonuria, 412, 436n
  PKU test, 412, 426
Phenylalanine, 412, 436n
PHisoHex, 221, 492
Phosphorus, 72, 150, 157
Physicians, Doctors, 9, 18, 20, 30, 110-11, 283, 387n, 444, 493
  choosing a, 13
  communicating with, 59
  consult with, 95, 118, 200
  convenience, inducing labor, C-section and, 46, 443, 485
  cooperate with midwives, 7, 23, 131n, 213, 448
  experiment, 153

Physicians (cont.)
  neglect hand scrubs, 494
  referral to, 106, 188, 189,
    213, 305, 413, 414
  respect for, 7, 12
  unthinking practitioners, 50,
    455
Physicians Desk Reference, 16
Pill, the, 40, 95-96, 154
Pineapple juice, 202
Pine bark, 525
Pitocin, 372, 375, 376
  anterior lip and, 291
  inducing, controlling labor
    with, 47, 51, 52, 199,
    285-86
  uterine lacerations, rupture
    from, 291, 487
Pituitary (gland), 52, 210
  reflex, 275, 454
  swelling, headaches from,
    195-96
PKU. See Phenylketonuria.
Placenta, 69, 70-71, 169, 327
  abruptio, 186-87, 305-6, 487
    management, 187, 305-6
    types of, 186-87, 306
  adhered, 367, 381
    management, 375, 379, 381
    inverted uterus and, 479
  anecdotes
    healthy, 387n
    nine-pound, 361
  circulation, 70, 242
  "Dirty" Duncan presentation,
    385, 386
  effect of harmful substances
    and, 46, 89, 96, 382
  examining (evaluating), 372,
    382-86
  healthy, 373, 383, 387n
  implantation. See also
    Conceptus, implantation.
    breech presentation and, 442
    cord length needed and, 339n
    miscarriage and, 191
    placenta previa and, 187,
    188
  insufficiency, 51, 96
  multiple birth and, 357,
    358-59, 457, 458, 459
  previa, 187-89, 487
    marginal, 187-88

Placenta (cont.)
  previa (cont.)
    multiple birth and, 457,
      458, 459
    proper, 188-89
    warning, 188, 189
  retained, 158, 360-63, 364,
    367, 368, 378
    fragments, 361-62, 368, 370,
      372, 373, 414
    infection and, 361-62, 363
    management, 361-62, 373
    management, 360-61, 362,
      367, 373, 374
    second placenta, 359
    reflex (foot therapy), 277
    second, 358-59, 384
    separation, 71, 355-67, 370
      blood loss, 357, 387n
      excessive. See Hemor-
        rhage.
    Polly-Jean formula and,
      155-56
    delay, cord pulsation and,
      350
    delivery management, 355-58
      precautions (kneading
        fundus, pulling), 357,
        361, 364, 366, 370,
        373
      inverted uterus and, 334,
        361, 479-80
    determining, 357-58, 373
    manual (retained portions),
      360-61, 362, 367, 373,
      378
    nursing helps with, 350
    premature, 88, 312, 384
    abruptio placenta. See
      Placenta, abruptio.
    from stress on cord,
      placenta, 312, 334,
      361, 370, 373
  retained portions. See
    Placenta, retained,
    adhered.
  shared (twins), 459
  "Shiny" Schultze presentation,
    385, 386
  souffle (uterine sound), 445
  trapped, midring constriction,
    364, 366-67. See also
    Uterus, retraction ring.

Plantain, 533
  for hemorrhage, 362, 376
Podalic version. See Version.
Pokeroot, 422
Poky birth, 237-38, 250
Polio, 99
Polly-Jean Five-Week Antenatal
  Formula, 155-58, 219
  advantages of, 54, 90, 127,
    155-58, 261, 287, 356,
    387n
Poly-Sitz, 165
Poplar bark, 525
Poppy seeds, 177
Positions, of fetus. See also
  specific presentations.
  determining, 229, 231-32
  occipital, 232, 233
Positions in parturition. See
  Labor, maternal position
  during.
Posterior occipital positions,
  232, 233
  back ache in labor, 254
  rotation with, 244, 245, 307-8
Posterior presentation, 307-8,
  339n, 371, 465
Postmaturity, 51, 94, 400
Postnatal exercises, 433-34
Postpartum instructions, 412-14
Posture, during pregnancy, 174,
  268
Potassium, 142, 150, 151, 157,
  195, 382
Poultice, 398, 421-22
Precipitous birth, 330, 371, 479
  Polly-Jean formula and, 155
Pre-eclampsia (toxemia), 88,
  117, 127-31, 363, 487. See
  also Eclampsia.
  diabetes and, 208, 211
  preventive care, 100, 120,
    130-31, 305
  signs of, 120, 121, 122, 128-
    30, 195, 196, 301, 302
Pregnancy
  ascertaining, 76-80
  celestial state, 37
  danger signs during, 185,
    186-203
  deficiencies in, 175-78
  due date, calculating, 81-82.
    See also Due date.
  hygiene, 182, 495

Pregnancy (cont.)
  interval between, 38-39, 90,
    487
  medication during. See Drugs.
  multiple. See Multipe birth.
  physical changes, complaints,
    168-83
  prenatal care. See Prenatal
    care.
  preventive supplementation,
    151-53
  psyche, 183-84
  sexuality during, 34-37
  surgery during, 194
  weight, mother's. See Weight.
Pregnancy, Childbirth and the
  Newborn: A Manual for Rural
  Midwives, 15
Pregnancy Tea, 193. See also
  LaVay's Pregnancy Tea.
Premature birth. See
  Prematurity.
Premature membrane rupture. See
  Amnion, rupture (premature).
Prematurity, 51, 94, 400
Prenatal care, 108, 116-31. See
  also Screening, home birth
  feasibility.
  essential, 116, 117
  examinations, 116, 117-31
  frequency, 117
  preventive, 21, 151, 369, 483,
    486
  records, 18, 117, 257, 411n,
    500-501
  tests, 108-15
Prenatal exercises, 158-64, 229
Prepping, 261
Presentation, of fetus, 229.
  See also Vertex presentation, Position, specific
  presentations.
  incidence of various, 461
  uncommon, 461-66. See also
    specific presentations.
Pressure points. See specific
  therapies.
Priesthood blessing, 377, 387n
Primigravida, 420, 457, 487
  breech presentation in, 229,
    442
  contractions, recognizing, 253
  dilation of, 261
  engagement, 233, 253, 294

556 POLLY'S BIRTH BOOK

Pritchard, Jack A., 16, 213n
Progesterone, 70-71, 154, 191, 415
Projection, of infant, 334
Prolapsed cord. See Umbilical cord, prolapsed.
Prolapsed uterus. See Uterus, prolapsed.
Proteinuria. See Urine, protein in.
Protein, 138, 175, 177-78
Psyche, 183-84
Psychophysiological intervention, 387n
Pubic arch, 60. See also Pelvis.
Pubis bone, 60. See also Pelvis.
Pubis, symphysis. See Symphysis pubis.
Puerpera, 391
Puerperal infection, 361-62
Pulsatilla, 528
Pulse (heart) rate, 368, 497-99, 502
 blood loss and, 368, 369
 internal (obscured), 118, 190, 372, 386n, 498-99
 fetal. See Fetus, heart rate.
 norms, 368, 411n, 499
Purslane, 203
Pushing (labor), 324-26. See also Bearing down.

Q

Quassia, 177
Quickening, 80, 81-82
Quotient, midwife's prediction, 324

R

Radcliffe, John, Hospital, 51
RDS (Respiratory distress syndrome). See Hyaline membrane disease.
Read, Grantly Dick, 16, 282
Recipes, Good Program, 504-21
 Apple Topping, 506
 Avocado Dip, 516
 Baked Soybeans, 511-12

Recipes (cont.)
 Basic Green Drink, 518
 Candy Bars, 517
 Carob Bread Pudding, 517
 Carob Nut Log, 516-17
 Extravaganza, 507
 Freezer Jams and Jellies, 520-21
 Fruit Malts, 509-10
 Grapenut Crunch, 506
 Golden Harvest Salad Dressing, 515
 Green Pepper Cups, 512
 Iris's Home Canning Method, 521
 Jeanne's Blend Green Drink, 518-20
 Lentil Loaf, 510
 Maple Syrup, 507
 Mustard Variation, 516
 Oil and Vinegar Dressing, 516
 Pancake Toppings, 506
 Petra's Auflauf, 505
 Pineapple Gondola, 507-8
 Ruby Delight Salad, 514
 Shortcake, 518
 Soybeans, Cooking with, 510-11
 Soy Mayonnaise, 515
 Summer Fair Salad, 514
 Thousand Island Dressing, 515
 Tomato Cups, 512
 Tossed Salad Supreme, 514
 Trail Mix, 518
 Vegetable Plate Pinwheel, 513
 Watermelon Basket, 508-9
 Whole Grain Cereals, 505-6
Records, 18, 117
 labor log, 256-57, 411n
 vital signs, 411n, 500-501
 ovulation, 41
Red Cross, 36, 346
Red raspberry leaves, 150, 156, 171, 182, 183, 198, 200, 219, 478, 522, 526
 anecdote, healthy placenta, 387n
 properties of, 150, 152, 157-58, 175, 177, 420
Redroot, 203
Refined foods, 144-45, 208, 478
Reflex points
 pituitary, 275, 454
 placenta, 277

Reflex points (cont.)
  uterine (foot therapy),
    273-77, 291n
  uterine (Neuro-Vascular
    Dynamics), 416, 417
Relax-Rhythm Method, coaching,
  280-82
Relief Society Magazine, 44n
Reproductive organs, female, 62,
  63, 64, 65-67, 68. See also
  specific organs.
  herbs for, 156-58, 522-24
Respiration, 496-97
  establishing, 341, 342, 344-
    47, 348. See also
    Suctioning.
  anecdote, 347-49
  cutting the cord and, 349
  distressed, 496-97. See
    also Hyaline membrane
    disease.
  evaluating, Apgar, 342, 343
  labor and, 257
  norms, 411n, 497
Respiratory Distress Syndrome
  (RDS). See Hyaline membrane
  disease.
Restitution. See Rotation,
  external.
Restraint. See Marriage act,
  restraint.
Resuscitation, 9, 93, 349. See
  also Respiration, establishing.
  Byrd's Method, 347, 348
  cardiopulmonary (CPR), 23,
    346-47
Retained placenta. See
  placenta, retained.
Retardation, mental, 96, 178,
  412, 436n, 469, 497
Retraction ring. See Uterus,
  retraction ring.
Rh-negative factor, 155, 204-8,
  384
  change in status, 207-8
  cutting the cord with, 206,
    213n
  hemolytic disease, 205-6, 426,
    436n
  home birth and, 94, 206
  RhoGAM, 84, 205, 206, 412
  screening, 84, 109-10

Rh-negative factor (cont.)
  sensitization, 84, 109-10,
    204-6, 412
  RhoGAM, 84, 205, 206, 412
Rice, 141, 505
Rice bran syrup, 291n
Right occipital positions. See
  Occiput, positions.
Rights, parenting couples, 12,
  17, 21
Rimming
  cervical, 271-72, 274, 297,
    307
  anterior lip and, 277, 299,
    369
  perineal, 297, 333
Rosebuds, 202
Rose hips, 178
Rotation
  assisting, 440, 445, 451
  external, 238, 241, 246-47,
    294, 335
  face presentation and, 244,
    307-8, 465, 466n
  internal, 238, 240-41, 244,
    294
  swelling of fetal head from,
    470
Royal, Penny C., 16
Rubella, 70, 110, 212
Rupert, Idaho, 321
Rupture of membrane(s). See
  Amnion, rupture.
Russian Roulette, 50
Rye, 141, 505

S

Sacral pressure points, 266-68,
  267
Sacrum, 60, 61, 62
  designates position in breech
    births, 232
  promontory, 60, 61, 62, 105,
    245, 309
  creating room at, 295-96
  rotation and, 245, 465
  therapies for. See Back,
    adjustments, exercises.
Sage, 180, 423
Sagittal suture, 230, 235, 258,
  308, 463

558 POLLY'S BIRTH BOOK

St. George, 340n
St. Johnswort, 226, 363, 415, 478
Salerno, M. Constance, 15, 410n-11n
Saline solution, 27, 379, 398, 406, 410n
Saliva, 428
Sanicle, 195, 526
Sanitary napkins, 180, 218, 366-67, 371, 374, 399, 524
Sarsaparilla, 154, 415
Scale, baby, 227, 400
Scalp
  care of newborn's, 404, 405, 406
  wrinkle in, 339
Scalpel, 215
Scar tissue
  from episiotomies, 92
  foot therapy and, 92, 276
  suturing and, 92, 394, 397
  uterine
    abortion and, 27, 95
    C-section and. See Cesarean section.
Scharffs, Gilbert W., M.D., 25, 29n
Scissors
  bandage, 224, 225
  kitchen, anecdote, 340
  sharp/blunt, 224, 225, 328, 331
  umbilical, 227
Screening, home birth feasibility
  pelvic and vaginal assessment, 102-7
  prenatal questionnaire, 83-87
  commentary, 87-102
Scrubs. See Hand scrubs.
Scullcap, 202, 477, 523, 530
Seasonings, 141
Secondary inertia. See Uterus, inertia (secondary).
Seeds, 141
Seizures. See Convulsions.
Sensitization. See Rh-negative factor.
Sepsis, 408. See also Puerperal infection.
Serology test, 110
Sesame seeds, 141, 505
Sextuplets, anecdote, 456

Shave grass, 131
Shaving ("Prepping"), 261
Shepherd's-purse, 226
  for bleeding, 188, 189, 192, 193, 305-6, 338, 359, 362, 371, 372, 374, 375, 376, 379
  properties of, 151
"Shiny" Schultze placental separation, 385, 386
Shock, 367-69, 501-3
  anaphylactic, 100
  solutions, 215, 503. See also HVC.
Shoelaces, 220, 351
Shoulder(s)
  arrest, 309-10
  delivery of, 241, 247, 331, 335, 338
  in breech birth, 452, 453, 454
  presentation, 229, 445, 461-63. See also Transverse lie.
  soreness between, 268-69
  therapy for convulsion, 304
Sickness, holding infants, 432
Sickle cell anemia, 110
Silent killer, continuous bleeding, 371
Silent Knife: Cesarean Prevention and Vaginal Birth After Cesarean, 15, 131n, 132n
Silver nitrate, 213, 226, 406, 410n-11n, 413
Siring son, daughter, 43
"Sitting bones," 62, 102. See also Ischial tuberosities.
Sitz baths, 37, 165, 166, 167, 229, 235
  for calming nerves, 101, 169, 172, 266
  for relieving soreness, 106, 330, 398, 527-28
  for toning, 102, 180, 229, 235, 340n, 476, 487, 527
Skin-brush, 160
Skunk cabbage, 530
Slant board, 444
Sleep, 80, 160, 170-71
  newborn, 413, 427, 430, 432
Sleepytime herb tea, 201-2
Slippery elm, 172, 523
Slushes, for nausea, 198

Index 559

Smith, Charles, M.D., 138, 167n
Smith, Paul, M.D., 138, 142-43, 145, 167n
Smith, Prophet Joseph, Jr., 55n
Smoking, 86, 89, 93, 96-97, 146-47, 486, 497
Sodium, 151, 195
Solid foods, for infants, 428
Sores, 213
Sore throat, 202-3
Sorrel, 208
Soybeans, 137, 141, 510-12
Soybean Cookbook, 510, 521n
Spearmint, 151, 202
Speculum, 107, 222, 366, 393, 475
Sphingomyelin, 346, 482, 483
Sphygmomanometer, 118, 499
Spikenard, 154, 286
Spinal defects, injuries, 402, 455, 469-70. See also Back.
Spleen, 112
Spontaneous abortion. See Abortion, spontaneous.
Spontaneous version. See Version, breech.
Squatting
  exercises, 159, 163-64
  for delivery, 321-22, 338, 360, 463
Squawvine, 127, 156, 158, 198, 522
  properties of, 157
Starvation, 196-98
Stations of progress, 239, 243
  zero station, 243, 244, 307, 319-20
  expansion, 295-96
Sterilization. See also Aseptic technique, Germicidal solution.
  birthing linens, 220-21
  instruments, 222, 223, 493-94
  umbilical ties, 386n
Stethoscope, 119, 222
Stillbirth, 83, 88
  anecdote, 347-49
Stinging nettle, 151, 177
Stitches. See Suturing.
Stomach. See Abdomen.
Strawberry leaves, 177
Stretch marks, 168-69
Stroke, the Pill and, 95

Suctioning, 335, 338, 341-42. See also Bulb syringe.
Suffocation, 386n
Sugar (blood). See Blood, sugar.
Sugar (refined), 144-45, 181, 207-8, 504
Sunflower seeds, 141, 505, 532
A Superior Alternative, 6, 15, 17, 23, 28, 29n, 131, 132n, 339n, 347, 485
Supplements, 151-53, 155, 483
Supplies. See Birthing supplies.
Suppository, glycerine, 429
Suturing, 390-99
  anesthetics, 392-93
  materials, 225, 391-92
  vaginal, perineal lacerations, 371-72, 374
Swaddling, 402-3, 404
Swamp balsam, 398
Sweet acorns, 177
Swelling. See Edema.
Symphysis pubis, 60, 61, 63, 65
  See also Pelvis.
  inferior symphysis pubis touch, 295, 299
Syphilis, 212. See also Venereal disease.
Syringe. See Bulb syringe, Suctioning.
Systolic pressure, 118, 119, 499-500

T

Tachycardia, 310
Tailbone. See Coccyx.
Tansy, 208
Tannic acid, 146
Tears. See Lacerations.
Temperature norms, 411n
Tension, 55, 148, 169, 195, 272-73, 421
  interferes with labor, 11, 184, 266, 282, 387n
  muscle, 268-69, 279
Textbook for Midwives, 16
Thalidomide, 49
Thermometers, 222
Theobromine, 145

Thiamin. See Vitamin B1.
Thiouracil, 419
Third stage labor. See Labor, third stage.
Thirst, 211, 502
Thompsonian era, 11
Thorax rub, 342, 344
Thromboembolism, the Pill and, 95
Thrush, 430-31. See also Yeast infection.
Thumb therapy, varicosed legs, 181
Tilia flowers, 202
Tipped uterus. See Uterus, anteflected.
Tiredness, 151, 170, 197, 291n. See also Fatigue.
  in labor, 47, 266, 278
Tobacco, 146-47. See also Smoking.
Toxemia. See Pre-eclampsia, Eclampsia.
Toxins, 98, 100, 128, 197
Tranquilizers, 47, 146
Transfusion
  after serious bleeding, 381-82
  hemolytic disease and, 206, 436n
  syndrome, with twins, 458
Transition, 284, 293-94
Transporting, 189, 237, 368, 381. See also specific conditions.
Transverse head arrest, 307-9, 463, 464
Transverse lie, 229. See also Shoulder presentation.
  correcting, 289, 445, 459-60
  C-section and, 463, 487
Triplets (or more), 460-61, 486
Triticale, 505
Tubal pregnancy. See Ectopic pregnancy.
Tub baths. See Baths.
Tubs, sitz, 165
Tuberculosis, 422
Tumors, 89, 95-96, 126, 488
"Tunnel" canal, 90. See also Pelvis, build (narrow).
Turkey rhubarb, 171, 526
Turning the fetus. See Version.
Twins, 125, 126, 456-60
Typhoid fever, 90

U

Ultrasonograms, 77-78, 110-11
Ultrasound, 110-14, 131n
  anecdotes, 111-12
Umbilical arteries, 72-73, 353, 354
Umbilical clamps, ties, 215, 226, 318, 354, 386n
Umbilical cord (funis), 68, 70, 72-73
  around neck, 313
  checking for, 246, 312, 335
  death due to, 339n
  breech version and, 445
  clamping, cutting the, 335, 349-52, 354, 386n
  circulatory changes after, 352, 353
  with cord stress, 312, 335, 349
  early, disadvantages of, 349, 386n
  with multiple birth, 459
  of Rh-negative mother, 206, 213n
  "stripping," 213n, 350-51
  compression, in breech birth, 453
  knots, 73, 314, 488
  death due to, 339n
  length of, 339n
  anecdotes, 313-14
  no nerves in, 73
  prolapsed, 314-20
  within amnion (sausage-shaped protrusion), 289, 315
  amnion rupture and, 200, 253, 314, 315, 319, 328, 458-59
  breech presentation and, 315, 442, 450
  C-section and, 488
  checking for, 255, 262, 315-16, 458-59
  hydramnios and, 209
  multiple births and, 315, 458-59
  pulsation of, 289, 317
  treatment, 315-20
  anecdote, 340n
  early labor, 315-19

Index 561

Umbilical cord (cont.)
 prolapsed, treatment (cont.)
  with head at or past -0-
   station, 319-20
  knee-chest position, 253,
   315-16, 317, 320, 340n
  pelvic rocks, 316, 318,
   320
  reinsertion, 317-19
  risks, 317, 340n
  transporting, 316-17, 319,
   320
 stress, 88, 151, 310-14, 349
  anecdotes, 313
 vessels, 72-73, 352, 353, 354
Umbilical vein, 72-73, 353
Umbilicus (navel), 73, 353, 453
Unwanted children, 25, 95
Ureters, 172-73
Urethra, 63, 64-65, 288, 409
Urinalysis, 117, 120-22
Urinary tract, bladder infections, 121, 133, 173, 178,
 194
Urination, 161
 frequent, 80, 172
 herbs for, 156, 158
 obstructed, newborn, 409, 413,
  423
Urine, 120-22
 labor obstruction, 264, 288
 protein in, 116, 120, 121,
  128, 129, 130, 197
 sugar in, 120, 211
Uristix, 120, 121
Urologist, 13
Utah, Bureau of Health
 Statistics, 29n
Uterine reflex
 foot therapy, 273-77, 291n
 Neuro-Vascular Dynamics, 416,
  417
Uterine sounds, Uterine (placental) souffle, 123, 125, 427,
 445
Uterine (fallopian) tubes, 66,
 67, 190
Uterus, 63, 65-67, 68, 69, 365.
 See also individual parts.
 activity in parturition,
  66-67, 365
 anteflected, 66, 415, 474-76
 confused function, 41, 90,
  91-92

Uterus (cont.)
 contractions. See Labor,
  Afterpains.
 stimulating, 151, 362, 372,
  376, 386n, 407, 415.
  See also Fundus,
  kneading.
 corpus, 66, 67
 fundus. See Fundus.
 immaturity, incompetence, 89
 inertia, 384-87, 387n, 487
  breech birth and, 275, 454
  excess weight and, 94,
   169-70
  fear and, 91, 387n. See
   also Tension.
  labor management, 285, 286
  Polly-Jean formula and, 287
  pregnancies close together
   and, 90, 487
  primary, 284-85
  secondary, 285-87, 292n,
   386, 454
 inverted, 476, 479-81
 involution, 414
 laceration of, 291, 330, 362,
  367, 375. See also
  Cervix, laceration of.
 lower, upper uterine segments,
  66-67, 364, 365
 perforation, abortion and,
  27-28
 retraction ring, 363-67, 460
 retroflected, 474
 rupture, 27, 373, 487, 488
 scarring of
  from abortion, 27, 95
  from IUD, 95
 screening, 19, 83, 90, 91, 94,
  95, 99
Utrophin, 287
Uva ursi, 131, 522

V

Vaccination, 212
Vagina, 59, 62, 63
 bleeding (uterine, vaginal)
  in parturition. See Placenta, separation (blood
  loss), Hemorrhage.
 postpartum. See Lochia.

Vagina (cont.)
 bleeding (cont.)
  in pregnancy, 185, 186, 191.
   See also Abortion,
   spontaneous.
  with threatened miscarriage,
   193-94
 condition of, assessing, 92,
  102-6, 307
 discharge, 182. See also
  Leukorrhea.
 postpartum. See Lochia.
 exams. See Examinations,
  vaginal.
 floor, 106, 161, 165
  curve of, 106, 246
  unhealthy, 62, 329, 523-24
 hygiene, 182
 itching, 182
 laceration of, 62, 306, 307,
  329-30, 371-72, 389-90
 mucus, fertility cycle, 40-41
 pH, 41, 182
 toning, stretching, 165, 228-
  29. See also Crowning,
  therapies to assist
  stretching, Sitz baths.
 kegels, 161
 rimming, 297, 333
 venereal disease. See
  Venereal disease.
 yeast infection. See Yeast
  infection.
Vaginal delivery
 after cesarean, 92-93, 485-86
 diabetes and, 211-12
Valerian, 226
 properties of, 154, 208
Varicosed legs, therapy for, 181
Varicosities, 86, 99, 106,
 178-81, 524, 527
Vascular system. See Circulatory system.
Vasoconstriction, 167n
Vegetarianism, 38, 44n, 136,
 137-38
Venereal disease, 86, 97, 106,
 212-13
 blindness and, 213, 408-9, 413
Vernix caseosa, 400, 401
Version
 breech
  manual (external cephalic),
   444

Version (cont.)
 breech (cont.)
  spontaneous, 229, 442,
   444-45
  transverse lie (internal
   podalic), 289-90, 445,
   459-60
Vertex, 229, 230
Vertex presentation, 229, 461
 mechanism of labor, 230-40,
  241, 242, 243, 244-45,
  246, 247. See also Labor.
Vervain, 208
Vinegar, 182, 183, 202
 in HVC, 291n, 503. See also
  HVC.
Vision
 disturbances, 185, 195-96, 302
 newborn, 213, 408-9, 413
Vital signs, 496-503. See also
 Blood pressure, Pulse,
 Respiration, Temperature.
 in labor, 128, 237, 250,
  257-58, 285, 305, 408
 norms, 411n
 records, 500-501
Vitamin A, 146, 150, 151, 203
Vitamin B
 B1 (thiamine), 146, 199
 B2, 146
 B6, 171, 196, 197, 198
 B12, 150, 178
 complex, 101, 122, 150, 152,
  170, 172, 197, 198, 199,
  431, 504
Vitamin C, 88, 140, 150, 151,
 152, 176, 178, 189, 191,
 198, 199, 203, 431, 520,
 521. See also Calcium
 ascorbate.
Vitamin D, 150
Vitamin E, 122, 130, 169, 189,
 203n, 226, 397
 assists oxygenation, 150, 152,
  312, 346, 349
 hyaline membrane disease and,
  152, 346, 349, 483
Vitamin K, 150, 152
Vomiting, 27, 80, 423. See also
 Nausea.
 diabetes and, 209
 eclampsia and, 302
 ergot and, 386n
 inducing, 530

Vomiting (cont.)
  persistent, 185, 196-98
  urinalysis and, 121, 197
Vulva, 63, 64, 65, 80
  crowning at. See Crowning.
  lacerations, 371, 389, 394, 395
  newborn, 401, 402, 409
  varicosities, 99, 116, 179-81, 524, 527

W

Walks, walking, 37, 159, 160, 172, 287, 403
Warts, 106, 528
Water, 148-49
  retention, 195
"Water breaks." See Amnion, rupture.
Watermelon seeds, 131
Weaning, 423
Webbed feet, 101, 402
Weight
  maternal, 84, 117, 231
    gain, loss in pregnancy, 110-11, 138, 169-70, 211
    toxemia and, 122, 128, 130
  problems caused by excessive, 94, 209
  newborn, 169, 170, 400, 429, 484
  of previous babies, 84, 93, 210
Wharton's Jelly, 73, 351
Wheat, 177, 180, 203, 208, 505
Wheat grass, 177
White flour, 181, 208, 478
White oak bark, 180, 476, 477, 523, 527
  tincture recipe, 524
Whitney, Orson F., 37
Widtsoe, Dr. John A., and Leah, 137-38, 167n
Wild alumroot, 423
Wild amaranth, 203
Wild ginger (Canada snakeroot), 156
  properties of, 157
Wild yam, 156
  properties of, 154, 158
Williams Obstetrics, 16, 205, 213n, 339n, 492, 495

Wind flower, 528
Wintergreen, 529
Witch hazel, 529
Womb. See Uterus.
Wood, Dr. Camilla S., 411n
Word of Wisdom, 137, 167n
Work, after evening meal, anecdote, 37
World Health Organization, 24
Wormwood, 523, 529
Wound healing, 396-97

X

X-rays, 77, 79, 127
Xylocaine, 332, 392

Y

Yarrow, 526
Yeast, 178, 532
Yeast infections
  in mother, 182-83, 329, 528
  in newborn, 430-31
Yellow D sugar, 504
Yellow dock, 475, 524
  properties of, 177, 194-95

Z

Zikria, Bashir A., M.D., 391
Zinc, 198, 199, 420